THE CANCER FILES

**A Biochemist's Story:
How the Answer to Cancer was Suppressed**

GW00601826

Renee M Henry BSc

Cover photograph: Author as she was in this battle ©

The right of Renee Henry to be identified as the Author of this work has been asserted by her in accordance with sections 77 and 78 of the Copyright, Designs and Patents Act, 1988.

This book may include words, brands names and other descriptions of products that are or are asserted to b proprietary names or trade- marks. No judgement concerning the legal status of such words is made or implied thereby. Their inclusion does not imply that they have acquired for legal purposes a non-proprietary or general significance or any other judgement concerning legal status.

The views expressed in this book are those of Renee Henry and not necessarily those of any other person or organisation unless explicitly stated.

The diagnosis and treatment of medical conditions is a responsibility shared between the patient and their choice of medical advisors. No recommendations are made by the author and all diets should be discussed with the patients chosen medical advisors.

ISBN 978-0-9529567-5-4
First printing 2011
Printed and bound by CPI Group (UK) Ltd, Croydon, CR0 4YY

THE PLATONIC MAXIM IS 'BEFORE YOU CAN CURE A MAN'S BODY YOU MUST CURE HIS MIND AND BEFORE THAT HIS SOUL.'

THE QUESTION BECOMES HOW DO YOU CURE A MAN'S SOUL?

THIS BOOK IS DEDICATED TO THOSE IN ALL AGES WHO HAD THE COURAGE TO FACE THE TRUTH AND SPEAK OUT

The works of this author can be ordered from all good bookshops as well as Amazon. It may also be purchased directly from CPIBookDelivery.com via a hyperlink from the publishers website at *www.answer2cancer.co.uk*

Seminar Workshop

'A Revolutionary View of Cancer'

(*A course that could save your life*)

For more information on these courses please contact us at
alphaeducation.infinity@gmail.com

I very gratefully acknowledge the contribution of all quoted authors cited in the text of this book and in reference and bibliography. I am particularly indebted to Colonel Barry and Mrs Turner for prompting me to publish this book by forwarding a copy of 'Living Proof' by Michael Gearin-Tosh and relevant clippings. I am also indebted to Michael Gearin-Tosh for his honest account of his experience and fears he experienced on the Gerson Therapy – so unusual for a man. I am also totally indebted to Rufus and Barney for their continued help and support over many years.

"Actuality means 'what is'...Are you facing in yourself what actually is going on...You don't take actuality and look at it."

"Man has been concerned throughout the ages to discover or live in 'Truth'."

(Taken from a series of discussions between Krishnamurti and David Bohm, Professor of Theoretical Physics at London University. In Truth and Actuality by J.Krishnamurti – London Victor Gollancz Ltd., 1986)

CONTENTS

PART 2 – THE AUTHOR'S RESEARCH – THE CANCER FILES

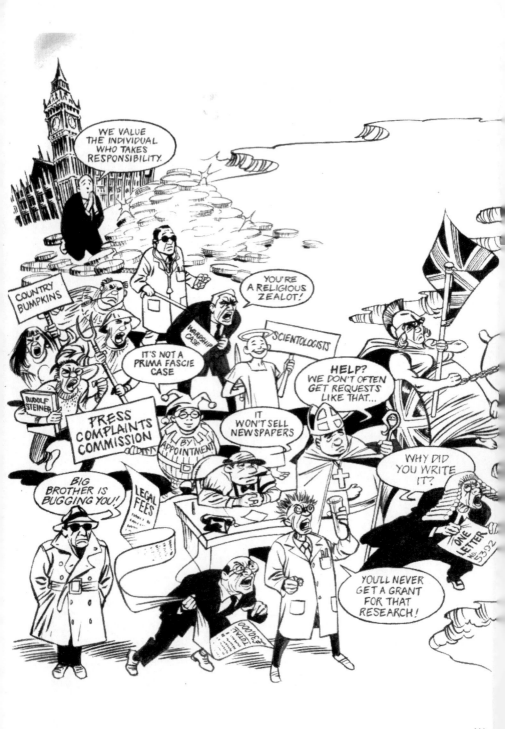

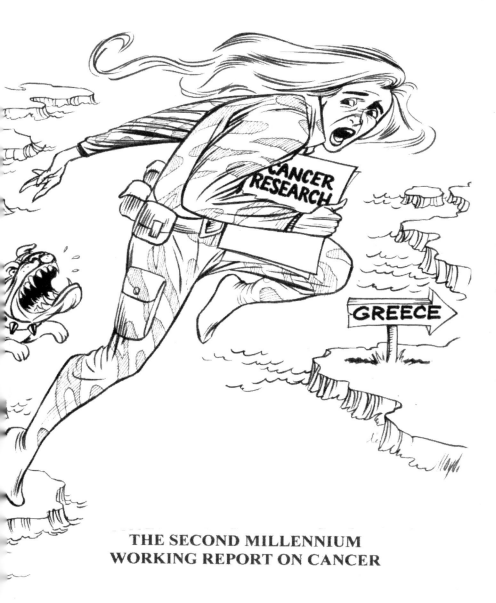

THE SECOND MILLENNIUM
WORKING REPORT ON CANCER

R Henry Copyright 1991, 1995 & 1996

Introduction

Cancer is a tragic problem. $13.5 billion is now spent on research each year, and this is on top of vast investment over the past 30 years. But is cancer being cured? No. Mortality "has barely changed since 1971" wrote Professor Michael Baum in the July 2000 issue of '*Prospect*': "About one in four people in Britain now die of cancer. The incidence of most cancers is increasing".

Why so little success? According to Professor Baum there are the villains of the "thought police" at work inside the medical profession. Baum should know he is an emeritus professor of surgery at UCL. The problem however is much deeper in my experience than anyone could imagine.

When I was diagnosed with breast cancer in 1986, my world suddenly collapsed. Cancer is a word that strikes fear into the hearts of anyone who has been given this diagnosis. My father died of bowel cancer in 1985 and I witnessed his traumatic and painful last months, feeling helpless to do anything.

I had two young children when I was diagnosed, one just 12 months and the other 4 years old. Like many newly diagnosed patients I was rushed by my oncologist to have orthodox treatment. It's rather like an express train you board and once on, the thing goes so fast there is no point to disembark or think about the road you are travelling along. After the initial shock I found myself boarding the train with thousands of others and following millions who had boarded that train before. It did not occur to me to ask how many came back, from the 'holocaust'- the cancer survival rates. For a time medical advice was followed as my gospel – surely they knew what they were talking about. Looking back I feel my vulnerability was taken advantage of – how I ever (as a Biochemist) let them convince me to undergo radiation is still something I kick myself over. The risk of damage to DNA is high and there is a risk that even after 20 years the radiation itself could cause cancer, apart from the serious side effects. The smiling Pollyanna smiles and assurances that: "everything will be alright, just close your eyes and you will get through it" are soothing words you want to believe.

One patient described a familiar experience: "Basically, I was in shock from the diagnosis. I was sitting there, with the doctor saying that this treatment was the best available and that it was actually a matter of life or death that I received it. My husband was sitting next to me, telling me that I needed to go along with it. I kind of went into a trance and although something didn't feel quite right, I found myself nodding to chemotherapy". A lot of cancer patients report that although they have an uncomfortable gut feeling that there must somehow be a better way forward, they still find themselves returning to their oncologist for more of the same. Undoubtedly there is a hereditary submissive attitude to the medical orthodoxy and its archetypal symbolism – the white coat, the stethoscope, the years of knowledge represented in those framed diplomas and the comforting feeling that this expert is going to look after you, where life has not. No doubt there are thousands of doctors who have their patients' best interests to heart, but under the various medical bodies that supervise the profession they are limited to *policy*, when it comes to treating cancer. It is the small print of *policy* that as a newly diagnosed cancer patient you are not informed of.

The medical profession and cancer charities quote their cure statistics, but the statistics are very open to manipulation or "massaging". If you survive cancer for five years you are counted statistically as a cure. Die in year six and you are still statistically cured. Further if you die from the effects of toxic chemotherapy such as heart problems or kidney problems this is not factored into the cure statistics.

In 1940, according to Prof. Hardin B. Jones at the University of California, Berkeley: "Through re-definition of terms, various questionable grades of malignancy were classed as 'cancer'. After that date, the proportion of cancer cures having 'normal' life expectancy increased rapidly, corresponding to the fraction of questionable diagnosis included".

Michael Gearin-Tosh – a cancer survivor using an alternative method, who wrote *Living Proof* [1], recounted in *The Times* newspaper [2] how he received a number of letters from GPs and quoted Dr Mollie Hunton:

'I have recently retired from the NHS and the sort of experiences you describe (in *Living Proof*) were one of the factors that encouraged me to retire early...The last patient I had with myeloma' (cancer of the bone marrow) 'took ages to diagnose, because she complained of pain in her ankle and, as a GP, I

2

had to refer her to a consultant for a scan and a succession of junior doctors missed it. When it was finally diagnosed, she had repeated courses of chemotherapy over which I had no control, as she never saw me, only the haematologist. I got to see her only in the last stage of her illness when she kept getting repeated bronchitis. The steroids she was on not only lowered her immune system but collapsed her vertebrae so that her spine curved and her chin was on her chest and she could not breathe. She really died of respiratory failure due to her curvature of the spine, due to her steroid treatment, but I signed her death certificate 'myeloma'. It made me wonder at the time how often the true cause of death is recorded, i.e. the treatment not the underlying illness. Before she died, I realised what was going on and wrestled with my conscience about what I would put on the death certificate, but I did not have the courage to put the real cause of death on it. I don't know if the haematologists audit the long-term outcome of their treatment in this manner, i.e. to find the true cause of death. If they do, I would be surprised. I get the impression that they have their meetings about how they feel each stage should be treated, but I am not sure that the outcomes are recorded honestly'.

The interesting thing is that the GP was in *fear* of her own profession and did not have 'the courage' to confront it and probably what she recognised would be formidable consequences to her employment or even career.

As I have come to realise in my own story, truth is a lonely path as one suffers loss of employment, loss of access to justice, loss of fair trial – Article 6 and constant harassment over Article 9 & 10 of Human Rights law as one is hounded.

Article 6: the right to a fair trial is fundamental to the rule of law and to democracy itself. The right to a fair trial is absolute and cannot be limited. It requires a fair and public hearing within a reasonable time by an independent and impartial tribunal established by law.

Article10: provides the right to freedom of expression, subject to certain restrictions "in accordance with law" and "necessary in a democratic society". The right includes the freedom to hold opinions, and to receive and impart information and ideas.

And because my research particularly in the Theatre Earth series included discussion of certain religions Article 9 was constantly violated:

Article 9: guarantees that you can think what you want and can hold any religious or

3

non-religious belief that you wish. It therefore protects religious belief and the beliefs of atheists, agnostics and those that are indifferent to religion, alike. You cannot be forced to follow or practice a particular religion and cannot be prevented from changing your religion. You are also protected from indoctrination by the State. This part of Article 9 is an absolute right and can never be interfered with.

As I was to discover British courts do not uphold these basic rights, where they are trampled underfoot by barristers and judges who turn a blind eye. For the sake of this research inclusive of my other books, my family and myself suffered many Human Rights violations in Britain over a period of twenty-five years, most of which occurred *after* The Human Rights Act of 1998 was passed into law and even astoundingly many were contravened *in actual courts of law*! If anyone finds that statement too unbelievable I might add I have recorded and archived all evidence to prove that.

After a partial gruelling bout of radiation, which later I was to totally regret having suffered personal injury through it, a single moment in a hospital, whilst I waited for the first dose of chemotherapy, stopped me in my tracks and opened my eyes wide, as if from sleep. I disembarked from the express train and metaphorically wandered off, into the meadows full of life and flowers and where among nature many years later I would see very clearly how cancer develops.

And so it was whilst waiting for the first chemotherapy session, I sat next to a woman who was waiting for her chemotherapy. She looked tired, grey and her eyes were the familiar sad expressionless eyes of cancer patients. She explained that like me she had breast cancer a few years ago, she had surgery including lymph node removal, radiation and then a course of chemotherapy. But then the cancer had *returned* and she had her ovaries removed and was now back for *more chemotherapy*. Why, if they had "got it all" to use the so familiar phrase, was she back?

After hearing this, I went straight to the hospital toilet and threw up. I felt I was in some casino game, where luck decided who wins and who loses. As I composed myself I looked in the mirror as if to face the truth – for one can never lie to oneself. I simply said: "this doesn't work, how many more bits will they have to remove and how many more courses of chemotherapy will I have to take, before they tell me it's no use?" I turned on my heel and walked straight out of the hospital and didn't go back. In 1986, this was an unusual action for anyone to take, where it was unheard of to question orthodox treatment. As a Biochemist trained in orthodox scientific methods and research, it is even more unusual that I turned my back on years of indoctrination: the idea however of pumping my body full of toxic chemicals seemed to make no scientific sense, but more a desperate throw of dice. As Einstein remarked "God doesn't play dice".

Thus started my journey, where my first task was to find out everything I could about cancer and alternative treatments. Back in 1986 and long before Michael Gearin-Tosh developed cancer this was an age where information was hard to come by, with no Internet. I engaged in a great search in London from reflexologists, to homeopaths, to herbalists, to spiritualists, to acupuncturists and even walking lines with Buddhist priests in a temple in Wimbledon. It is perhaps poignant that in the dark stillness of the temple as we walked forward on an exact line, the bell would ring and we would walk backwards on an exact line, until the bell rang again, then repeating this action for what seemed hours. I have no idea to this day what the priests did this exercise for, since I just walked in and joined in and no one objected. However a thought arose in my head that it was easier to walk forwards in life than to walk *backwards* and yet if I did not go backwards on an exact line, I could not go forwards. It is strange how one comes to these spiritual epiphanies, but it was the start of a spiritual journey, to find out 'who' I was and it would therefore be necessary to go back.

The immediate and pressing problem however was the body and the medical condition. As a Biochemist, I was searching for a therapy that would make sense to my scientific mind, but I was also looking for *more* – quite what in fact that *more* was, I did not know, but I *knew* there was more to this illness than just malfunctioning of cells. Finally I discovered the Gerson Therapy and for two years completed the arduous nutritional programme.

During that time I read a great deal, researched endless mechanisms of the mind and body and later set up a charity – Karnak and undertook a limited clinical study with terminal cancer patients finally formulating a mechanism for cancer, which involved mind and body. Twenty years down the line and still the medical profession can't accept a mechanism of mind and body and I doubt whether the role of the Spirit will ever be accepted. If it won't go into a test tube then you can't test it, is the mentality I'm afraid.

5

In 1989 I published the research study on a proposed mechanism for cancer in the journal *Complementary Medical Research* [3]. The paper was entitled '*A Theory for Cancer, using the Gerson Therapy in conjunction with psychological counselling*' [*Appendix 1*]. Sheila McLean a nurse specialising in the Gerson Therapy co-authored the paper with me. The mechanism proposed, linked a **specific biochemistry** of cancer to a **specific psychology**.

Perhaps the information on the politics of cancer will come as a shock to you as the data did to me 24 years ago. In 1986 I was told by an alternative (homeopathic) doctor: "The only thing standing between cancer and a potential cure is the profit the drugs industry stands to make by keeping people sick". As an orthodox trained scientist – a biochemist, it was in 1986 very difficult to accept that statement, or even realise the depth of what was meant. It soon became apparent however that doctors who treated cancer patients with alternative methods were put in prison, discredited, invariably harassed, swamped with tax problems and even had their wives and families taken from their homes. It painfully dawned on me in 1986 that money and profit for blue chip pharmaceutical companies was at the root of all the suppression. Governments are dependent on these companies to provide jobs, pay taxes and also pay dividends, which in turn pay things like pension funds. A dog chasing its tail in a revolving round of deception is only the first barrier in crossing the abyss. The lie is that with just a little more money and investment, they can crack cancer. I had a £400 donation to the Karnak Charitable Trust and did it on that, although my personal financial contribution to Karnak was more than a hundred times that figure, if not more if you factor in the loss of employment through attacks over my research and books.

As a Biochemist I was more fortunate than the lay person, who asks advice on alternative therapies: such questions are usually met by the medical profession with the stock answer that alternative therapies have no indication by way of research or trials that they work. The same might be said of orthodox methods, where one person may survive and another succumbs. Generally doctors and Scientists are indoctrinated into their profession at University and I can assure you alternative methods are not on the curriculum. Doctors only practise what they have been taught at medical school and no doubt they were told that alternative medicine was quackery. When I mentioned to an oncologist that I was going to do the Gerson Therapy, he fairly frothed at the mouth and predicted I would die. As a Biochemist I could make my own decisions, but what of the layperson who undoubtedly would find such a response

6

intimidating? The truth that doctors should be giving, is that many people have survived using alternative methods, but as a doctor he cannot recommend such an approach as he is governed *legally* by a medical body – The British Medical Association and rigid policy laid down by that association and the main Cancer Charities, which align with government *policy*. The position is the same in virtually all countries. Is the policy correct? Well that was the question I was left to decide in my own journey. There is also no doubt I discovered that the patient undergoing orthodox treatment, is subject to a regime diametrically opposed to that which is needed for survival and therefore I concluded the policy was wrong.

I never had any intention to publish this book and my biography of the 'cancer years,' which had sat on my bookshelf as a manuscript for twenty years along with the research material in my notes and files, which outlined the entire mechanism of cancer. When I left the field of cancer in 1997, I decided it was an insane battlefield and I certainly had had enough of it. In order to save your own sanity, you have to walk away, just tiptoe through the battlefield of the two opposing sides orthodox and alternative and ride on out as fast as you can! I had also suffered violations of Human Rights even in Courts of Law for twenty-four years because of the research and eventually could not withstand the forces. There is a saying that the nail that sticks up, will be hammered down and I can assure you that if you stick your head above the ever- watchful radar scanner, you will be attacked. – It is a ferocious attack and proves pretty formidable barriers in crossing the abyss.

The fact that ordinary people also threatened my employment and my children's education and were even willing to lie in courts was particularly repugnant reminding one of how individuals like this keep all Kafkaesque states in power. Kafkaesque can also describe an intentional distortion of reality by powerful but anonymous bureaucrats. Lack of evidence is treated as a pesky inconvenience, to be circumvented by such Kafkaesque means as depositing unproven allegations into sealed files. Another definition would be an existentialist state of ever-elusive freedom while existing under immitigable control, characterized by surreal distortion and a sense of impending danger. The Kafkaesque terror of the endless interrogations, false trials – and threats to employment, in some nightmarish fashion my family experienced all of this. One could only compare the justice system in England to Stalinist Czechoslovakia – where outcome is decided irrespective of what evidence you provide and before the case starts. Who would not leave it all behind?

Then a friend Colonel Barry Turner years later, sent me a book by Michael Gearin-Tosh entitled '*Living Proof – A Medical Mutiny*' [1] and some newspaper clippings from *The Sunday Times News Review* [4]. Michael was an Oxford don in Literature and was diagnosed with myeloma (bone cancer) in 1994, a year after I had fled to Greece, and had been told that without orthodox treatment he would die, but with it he could expect to live from anywhere between 6 months and 3 years. Michael had opted out of orthodox treatment and completed the Gerson Therapy and 8 years later was still alive. Good for him! I thought, not being tempted to read his account or the newspaper clippings, less I be dragged down the black abyss again; I popped the book on my bookshelves next to my aging manuscript and the clippings were filed away in the 'Cancer Files'. I certainly had no desire to pull down my biography of the 'cancer years' and go over the painful account: neither was there any desire to rattle the research in front of media, politicians or oncologists – I had done that in 1997. In fact I was fairly jaw-hung, when I asked one oncologist to read my research paper, he replied: "If I read what you are saying, I might have to question what I am doing and I am not prepared to do that". Ostrich doesn't describe it! Several doctors had described the research as "brilliant" and had urged me to make the research known – but by that time I was exhausted with the whole battle.

I noted however that Gearin-Tosh's survival had set off the 'thought police,' where it was argued that he was no more than an exception. 'Nearly every week, someone wins the lottery jackpot, but many millions do not,' wrote a consultant haematologist (Dr Andrew Will) in *The Sunday Times*: 'Gearin-Tosh is not just lucky. He is very lucky indeed'. Gearin-Tosh noted: 'classify someone as lucky or an exception to the rules, and you do not have to worry if the rules are wrong'. But hadn't I questioned orthodox cancer treatment as a lottery of luck?

Gearin-Tosh wrote *Living Proof*, at the suggestion of Sir James Gowans FRS. A research professor of the Royal Society, Sir James was also secretary of the Medical Research Council in Britain for 10 years. He is a pioneer of immunology and Gearin-Tosh's cancer was one of the immune system. Sir James whilst believing that exceptions should be studied and not dismissed evidently was totally unaware of the forces that are thrown at you when you try to do that. According to Professor Baum, 'the ear against cancer is bogged down by undeclared special interest, petty mindedness, political quick fixes and slavish adherence to out-dated paradigms'. Indeed new thought and paradigms as I was to discover, are considered heretical rather than a breakthrough.

Then in 2005, I read an obituary for Michael in a national newspaper. I wondered what psychological event had triggered his demise – after all he had survived for 10 years - far beyond his prognosis. Even so I resisted pulling down Michael's biography. Don't go back into *that* battle I thought. Then in 2008 I met a young woman whose husband had died of cancer – nasal-pharyngeal – or cancer of the linings of the nose and back of throat. I asked her whether anything had happened to her husband's nose in the 12-18 months prior to diagnosis. She thought for a moment and then said "Oh well he had a bad fall on it". There was *the trigger* right there. The fall did not *cause* cancer but triggered a subconscious memory of a past significant loss: it was a *"key in"*. The accident with the nose was perceived as a loss in the subconscious primitive mind, but not recognised as such by the conscious analytical mind. The fall was not *causative* of cancer only a psychological *trigger*, and so I asked her whether she could think of any other earlier incident in his life, which had involved the nose. She thought for a moment and then told me his Chinese grandmother used to waft opium under his nose as a baby to get him to go to sleep. The husband died after gruelling rounds of radiation and chemotherapy and thus one will never know what *command phrases* of the grandmother, were locked into his subconscious mind during these opium incidents. I will expand on this in the section entitled *The Mind in Cancer*. The battlefield between orthodox and complementary medicine is fierce enough when it involves the body, but I can assure you that once you approach the mind in cancer, the psychotics crawl out of the proverbial woodwork to attack you!

After that a nagging question came into mind, as to whether if I had published a book, put down what I knew, whether the husband might if he had read it, still be here today – would Michael Gearin-Tosh be here today? I resisted the nagging question, telling myself I had published a scientific study, tried to disseminate it, and virtually bankrupted myself by bankrolling the research. I had finally gained the help of my MP the late Tim Rathbone who in 1997 agreed to Table Questions in The House of Commons UK Parliament, based upon the Ancient Right of Petition, which had taken a month to research and complete [*Appendix 2*]. When that was predictably scuttled as one might expect in Britain's laughable ruse of democracy and "transparent government" – the research was sent through the so-called lines of "*open government*" to the major charities who fund cancer research in the UK including the Medical Research Council and the National Health Executive who direct policy. Despite then, the Human Rights Act was about to materialise the following year, evidently Article 21 – The Right to Democracy (everyone has the right to take part in the government of his country) and Article 29 (Responsibility) had yet to impinge on the British government. They were still with courts of law fighting Article 10 – free expression of ideas.

Following that in 1998, I washed my hands of the whole business, shocked to my core by it and the undemocratic workings of our government, not to mention 'law' courts. At the time of my petition the Prime Minister (John Major - Conservative) was prattling on about: "we value the individual who takes responsibility" (whilst it emerges having an extra-marital affair) and today the Prime Minister (David Cameron – Conservative) is prattling on about responsibility in "The Big Society". The Blair years were silent for me, no point approaching a man with research aimed at saving lives, when he appeared intent on the reverse. In fact the Blair years marked the biggest decline in civil liberties in the Britain, years in which my family went through Human Rights violations in courts, which the government turned a blind eye to.

In 2009, following another incident such as the one with the husband I recounted, a woman said to me: "Oh I just wish we could have known about you and your research". I eventually pulled down Michael's book from my shelf and read it, along with the newspaper cuttings from 2002. Turning to the clippings and a spread in *The Sunday Times* [2] I noted a quarter page was allocated to letters from readers in response to the previous week's coverage of Michael's story entitled '*Readers ask: How dare he challenge the doctors?*' I sighed as I read them – same old scene I thought nothing in this field changes as I remembered the gamut of anger and hostility I ran in 1986, when The Gerson Therapy was virtually unheard of and the only survivor I found in the UK was Beata Bishop who wrote *A Time to Heal* [5].

Reading through the letters – here is an example of the reaction to Michael's story and his decision to forego orthodox treatment and complete the alternative Gerson Therapy:

'I hope you thought long and hard about the effect on other myeloma sufferers and their family and friends, particularly those starting, in the middle of or completing "traditional" treatments, of Michael Gearin-Tosh's account of his myeloma experience. I am of course delighted he is still alive and, it is to be hoped, well, but it seems irresponsible and possibly cruel to print, even as reported conversation, something like "If your friend touches chemotherapy he's a goner'.

According to the government's own figures, in the 1991 *Health of the Nation Report*: around 2 percent of chemotherapy recipients are still alive after 5 years. It seems that some can confront the facts and others are quite incapable of doing so.

Another example ran:

'It was with growing disbelief and later anger that I read last week's excerpt from Michael Gearin-Tosh's book *Living Proof*. Desperate people will try anything and cancer patients are often desperate, therefore easy prey for woolly-brained mavericks at best, and at worst, unscrupulous unethical charlatans....' And so on.

The five year survival rates for the different orthodox treatments were given in the *State of the Nation's Health Report* in 1991: Surgery 22%; Radiotherapy 12%; Surgery/radiotherapy combined 6%; chemotherapy plus others 2.5%; chemotherapy alone 1.6%. These figures however have not stopped the cancer business carrying out the same procedures over decades, with the same inevitable and deadly results.

Here's another letter:

'To encourage patients with myeloma or any other form of malignant disease to disregard medical advice is grossly irresponsible...' and so on.

Are you getting it, or not – I mean the reason I walked away and these are only readers, wait till you reach the medical hierarchy and in my case the law courts, where my research was constantly used against me, even in the simplest of cases such as a trading standards case. How my research could be connected to a leaking roof, care of a cow boy builder, is anyone's guess, but as I pointed out once you put your foot into this insane field you are considered 'open season' – a case of 'shoot the messenger' as poor old Galileo was to find out.

Now let me say right here that if you agree with the above letters, don't read this book. I decided to record what I know, some will totally get it and it is for them I did so. I really don't want any angry letters from those who went past this warning and then did not like what they heard.

....

O.K so if you are still here you have made a decision to continue and you should recognise that I advise no one and make no recommendations. Healing and the methods we choose are a matter of *personal choice.* This book is simply **my story and the way I chose** *to heal my mind, body and spirit,* through my own research. There is no doubt in my mind that I was able to discover the mechanism of cancer through that research, whether that is true for you, is *your choice.*

I never saw cancer as merely a medical problem, I was always aware that healing - true healing is a much deeper story of mind, body and spirit. The journey (Part 1) recounts my story - 'the cancer years' and my research is covered in Part 2, which also covers the politics of cancer and meta-politics (politics of the spirit).

A few up-dates and contemporary notes have been made but the basic research and theory for cancer is the same as when I compiled an initial manuscript in 1989. Some names have been changed to protect privacy.

PART 1

MY JOURNEY

THE CANCER YEARS

*The highest reward for a man's toil is not what he gets
for it but what he becomes by it.
(John Ruskin 1819-1900)*

1 Cinderella and Prince Charming

In early June 1985 I was walking down from the Palais de Croisette to the Carlton Hotel in Cannes in a white lace dress I nearly had on, plunging as it did down my back, having convinced myself that this was all I had ever wanted out of life.

A childhood in the fifties coloured by heavy dark brown furniture, brown linoleum floors, austerity and chronic eczema and asthma in a home where there was a rather despondent atmosphere, had caused me from an early age to escape reality. I had my head permanently stuck in a book. Brother Grimm fairy stories were an early favourite; where beautiful princesses dressed in white lace dresses, would be rescued from unimaginable fates by knights in shining armour. One of my first toys was a wind-up Cinderella, dancing with Prince charming and an old jewel box where I would keep my 'jewels'.

I would put on my mother's dance dress and career around the room. I loved the orange taffeta one with its gold embroidery and the black velvet one with the pink ostrich feathers and long white kid gloves with pearl buttons. Pouring imaginary tea in the wheat fields behind mother's house on our annual holiday in Yorkshire from an antique black and red coffee Wedgwood set, dressed in a plumed black hat with netted veil – I could have easily been in a palace.

I soon graduated to the Famous Five books where children seemed to have the most wonderful adventures. Weekly I would walk the mile from our family home to Richmond-upon-Thames town centre and climb the stairs to the public library on Richmond Green. I can still smell the fusty air that led my way to the shelves of books, which offered complete sanctuary. The Turner picture 'The Millpond' on the first landing became a comfortable familiar encounter, in a world that seemed far from secure. The library would become a second home, where because there were no studying facilities at home, I would spend weekends studying for A levels there, going on to graduate in Biochemistry and Physiology. Afterwards I had worked in academic research for fifteen years and had lectured at a Polytechnic.

Having failed the 11-plus, after a childhood in and out of hospital with eczema and asthma, I was considered highly unusual in that I had gone on to

University. It may seem incredible now, but I had to lie about my father's profession on my University Entrance forms – class barriers were still very evident even in the so-called 'swinging sixties' and even today are still evident in a very unequal society, if not more so as at least I gained a grant to attend university and would not otherwise have been able to go.

As I walked by the Cannes seafront now with Max, the father of my children and a successful advertising executive, perhaps I felt that he was my knight in shining armour I dreamt I would meet as a child. This evening we were having dinner at the Carlton Hotel. Max had a white baggy jacket on, sleeves rolled up in feigned casualness, his silver flecked hair hinting that he was ten years older than I. He had a sort of fashionable, gaunt, strong, left over from-the night before look, which resulted from long years visiting the notorious watering holes of the Advertising Industry dotted over one square mile of Soho and Mayfair in London.

As we walked into the restaurant, three waiters rushed to pull my chair out to seat me, and I was aware of the eyes following the lace down my back. I was also aware that most people in the restaurant were looking at us, perhaps wondering whether they should recognise us.

I flicked my gold cigarette lighter, and lit his cigarette and mine. I held it, turning it around in a lightly tanned delicate hand, edged with shaped cerise fingernails, and entwined in a pearl bracelet. Looking around the elegant restaurant with its soft velvety anaesthetizing atmosphere, feeling the soft carpet in tones of beige, grey and pink beneath my delicate shoes, if there was a glimmer of pain and loneliness that evening, I had pushed it far from my mind. I convinced myself that this was the real world – there was no brown linoleum or tin baths of my childhood here.

The outwardly attractive confident woman of the world image I presented was a far cry from what was happening in the turbulent inner me, where feelings of self-doubt panic and above all loneliness and pain were constantly threatening my very existence. I had often thought of raising the subject with Max, but he was indoctrinated into the so-called 'Golden Age' of advertising and the fifties idyll of smiling housewives showing off the gadget filled kitchens of their idyllic houses, which they shared with handsome attentive husbands and perfect children. Loneliness and misery were not part of the advertising world's construct of happiness, seen as fulfilled in the pursuit of material possessions and the right to individual happiness through that.

I sipped my champagne and lit yet another cigarette. I noticed Max's cool gaze, and another arrow bounced off my already armoured chest. I picked at my lobster, which I had calculated at £30 per mouthful was ridiculous. I sat silent less my lobster should be removed and replaced by brown linoleum under my feet, less Cinderella be returned after the ball back to rags and her coach back into a pumpkin, less I should awaken from my dream and discover I was dancing with Dorian Grey, not prince charming. Like 'A Picture of Dorian Grey' by Oscar Wilde, there was a hidden picture that seemed to be ever present in the attic of our minds, some forgotten memory but which was ever present. Years later in my journey I would discover the picture, but that evening in the Carlton Hotel neither of us knew that we were merely actors on a stage, compelled by a past life, to re-enact the scene again in a different setting but with the same actors. The closing curtain was about to drop.

Max was speaking, what was he talking about? Ah yes, advertising. I tried to seem interested, but the truth was, after seven years, I wasn't listening anymore. I failed to connect with the power battles fought in board rooms, the names of people who I had not met, it all seemed so irrelevant to me. Seven years of sitting through stories of advertising shoots with advertising people had made me yearn for a deep meaning to my life – something more real than this. The brittle people, ferociously ambitious, who ruthlessly knifed each other in the back, simply held no meaning for me. The dog eats dog culture where as Max once told me: "you're only as good as your last ad". Their reckless lifestyles, with outrageous heavy drinking and ability to keep affairs hidden, through explanations such as: "I had to work late as the presentation to the client is this week" - or the location shoots in other countries. There was a sense of a life of empty pointlessness and systematic betrayal. Betrayal although I did not recognise it then, had stirred a number of deep betrayals in this and past lives, where Max and I had tussled before on issues of social equality and male power.

Here I was once again dusted from the kitchen cupboard, to be paraded at the advertising film festival in Cannes where Soho would migrate to for one week every year. Some of the faces behind the names would become real, the champagne would flow, the laughter, the stories, the never-ending stories. I would smile and listen, smile and listen. Sometimes I wanted to interrupt the

16

conversation and ask whether advertising had exploded consumerism to the point where people had developed greed to an extent where they felt they could have whatever they wanted. Or what about the idea that unlimited opportunities posed by material wealth had fuelled the culture of individualism: where moral authority, duty and responsibility were no longer ideals instilled into children.

"For God's sake Renee!" Max looked cold and irritated. I jumped.

"Oh yes...I'm listening".

Surely, I should be happy I thought, sitting here in Cannes. I looked at Max and could only feel deep resentment that this man could not see that material achievement and power counts for nothing – what matters are the needs of others and relationships with them. I felt resentment that somewhere in this man's world I had lost myself completely. There was no purpose and yet I felt almost a desperate need to find something beyond the self, I felt a pressing commitment but had no idea of what it was. I could not explain my suffering really, it was inarticulate, but somewhere I could feel a sense of foreboding – that I was being forced to confront something I had carefully avoided for a long time.

Max looked relieved as the others came to join us, we had ceased lately to communicate past a basic level and somewhere I no longer wanted to talk to him. I wanted desperately to communicate with him, but the likelihood of that seemed remote and so I surrendered to silence. I was glad too that the others had arrived, it let me off the hook, I no longer had to listen but just smile and nod and for another evening we would not confront the tiger in the living room.

I wanted to jump up and shout: "Does anyone here have feelings of helplessness, hopelessness – Is anyone here deeply unhappy?" Perhaps the conversation would have stopped dead as they stared in disbelief that anyone could be anything other than happy in the bright and colourful world created by media. Unhappy, how can that be? Had they convinced themselves that the mythical world that they had created existed? Or was it more that there was something wrong with me? I felt at the time that the latter was the best solution.

17

The Princess in her Cinderella dress in Cannes, and I was no more real than the clockwork Cinderella of my childhood. Sometimes when spoken to, I would have to concentrate very hard. The names would blur in my mind, and I would muddle names of chairmen and managing directors. I would key into conversations picking up bits and pieces and yet this did not forewarn me, of a decline in my emotional state, after which serious illness arises. And so it was that night in Cannes in June 1985, I sat motionless waiting for the guillotine axe to fall.

2 The Awakening

It didn't take long for it to do so. In March of 1985 I had given birth to my second son, Barnaby and a few months later my father died of cancer. Up until his death, I watched him slowly and painfully wasting away, but felt helpless to do anything. The doctors declared that no more treatment would be effective and told me to take him home and wait for his death. Just before he died, he said philosophically, "some people do great things with their life and others do nothing at all". If he was reflecting on his own life then he judged himself harshly. He had fought in North Africa, recovered from typhoid and was hit with a bullet on D-Day in his leg, which caused problems later. He returned from war with what would be termed today post-traumatic stress disorder. My mother told me he used to jump out of bed, believing he was in a trench and once when the children went to the war museum, he would not go in, but sat quietly on the bench outside. He never spoke about it and for my generation growing up in the late 50's we were for the main unaware that our parents had survived a war – nobody spoke about it, as if they shared silently a collective trauma of loss and grief.

The general air of despondency in the fifties matched the brown linoleum. When radio programmes covered dedicated songs to "our troops in Germany" I sometimes wondered why they were there. Mother had been a land army girl and she was made of strong Yorkshire mentality. The land army girls had taken over food production on the land for the British people, whilst the men were away at war. Despite the austerity of post war Britain, she managed to feed us well, where Yorkshire puddings, pies and dumplings figured heavily on the menu. As an extraordinary pastry cook she would have done well if she taken up my father's suggestion that they start a pie shop: but having lost her father at thirteen through hypothermia in the coal mines and having then to work in service, to help support her mother and younger brother, she was afraid of risk. She once told me that she had to sell vegetables from her father's allotment from a wheelbarrow before she went to school, so that the family could survive. Despite our diet we were not overweight as without computers, Richmond-Upon-Thames the town where I was born provided an enormous child's playground with numerous activities. It was a royal borough and from an early age I was very cognisant of a class divide and I was also aware that I was not to ask for anything. To ask for anything was seen to jeopardise the family's survival.

As a child I would walk for miles through Richmond Park searching for the herds of deer or listening to the band playing at the bandstand on weekends. I would think nothing of walking along the Thames ten miles to Brentford and then back. A love of horticulture was nurtured in the many hours I spent wandering in Kew Gardens, where I would stare in awe at the trees hundreds of years old. Fishing for frogspawn in the 'Mini-ha-ha' in spring was a yearly ritual along with conkers in the autumn. Our parents saw nothing much of us at weekends, where packed off with jam sandwiches and a bottle of home-made ginger beer we would spend our days, experiencing the season's activities. Parents never concerned themselves over whereabouts or safety, we were expected to "go out and play".

In the summer the gardens overlooking the Thames, a scene made famous by the painter Turner, would be the stage for plays by Shakespeare. Not being able to afford the ticket, I smuggled myself into the bushes, to watch 'A Midsummer Night's Dream' and sat entranced for the whole performance. Without television until the late 50's, our treat as children was Saturday morning pictures. Children would cram into the Odeon where an organist playing his organ would emerge from the floor, heralding the start of the programme. I don't regret that my parents only lately brought a television, as games and books developed my imagination but I was always very innocent of the workings of the world. I was a great fan of the BBC world service and Radio 4, which taught me the art of listening. Time moved more slowly then and there seemed to be more of it.

My father's passion was swimming and before he died he set up the Richmond Water Polo Club. I trained with my father and every year we would enter the mile swim along the Thames and after the swim we would have a barbeque on one the Thames islands. Taking a rowing boat along the Thames, one could moor up at little teahouses and experience the delight of home-made scones and teacakes. The Thames held many memories for me and I still remember the book 'Three Men in a Boat' by Jerome K Jerome as being a favourite.

Mostly Richmond-upon-Thames, gave me a sense of history. My favourite walk was through the old palace, where Queen Elizabeth 1, had stayed. Hampton Court palace was another favourite, where I would wander through

20

the rooms fascinated by the ancient faces who stared down from their portraits.

Max was a Fulham boy, very street savvy and having worked in the Advertising industry for years, was versed far more than I in the ways of the world. I was his third wife and a decade younger, but it never occurred to me question the reasons for the break-up of two marriages, naively accepting one side (his) of the story.

The day I buried my father, I remember sitting at the window unable to cry, unable to feel anything. I felt numb. Although I wondered about this, I was not then aware that I was not able to cry because of an early childhood trauma hidden in my mind, where I had learnt to contain grief and anger.

I was sitting in the restaurant at Gleneagles Hotel in Scotland; a huge dolphin cut from ice was on the trolley beside me as the waiter delicately lay the little caviar eggs on my plate. Dressed in a chic white jacket crossed over at the front and clasped with a blood red ruby brooch over my heart, my fair hair flowing down over my shoulders, I looked down at the large white plate with the little eggs on it, the lump in my left breast was perhaps a little bigger, it was hard and it moved slightly when I pushed it. When did it arise? What was it? Why was it there? What does it mean?

"For God's sake, if you're going to sit around here, with a face full of misery, feeling your breasts all weekend, I'm going home!"

Feeling Max's irritation, I removed my hand from under my jacket like a child caught doing something naughty. I started to eat the caviar, which I had calculated at £60 per small mouthful as utterly ridiculous.

The lump had become taboo, it did not fit into Max's idea of the perfect family and emotional pain was not a subject Max could or would confront. His only concession was that I should get our GP to have a look at it when we flew back after the weekend.

The ice dolphin I noticed was beginning to melt, little ripples of water that looked like tears, tears for the unborn caviar eggs or tears for me? A foreboding entered my whole being and as I looked around the restaurant, the fire flickering all was peace, but inside me, was turmoil.

21

3 The Magic Roundabout

It was Tuesday morning when I found myself in the waiting room of Dr Raymond our GP in Esher.

"Hello Renee, we haven't seen you for some time, what can we do for you?" He spoke whilst writing at his desk.

"I've got a lump in my breast," I replied flatly.

"I see, well let's have a look at it", he replied leading me to the examination couch.

I lay there on my back, staring up at the ceiling, whilst he examined me. His breath smelt strongly of cigarettes. I noticed it was 11.00 am, and he had probably just had his mid- morning cigarette.

I had my arms up over my head; my breasts looked rather small and girlish. Compared to the rest of my family, my breasts appeared to have stopped growing at puberty. I often used to wonder whether as a girl I had been too worried about the business of surviving to develop the luxury of reproducing myself. Perhaps in some way I had remained stuck in something in the past. Years later I would discover the hidden traumas of childhood.

"It's a cyst, nothing to worry about at all".

"Are you quite sure?"

"Yes," he replied reassuringly.

"Do I have to come back and see you about it?"

"No, it's perfectly all right; it will probably go down soon".

"What if it doesn't?" I asked, wondering whether I would have to permanently put up with a cyst in one of my offending breasts.

"They usually come and go," he replied matter- of- factly.

I thanked him and left. I wasn't assured and that evening tried to voice my feelings that maybe Dr Raymond wasn't right, maybe it wasn't a cyst. Max seemed irritated.

"Look if the doctor says it's a cyst, it's a cyst, why do you have to question everything?"

But I did question and visited a doctor privately at the Lister Hospital to gain a second opinion. I was again assured it was a cyst.

"There you are!" Max exclaimed with some relief that once again we did not have to confront too much reality.

Sometimes Max would catch me feeling the lump, his eyes would roll heavenward and he would sigh and give me one of his famous withering looks, which had often turned many a yuppie account man into a quivering wreck; as one once confided in me at a cocktail party: "You know I have to have a stiff drink before I go into a meeting with your husband". I knew the feeling well.

Advertising is a cutthroat business, where one has to continually look over one's shoulder lest the knife from a smiling assailant be plunged neatly between your shoulder blades, by a so-called 'friend.' Perhaps if Max had gone into another career he would have been different. My hopes of a warm, fulfilling, safe and secure meaningful relationship seemed to diminish daily. Where there had once been love now there was bitterness and resentment, but above all the betrayal consumed me. I wondered whom Max really was, who I really was. I knew he probably didn't even know himself anymore. It would take some years before I would in regressive past life therapy remember.

On the rare occasions that we now went out together we sat in strained silence or antagonism. I couldn't remember when I had stopped smelling the spring. Spring brought hope, rebirth and growth. This spring seemed like a cold perpetual winter. I felt my breast a lot when I was alone. Was it getting bigger? Yes, it was. I knew every minute detail of 'the lump' now. It had stopped moving and was quite large. It was irregular and no longer spherical. It was solid.

In February 1986, Max went to a wrestling match in Ireland with his friends. Leuinne a South African friend, who I had met on the school run, had invited me and the children to Sunday lunch in Oxshott, with some of her friends and their children. Leuinne for some time had been worried about the lump in my breast and over lunch, she had the bad practise, but for my sake, the sheer good fortune, to mention my lump to her GP friend, who was married to a gastro-intestinal surgeon. Both she and her husband looked aghast, when they discovered that the lump had not been aspirated to determine whether or not it was a cyst. "Cysts" maintained the GP "always have fluids in them". The surgeon then asked me if I had had a biopsy. I shook my head in what felt like slow motion and in those split seconds my whole life juddered to a halt, when I realised I had cancer. The GP recommended a specialist in Harley Street, where I could receive a biopsy immediately.

There is no recollection of the following period as I was in a state of shock; only my diary reveals the events.

24th February

Made an appointment with Harley Street specialist.

27th February

Saw the specialist at 8.00am. Had mammograms taken and aspiration attempted. Told it was not a cyst. Took slides for pathology. Feel angry – NOT A CYST!

28th February

More tests. Max has invited Leuinne and her husband Herman to supper with David, Myuki and Susie Henry and Alex. Max continues as though nothing has happened. Too worried to speak much. Shock, fears realised. In my heart I know what this means. Angry for allowing Max to subdue me into acceptance that it was a cyst. Angry ... with Max and being forced to accept his behaviour... Angry that I should have double-checked.... Anger at myself.

3rd March

Specialist says lump will have to come out. See another specialist Dr Gazet at 7.30 pm at Parkside Hospital in Wimbledon. He took slides for pathology. Feel more comfortable with Dr Gazet than the other specialist.

4th March

I change surgeons over. Everything set for next week. 5.30pm in the evening, bathing the children, first surgeon rings to say: "it's malignant". That's all he says, he does not ask if I have anyone with me. Legs go weak – collapse and give phone to Max. Lie on bed. Max finishes the children's bath. Feel totally cut off from everything and everyone – not a part of this world anymore. Later Dr Gazet rings to tell Max it is malignant and he will operate next week on Thursday. Max is genuinely shocked. Thursday is Thor's day the god of thunder and wrath – I do feel angry.

5th March

Arrive at Parkside Hospital. Can't see or hear anything. Just time passing. Has it spread? Will I see my babies grow up? Go upstairs to my room and get undressed for bed. I pull up my nightdress in front of the mirror and think: "I won't ever feel or look this way again". Dr Gazet comes in and I give him explicit instructions that he is only to remove the tumour and not the breast. He looks doubtful. I make him give me his word of honour. He gives it.

6th March

Thor's day has arrived. Nurse arrives in operating gown and 'jay cloth' cap. I ask for socks, because my feet are cold. The nurse tells me I won't need them because they strip you naked on the operating table. "There's no dignity," she says.

I wake up and it's over. Bandages all over my chest, very tight squeezing the life out of me. Can't breathe. Memories of childhood and asthma attacks come flooding back. Faces drift in and out. I wonder what's happened. They tell me it has spread to the lymph nodes but I still have my breasts. I don't care anymore.

10th March

Leave hospital. Empty shell.

21st March

Radiation treatment starts at The Royal Marsden Hospital -very apprehensive and nervous. I ask the radiologist a question he replies that time means treatment: "If I'm not treating you I could be treating someone else". That's when you realise how inhuman you are to them just a piece of meat on a conveyor belt. Rude people are cruel people. As a scientist I had asked him about the damage to DNA by radiation and the effect of mutation. No answer – so what is the answer? If this is private medicine then God help those on the NHS. Like peas on a conveyor belt, processed by this wretched machine – this monstrous machine. Spends its entire day burning people – busy little machine. Surely this can't be the way to treat cancer – can it? He draws marks on my chest with a marker, which now looks like an ordinance survey map. He says: "Have got to get it right". Yes I think, do get it right this time, because I can't afford any more screw-ups on my body or mind. The buzzer goes they all run out of the room – I have to stay alone with the wretched machine, blasting out lethal radiation. A xylophone "ping, pong, ping, pong," breaks the silence – the quiet little sounds of lethal radiation hitting you. I wonder if they played "ping, pong, ping, pong" when they dropped the bomb on Hiroshima. A picture of Frank Sinatra singing *My Way* comes into my mind, whilst World War III or Armageddon is raging to the ubiquitous notes of "ping, pong, ping, pong".

The buzzer goes and they all rush back in. They swing the machine over. I am looking down the barrel now. The buzzer goes they all rush out: "ping, pong, ping, pong, ping, and pong". A picture comes to mind of a table tennis tournament and I imagine I am batting the lethal waves back to my opponent. A picture of Frank Sinatra singing *My Way* comes to my mind again – is this *my way* I think?

They tell me it's not harmful, but then that can't be true. Oh help me – what is the truth? I've got to stay, I've got to go, I want to go, I can't stay – what shall I do!

22nd March

Rufus and Barney's birthday party - Tried to make it happen. I smile and act cheerful because Max expects it. The children feel safe and happy. It is as though nothing has happened. "Make an effort" Max says. I do, but how does that solve anything? You can't pretend to yourself that this illness is not a warning - a warning of what? One parent arrives with their child and looking around the great hall says: "Oh, I never knew". Knew what? God these people in Oxshott and Esher are such snobs.

23rd March

Sunday, but feel too tired and exhausted to do much. The radiation area is incredibly sore. Feel depressed. Woke up this morning with sun coming through the window and for one moment I forgot I have cancer – then the reality again dawns and this totally all enveloping black desolation overrides me and I realise it's all true. A voice in my head says: "do something Renee!" What should I do? – I know I am going down the wrong route, but which is the right one? There are no signposts only forks in the road.
I must get back to the road before the fork.

I had a dream last night. I don't think it was a dream it seemed more a real event. I dreamt Max was standing with another woman. It seemed inevitable in my dream, an inevitable strangeness. I was burnt and wrinkled like an old woman. I was holding out my hand and he was standing next to this woman. Her face was blank – there was no face but she had blonde hair and she was standing with my children. My children were looking at me with such pain and loneliness in their eyes as if to say: "Don't go," and I held out my hand to them and it was withered and burnt, and I looked down at my hands and I was shocked. I woke up crying. Max asked me what was wrong and I told him I had a bad dream, a horrible dream. I don't think it was a dream.

24th March

Denise rang to cheer me up. They took a mould of my chest today. They said they were going to feed information into a computer to see whether I was getting overall radiation for the area – "to make sure it wasn't going too deep to my lungs." What the hell do they mean, not going too deep to my lungs!

Are they killing me? God what shall I do – can't go, must go. Do they know what they are doing? Do I know what I am doing?

25th March

Had to sit through forty minutes of buzzer and "ping, pong, ping pong" before it's my turn: like a conveyer belt, a machine at it all the time. I am the youngest woman there as most days. I wonder if my life has contributed and whether all those lonely nights waiting for Max to come home from London and his reckless social life have caused this.

27th March

Jo the cleaner came, and told me the story of Sarah, her sister, having died from breast cancer and it travelled to her spine and she died in agony. I'm not sure I felt grateful for this story, which she related by following me from room to room as I tried not to listen. I am realising that a lot of people don't make it despite the doctors' assurances. What shall I do?

I am early and go to the hospital cafe - there are some pitiful sights. I try not to take it in but think, 'thank God that's not me' and look with pity as the healthy do on you. There are degrees of anything. A group of people were gathered around a woman in a pink dressing gown with a pink turban on "well you would wouldn't you?" was all I caught. 'Would what?' I thought – wear a pink turban when my hair falls out? One teenager in a wheelchair with a very grey face and tufts of hair was staring into space, his eyes almost completely dead – those dead eyes again. I made a note that I must not drift off anymore less I develop the dead eyes. His father was wearing tight jeans and had tattoos all up his arms. His mother sat silent with dead eyes. "There you are son," said the father lighting up a cigarette for his son despite the 'No Smoking' sign. He poked it into the mouth of the lifeless boy. I move to another area – I have given up smoking.

Sitting down with another group I hear one say:

"It's wonderful here".

'Wonderful?' I think.

28

"They told me I would be alright".

I wonder if she will be all right.

"I love coming here you know" says the women next to her.

'Love coming here?' I think.

"I have to go downstairs for high voltage," she continues.

I unkindly think she needs high voltage to her brain.

"You don't feel it do you, I mean you feel on top of the world don't you?"

'On top of the world?' I think. I wonder whether she realises she has cancer, I wonder if she realises what it means. I wonder if she will be all right and I won't, because she does not think about it. I decide not thinking about it, is the way to get through. Just blank your mind off and hope that it won't come back in your spine or somewhere else. Dismiss it like a wart on your finger, have it cut out ...but then warts *do* come back. I feel as though I have aged a lifetime, "I am older than that now".

Good Friday 28th March

Max and I take the children down to Devon for Easter. It was warm and lovely. I try to hang onto good memories. Rufus eats his way through room service and he's only 4 years old. When he was 18 months we took him to Venice and stayed at the Hotel Daniellie. The room service bill for him came to £600 because they insisted on serving his pasta on a trolley with silver tureen. Barney would love Italy – he only likes pasta.

29th March

Took the children to Clough Valley. Barnes and Rufus loved the donkey rides. It was a happy day – a good memory.

1st April

I was told to go and see the breast specialist because, "You don't seem to be accepting treatment well". What does that mean that I am not enjoying being blasted with lethal radiation? Evidently they are used to comatose women who say: "It's wonderful here".

The hospital is very busy- a nurse informs us there is a "backlog" as they call us, after Easter, like sacks of mail waiting to be shifted but apparently: "the transport never came in this morning," she adds. I imagine a large battle, with wounded lying on the battlefield with no trucks to transport them.
It does look like the front line of a battlefield, with wheelchairs everywhere and people covered in blankets, people on trolleys; everywhere grey people, with those dead eyes. One nurse parked a man next to me who then told me how he had spent a "rotten Easter weekend, vomiting on the drugs". I felt extremely sorry for him, but wished he would go away – I was still trying to hang on to the good memories. His breath had the distinctive smell and fetor of cancer and the vomit he spoke of. I get up and walk about. I hear a nurse moaning about: "everyone losing their marks" over the holiday. I go to the loo and pencil mine in with khol eyeliner. Maybe they won't remember exactly where the marks are, maybe somebody won't get it right ... maybe I'll be back here in the next five or ten years.

I meet a woman in the 'Theratron Unit'. She is in her late fifties. She has a lung tumour. She has to have several types of radiation, but no chemotherapy. She is frightened.

"But you are so young you have had no life at all" she says adding: "You don't look ill".

I find myself comforting her, telling her she will be all right. I don't for one minute believe she will be, but she seems better for the comment.

"You are very kind," she says.

If I was kind I think, I would tell her that she should escape because I don't think this treatment works – there is more to this. What shall I do?

6th April

Max does not want to talk about cancer, he says he wants to get on with his life and wishes that I could do the same. A rage arises in me, but I quickly pop the wild animal into a cupboard and lock the door. It won't stay there for long. I know that I am doing the wrong thing by undergoing radiation, but its Max not me who wants me to take it. Is he saying, "die quietly" and cause the least inconvenience? Let him get on with *his* life! But isn't that what he has always done? Isn't that why I am ill now? If I try to approach anything on the subject now, Max leaves the room: he is quite incapable of discussing feelings or confronting the crisis.

8th April

The wild animal is bubbling away in the cupboard, it's going to explode soon through the door; I fear the intensity of the rage I feel.

I am at the hospital for more of their lethal rays. I tell the doctor that I am exhausted all the time. He tells me that it is inevitable with the treatment and then adds it should not make me that tired. Well, again what does he mean? - Should I be tired "inevitably" with the treatment or not? In actual fact I am too tired to worry about the contradiction.

My mother has given me a gift of £2,000 to be frivolous with and I visit a favourite and expensive shop in Esher. I buy a tied died blue silk dress, with tied dyed soft kid leather flowers and pearls. It reminds me of the fairy in Midsummer Night's Dream. I don't know where I will wear it, but it reminds me also of my 'flower power' days and the freedom we all felt at the Isle of Wight Festival listening to Hendrix. I can still remember floating around in my flowers, bangles and beads watching others get stoned but for me I never took drugs – there had already been in my life too many things over which I had had no control. Drugs scare me.

I float around in my dress with my eyes closed, and I am back at the Isle of Wight, I am happy, very happy. I hear Max's car pull up, my vision of the Isle of Wight dissolves.

28th April

Max told me I could drive his Aston Martin to the hospital – he thought it might take my mind off the treatment. I don't want it – it's a man's car and anyway it doesn't make up for having to go alone again. How can he believe that material possessions are any replacement for human warmth and support?

I met a woman at the hospital today. She told me she had a lumpectomy like me. They had also removed her lymph glands and then she had to have her ovaries removed. She was given the all clear a year ago after chemotherapy and radiotherapy. Now she is back and the cancer has returned in her spleen and in her eye. As she told me this, a terrible fear arose in my throat. I went to the hospital toilet and threw up. This doesn't work I think. I tried to think and regain my composure. I decided that this is the wrong route and I walked out of the hospital. I felt strangely elated, as though I had jumped off the train and wandered into fields of flowers.

I went to Foyle's Bookstore in London and brought every book they had on cancer. I decide I will not tell Max that I am not doing chemotherapy it will only cause another argument. Anyway it's my life! Having said this I feel a strange power and a decision has been made!

5th May

I feel the wild thing rattling on the door - it wants to be free.

4 White Lace and Promises

The books gave cause for thought and I started to make notes on periods of my life, which could have affected my health. A poor student diet at University; a strenuous renovation of Stowford Farm in Oxford, where I had worked continuously long hours on the works, whilst taking care of Rufus just 3 years old and Barnaby just a few months old. I had not been entirely kind to myself.

I believed perhaps that if I could communicate with Max, our relationship could still be saved and there were the children to think of.

"I am going to Los Angeles on business soon and the Agency has said that they would pay for you to go along, as you have had a rotten time of it. Would you like to go?" Max casually asked one evening.

When I landed in LA, I forgot about cancer, drugs and hospitals and straight out of the blue after a couple of days Max asked me to marry him. Perhaps this would be the turning point – a commitment.

We were packing for the flight to Vegas and I was dabbing some perfume on my arms, when I stopped dead, a weak feeling that I knew very well consumed me. Yes there, under my left arm was a lump. Why hadn't I noticed it? It could not be more cancer no that was ridiculous- ridiculous. I took a long and deep breath and snapping my suitcase shut I decided that lump or not it wasn't going to spoil this day.

Max's writer, his girlfriend and the producer were with us on the plane and we drank champagne. We went to the courthouse to get a licence and booked the Candle Light Wedding Chapel and by 8pm I was wearing the blue tie-dyed chiffon dress that I wondered whether I would ever wear and we were driving down 'the strip.' We arrived at the Chapel to be asked by the minister whether we wanted music. A rather dubious character was pulled from the nearest bar and I asked him what his repertoire was.

"I know 'A Lady,' by Lionel Richie".

"That will do".

During the ceremony I realised he was inappropriately playing 'Memories' something he evidently did not possess. The words "too painful to remember, we simply choose to forget," rang out and I wondered whether it was an omen or a warning or just a grotesque parody that Cinderella and Prince Charming were marrying in Las Vegas.

After a meal in a restaurant, it was on to Caesar's Palace to hear Pati Boulai in concert. Arriving back at the hotel late I passed a couple that said:

"Hi bride, you look beautiful".

I sat for a while on the balcony looking out over the lights of Vegas, with the warm night air on my face. I read through the words of the wedding ceremony, taken from 'The Prophet' by Imram Halil:

'Love one another but make not a bond of love
Let it rather be a moving sea, between the shores of your souls
Fill each other's cup but drink not from one cup.

Give one another of your bread but eat not from the same loaf.
Sing and dance together and be joyous but let each one of you be alone.
Even as the strings of a lute are alone they may quiver with the same music.

Give your hearts but not into each other's keeping.
For only the hand of life can contain your heart.
And stand together yet not too near together
For the pillars of the temple stand apart, and the Oak tree and the
Cyprus grows not in each other's shadow'.

Max and I two trees perhaps, who did not grow well in each other's company. Perhaps I had all my life, given my heart when I should have thought with my head. The poem seemed to stir some memory – the last two lines fascinated me although it would take some years and a past life memory to see exactly why.

5 The Search

Too soon I was back in reality again with cancer, the English weather and Max who inevitably returned to his old haunts of the Zanzibar and Groucho club in London. The thought often arose that I should do something – but what? The lump under my arm was getting bigger.

A trip to Bushy Park with the children became a defining moment. I felt a deep tiredness over my whole body, I was still red in the area of the radiation and my left arm horribly ached. I would not be told until years later, that I had been overdosed along with one hundred other patients with radiation and the left arm was permanently damaged as a side effect – they could not even get that right.

As I lay on the grass watching Rufus play and Barnaby asleep in his pushchair, I closed my eyes and held my face to the warm sun, listening to the little peals of laughter. I must do something for their sake I thought. I cannot leave them.

I decided that I should attack the problem from a scientific point of view and as a Biochemist I would review all the research myself, in case the scientists had missed something. I would also find out what alternative medicine had to offer. Ever methodical I opened up 'The Cancer Files' - labelled them and put up a list that ended in the word 'CURED'.

I spent hours going through research papers, listed in the science citation index. The data is now voluminous if not mountainous and would require years to do a review even so a biochemical picture of cancer was emerging.

I spent a frantic few months travelling all over London, in search of alternatives. I would sit with Joseph Corvo a reflexologist, who would tell me:

"You are a beautiful rose Renee that has been neglected and allowed to wither and die".

Rose? – Neglected? Yes there seemed to be something there – two trees perhaps, or two sides of alternative and orthodox where one had withered and died whilst the oak, with roots that go deep underground took all the water and nutrients and had become strong and was now king of the woods.

I also visited the 'White Witch' as she was teasingly known, one of the best herbalists in London. Sitting in her office she paused when I ask her if there was a comprehensive alternative in cancer treatment.

"Well, there is the Gerson Therapy," she replied hesitatingly.

She continued to explain that it was a nutritional therapy for cancer and was in fact the most notorious and vigorous of all the nutritional therapies that had shown some success and she quoted Beta Bishop who was a recovered myeloma patient who had used this approach. I did not know much about myeloma at that time other than it was a particularly fast spreading and usually lethal form of cancer.

I rang Beata the following day and she told me I was fortunate in so far as there was a Gerson Seminar to be held in Kensington - London the following week, to be given by Margaret Strauss the granddaughter of Dr Gerson. Beata was non-committal about the therapy only saying that it was extremely difficult and that with two small children she thought it would not be appropriate, unless my husband was committed and I had help and support.

Margaret Strauss the granddaughter of Dr Gerson was a tall well-groomed, confident and healthy looking woman with a well-spoken American accent. I learnt that she and her mother Charlotte Gerson were responsible for continuing the work of Charlotte's father Dr Gerson, mainly through a Clinic in Mexico. Two years later I would meet Charlotte, who was astounded that I had tackled the Gerson Therapy alone, with two very young children telling me:

"It is unheard of, I would have said it could not be done – but then you have done it".

I sat entranced for the whole day listening to details of the therapy and its development in the 1920's by Dr Max Gerson a German doctor who died in 1959. Later dietary methods were all, "an adopted form of his therapy" claimed Margaret. Ah I thought I have found the road before the fork!

In the break whilst sipping herbal tea, I read some of the supporting leaflets and discovered that during his life, the orthodox medical establishment vigorously rejected Dr Gerson's therapy and theoretical explanations. I purchased a copy of Dr Gerson's book '*A Cancer Therapy: results of 50 cases*' [6] where he stated:

'What is essential is not the growth itself or the visible symptoms it is the damage of the whole metabolism including the loss of defence, immunity and healing power. It cannot be explained with, nor recognised, by one or another cause alone'.

The paragraph intrigued me, and the final sentence went round in my head for some time. I began to wonder whether cancer was not just a physical manifestation, but wondered if there was a mental component, as I knew from my research as a Biochemist when working on suicide cases, that depression was linked to low immunity.

Finally I managed to corner Margaret at the close of the meeting and ask her about my suitability for the therapy. She had stated during her talk that those patients who had undergone orthodox treatment of radiation and chemotherapy did not do as well, since their own healing power and immune system had been damaged.

"Have you had any orthodox treatment? She asked.

"Well I had some of a course of radiotherapy".

"Oh...radiation," she paused.

"Where did you have the radiation?"

"The neck, breast, underarm and sternum" I replied hesitatingly.

"The sternum - Oh I didn't know they did that any more".

"Why?" I asked feeling as though someone else didn't get it right. "Is that dangerous?"

"Well the thymus is there".

"The thymus - well isn't that non- functional in the adult?" I queried dredging up old biochemistry notes from my brain.

"Well that's what the doctors will tell you", she replied with a look of distaste.

"Oh," I replied feeling that somewhere there was a hidden communication line going on between alternative and orthodox medicine and that a university education had given me one side of the story – orthodox.

"Have you had any other treatment like chemotherapy?"

"No, I walked out of the hospital before that stage and I was told to take tamoxifen, but haven't".

"Well I'm not really sure whether you would be exactly right for this therapy," she replied in all honesty.

"I have to tell you that with people who have taken orthodox treatment the diet doesn't work very well, this is because the body's natural system of defence is damaged by orthodox methods, but in your case you haven't had the chemotherapy, so there may be some hope".

"I have got another lump under my arm," I said flatly: "And I am not going back to have any more radiation or chemotherapy, because I have met patients who went through the mill and still developed metastases".

"Well Renee, you must make your own decisions, but as a scientist you are more than capable of doing that".

She was right; I would have to weigh up the evidence. I made a mental note to go through everything and make a decision.

On the train home, I felt a burst of anger, with Margaret's words "The sternum? Oh I didn't know they did that anymore," repeating in my ears. I wondered if American medicine was more advanced, whether I had been an ignorant participant in an archaic form of treatment. The tube train was full; it was rush hour, motionless blank faces staring out of the windows. I opened Gerson's book and started to read.

38

Two days later, I closed the book. A sense of relief flooded over me that the rationale behind the Gerson Therapy made such good scientific sense. Here was a truth about cancer, I had not recognised elsewhere. In the same moment I felt a sense of huge betrayal that I had undergone damaging radiation therapy and been left with the consequences of that and damage to my left arm. I pondered on the fact that it was my left breast, left arm and wondered whether there was some significance to the 'LEFT' – I made a note and put it up on my 'to do' list.

The months of questioning seemed to be fulfilled; now I had an answer. I could not believe that this therapy had been ignored or the rationale behind it. In my days as a research scientist, had I been given this therapy to look at, I would undoubtedly have tested it. Why didn't people know about it?

The initial euphoria settled, when on re-reading the book several times, I realised why Margaret Strauss and Beta had thought it would not be suitable for me. It was a punishing schedule of food preparation, with 13 organic juices and 3 organic meals a day. The therapy was precise and arduous and I wondered how I could fit it all in, with the children still only one and four years old. Most of all I worried about Max who had stated in no uncertain terms, that he was heartedly sick of hearing about cancer, although he had shown some help recently. The entertaining schedule would have to go. Then there was all the organic produce, this was 1986 and you were considered weird if you ate organic food and supermarkets did not yet stock it. Where was I going to find the 50 pounds of carrots a week and 38 pounds of apples and 30 lettuces and the pounds of other vegetables? Where would I get the organic calves liver for the diet? Could I force myself to drink it as a juice 3 times a day? Then there was the special equipment, the juicer and certainly the cost. If someone then had explained to me the depth and terror of the healing reactions that would occur, I may have discounted the therapy altogether.

Feeling apprehensive that I would not be able to complete the rigours of the Gerson Therapy and sustain a relationship with Max, I looked around for many alternatives. The 'wild thing' I had locked in the cupboard accompanied the sense of urgency to do something, as the lump under my arm grew. The anger at having my life dictated by the actions of another had become increasingly difficult to contain.

6 Stopping My World

It was a crystal clear blue morning in September of 1986, when Max with one cold and sarcastic remark too far, unleashed my fury – the wild thing finally escaped; a furious row over, he left.

As if in a dream I gathered up Barnaby, put him in his pushchair and went down to the local greengrocer store in Cobham, buying up all the organic produce they had.

"Going to feed an army then?" the greengrocer laughed.

The price was astounding and I made a mental note that I would have to find somewhere cheaper. That day I started by making eight juices, with the centrifugal juicer. It was not what Gerson recommended, but I felt the need now Max was gone, to start the healing process. It seemed a never-ending session of washing and preparing vegetables, which in those days as organic, they came covered in mud and unwashed; as if proof they were organic.

Within two weeks of starting the therapy, I started to experience the 'healing reactions' that Gerson spoke of. Nothing in Gerson's book could have forewarned of the severity of those reactions, which at first were just physical: terrible nausea, vomiting, weakness, breathlessness and a continual headache. I was almost constantly retching and my stomach ached from this. Somehow I managed to continue with the juices, which Gerson claimed was critical during the 'healing reactions' and get Rufus to school in Oxshott.

I read and re-read Gerson's book and the section covering 'flare ups': 'A number of patients have remarked that within the first two weeks of the treatment that they cannot stand the diet and wish to discontinue it'.

Gerson reeled off the symptoms as nausea, headaches, in some cases vomiting even severe vomiting, cramps in the intestines, gas accumulation, no appetite, and inability to drink the juices and difficulties with the coffee enemas.

I had not yet got to the coffee enemas and in 1986 this was likely to have been sufficient to have you certified. Gerson's words rang in my head: 'It is better not to start than to only do a portion of the therapy as it could be dangerous'.

And:

'The reaction period...may recur almost every 10 days to 14 days and later once a month'.

True to his warning, I would feel extremely ill during the "flare ups" and on those occasions when I was too ill to leave my bed Rufus who was just five years old, would ferry things up and down the stairs to the bedroom. I did feel guilty, but far better that I survive than he and Barney end up without me.

I tried to tell myself that the healing reactions were a necessary part of my recovery, that during these periods, my body was detoxifying, that I would recover and if I could last two years, I would be healthy and would not have to worry whether the cancer would re-emerge or have another organ removed. It was hard as the days slipped by in the half- light of vomiting and diahorrea and the deep depression that comes with the "flare ups".

"Never mind mummy, I will look after you and Barnes" Rufus said, putting his little arm around my neck, with a little comforting pat up and down. A deep regret rushed over me, where I thought that it should not be like this for them. Rufus however, seemed to enjoy the responsibility during those periods.

In order to raise money for the full therapy and essential juicer, I had to sell most of the furniture and my family heirlooms. Even my jewellery was sold to an acquaintance in Wales. Rufus was upset and thus I tried to make it into a game. I explained that now the furniture had gone, the boys could use the house for more activities. Rufus brightened up immediately and Barnes seeing excitement ahead clapped his chubby hands. The Lea, our home had once been the Swedish Embassy in Esher, I was told. The house had an impressive 'Cecil-B-de-Mill' type staircase, with a minstrel gallery at the top. I explained now they could bike and skateboard around the minstrel gallery, without fear of damaging anything. As they became more adventurous they would abseil using climbing gear from the minstrel gallery. The loss of the furniture was forgotten. Rufus and Barney in later life would become good climbers and skaters and look back fondly on the activities in The Lea.

Anyone who saw the house would automatically think that I was not in need of charity, but maintenance cheques were variable and sometimes did not arrive at all: and did not allow for any part of the therapy. Throughout the therapy money was a severe problem, which did cause distress in itself. My first knight in shining armour came with Riccardo Ling, a man who had been charitably connected with the Gerson Therapy for over 30 years. He ran a trust whose aim was to help people who were in need of financial assistance. I was given the loan of a juicer and the juice press required for the liver juices, until such time I could afford my own. Ricardo showed me how to press the juices and I just felt overwhelmed at the extent of preparation.

"What a lot of preparation just to do one juice and then there are 13 a day", I said almost despairingly.

The days and weeks went by, my days occupied with having to prepare the juices and the phone, which had rung occasionally after Max left, now stopped ringing altogether. The therapy was isolating and I often felt like an alien from another planet, as I waited with other mothers to pick up Rufus from school in Oxshott – generally considered the stockbroker belt. I would catch snippets of conversation as they stood by their Mercedes, Porsches and Range Rovers.

"Lunch...love to".

"Tennis tomorrow ...love to".

Only Denise a Jewish woman, with three boys, who tied with Rufus and Barney for the title of the 'little rascals', was sympathetic to my predicament. Denise admitted she was "spoilt rotten". Her husband a hard working barrister in the City would often work long evenings on the dining table, preparing cases. Denise after having safely jailed the 'little rascals' in their bedrooms with a scream second only to Ethel Merman of:

"And don't come out or I'll murder you all!"

She would then retire to her bedroom, with chocolates and TV and spread across the bed would spend the evening increasing the telephone bill. Sometimes you would hear Peter in the background making sarcastic barrister type jokes of "the cost of your case". Where she would reply:

"Yes darling, I know darling, you are a wonder of support to me".

She would plead with me to give up the therapy.

"Oh Renee, I do wish you would stop driving yourself mad with all this. Can't you forget all this and take the drugs?"

I had tried so often to explain the rationale behind the Gerson Therapy and the deceit that had been woven by orthodoxy with regard to cancer, where the data now occupied two of my files, that it seemed pointless to once again explain it. To those on the outside one was considered a "conspiracy theorist" a label attached to avoid looking at the evidence. Later contact however with other scientists, such as Dr Becker, only confirmed to me that credible research had been *deliberately* hidden.

As I went through the healing reactions and 'flare ups', I began to re-experience the illnesses of childhood. One morning I awoke to find that I itched like crazy. Red swollen blotches had occurred prominently on my arms and legs. As the days went by and the healing reaction remained after 10 days, I could stand it no more and went to the doctor.

"Eczema," he pronounced.

After the children had gone to bed, I looked up Gerson's book and was jolted into remembering my notes from Margaret Strauss's lecture. I had made a note that: 'The therapy brings out old ailments to be cured, even childhood illnesses'.

I tore up the prescription for cortisone from the doctor, if the childhood eczema had to be re-lived in order to be healed then I would have to grin and bear it. However I made a note in my files that it seemed that the Gerson Therapy is able to cause one to recapitulate past illnesses asking:

'Does this mean that one recapitulates, the emotional and mental upset, that accompanies the illness?' and:

'Is the depression - and feelings of fear and terror, related to the recapitulation of past traumas?'
And finally in large capitals I wrote:

'WHAT IS THE MECHANISM? HOW CAN THE GERSON THERAPY DO THIS?'

The next morning I awoke with eczema and now the left side of my body where the radiation had been was bright purple and very painful. I lay in bed and looked down at the horrifying mess my body was now in, with chronic eczema and now looking more like an aubergine down the left side. And to boot my ribs in the area of radiation were horribly aching, as though I had been kicked repeatedly in the ribs overnight. Barnes started to demand his bottle and waves of desperation flooded over me, wondering how on earth I could continue, when I could not even stand up.

"Will you get Barnes his bottle love?" I said to Rufus, trying to hide the panic I felt. Rufus was always enthusiastic about being given responsibility and rushed downstairs "to" as he informed me "get breakfast". It was fortunate it was Saturday and not a school day.

By the evening I decided to ignore the cost and ring the Gerson Clinic in Mexico. I waited impatiently as the phone rang in some unknown room thousands of miles away. I spoke to a German doctor GarHildenbrand - rapidly describing my pitiful condition. He paused when I had finished and then said:

"You're doing great!"

"Great?" I answered in total disbelief that my miserable condition could be referred to as great.

"Yeah just great. You are getting some really good healing reactions. The eczema thing will clear up, the purple colour sounds as though there is a healing reaction, which has occurred in the area of radiation. There is probably increased blood flow in the area. The ribs and bones aching well, that sounds to me as though you had radiation damage to your muscle and bone".

Once again a feeling of being fooled and betrayed by orthodox medicine over radiation emerged as a steely anger – they didn't get it right.
"What about the orange colour?" I asked feeling a little more placated. I had by now also developed an orange tinge all over my body.

"Sounds as though you are a really colourful lady!" he joked and continued: "Don't worry about that, some of my best friends are orange and hey you are purple too!"

"Seriously" I replied "is this not due to carrotenosis from the orange pigment in carrots, taken in large quantities?" and as another thought added: "they say this could be dangerous".

"No, you will find that the orange colour will go as you continue with the therapy even though you continue to drink the same amount of carrot juice. It is just the liver sorting itself out". Then he asked casually "How many coffee enemas are you doing?"

"Err.... well I haven't exactly started them yet, I am still trying to get everything together" I replied sheepishly.

"Hey, that's bad, you must do the enemas, otherwise you won't get rid of the toxins and it sounds to me that you have got a hell of a lot of toxins going on right now".

The phone call calmed me down, and at least jolted me into the realisation that I would have to organise the whole therapy including the dreaded coffee enemas.

I was quite aware of the intense emotional feelings produced on the therapy, which were fear and often terror. I neither understood the feelings, but considered the therapy was bringing such emotions to the surface. I considered that it was essential to have an outside reference point, if I was to jump wholly into the black abyss. I was aware that my husband might try to take the children away, and he was sufficiently ignorant of the alternative field, to consider the Gerson Therapy as proof of insanity – which almost certainly a Court of Law would support. I decided to visit Barry Luxton a clinical psychologist, at the Charter Clinic in Chelsea once a week, which fortunately private healthcare insurer BUPA would pay for, and get myself certified sane each week, to stave off any legal proceedings my husband might bring. I wondered how many Gerson patients had to cope with the therapy alone *and* litigation at the same time and more importantly - if they survived. As it turned out it was a wise move, as litigation would be served for custody in 1989 after I had finished with the therapy, the year I filed for divorce.

Each week then I would tumble into Barry Luxton's office off the King's Road in Chelsea. After a week in the black abyss, fighting the demons of fear and terror, battling with the therapy and healing reactions, it was as though I had surfaced onto a different planet after being sucked down some dreadful wormhole.

Barry was medium height, although his shirt always fought at the fifth button to remain closed. His hair always neatly parted to one side, gave him an almost boyish look. He wore a check wool jacket and beige wool trousers and to top it off a statement about himself - a red paisley bow tie. His brown leather brogues were comfortably worn and along with his pipe laid on his desk, there was an air of English peace about his office. Barry had a good grasp of facts and once told me he had been a barrister, which always seemed a curious career change to clinical psychologist. I chose Barry for his reputation of communication, rather than drug prescription.

It was a relief to talk to someone about my life and particularly my marriage. Barry had always told me:

"Don't worry Renee your humour will always get you through".

I once recounted a story Rufus had told me. The boys were at their father's and there was a lunch party for a number of people in the advertising world, who had once sat at my Sunday lunches. As coffee was being served Rufus who thought it was the most natural thing in the world, shared the news that mummy has coffee enemas. Well in 1986 this caused extensive mirth around the table. Rufus said Max cracked a joke: "One lump or two" and circled his head with his finger, which obviously meant, I was two sultanas short of a fruitcake. As I quipped to Barry, "it's a good job Newton's apple did not fall on his head, otherwise we would have had 'ouch!' instead of gravity".

The weekly trip to Barry's office, off the King's Road, reminded me of the life I once had. Walking back to my car one night, I noticed a restaurant where we used to eat. I paused at the window, watching people so happy chatting and eating; yes eating all that glorious food that the Gerson Therapy prohibited. I felt a pang of loneliness and pain; I really felt like an alien from another planet. I felt much older now. I turned quickly on my heels and headed for my car.

I opened the car door and sat down fumbling for the keys. The passenger door suddenly swung open and in jumped a young man and sat down. The strange thing was I did not react - mugging would be the least of my problems.

"Your fantastic and I am totally in love with you".

I sat dumbfounded whilst he continued:

"I saw you looking in the restaurant, my name's Paul will you come and have supper with me?"

My thoughts of the way I met Max, came to mind:

"That's how I got into the last mess," I replied suggesting he leave the car.

"...But I love you, you see, you've broken my heart", he laid back opening his jacket clutching his heart," laughing and continued:

"Trust me and come with me and fly with me to some foreign land, but if not at least have supper with me".

"Trust?" I queried.

There was one sure way to ensure his immediate exit:

"Actually I have cancer, two small children and my husband has run off with an ex beauty queen from East Germany. I have just finished seeing my clinical psychologist, is that enough reality and trust on a Friday night for you?" Definitely it was, as he closed the door and I drove off.

I certainly had not only to rebuild my health, but also my trust in others again. Sheila was to help in so many ways. Sheila the Gerson nurse in the UK flew through the door in December of 1986, her huge presence inexplicably occupying a tiny frame, immediately filled the house. Dressed almost absentmindedly in a black cloak and trousers, her lilting Irish accent flowed confidently with energy and enthusiasm. I heard some years later, that she had helped Dirk Bogarde - but too late I assume.

Sheila had been an SRN in Ireland and then trained in Midwifery, but after working a great deal with children, whom she loved enormously, she had worked in the cancer wards; before heartedly sickened by the death of people she saw daily and feeling almost powerless to help these people she recognised the inadequacy of doctors and left to find an alternative method of treatment. Sheila had a very astute mind and was highly intelligent and it was a relief to finally find someone I could actually communicate with.

Sheila was aghast that I was doing the therapy alone.

"I just can't believe that you are doing this alone with two children, its crazy Renee, I mean your husband is earning £120,000 a year so why can't he pay?"

"I think he's made his position very clear and I can't demand he pay, you know what the lawyers will say, they will tell me to go take the drugs, accusing me of setting myself up against experts". Pausing I continued: "well didn't one woman do it alone... I thought I heard that?"

"No for goodness sake, she did have lots of help from neighbours and friends".

"Well I've started now and I am not going back to the hospital to take the chemo," I replied defiantly.

"Aye, well let's get on we' it" she replied practicably in her broad Irish accent.

Sheila told me to get all the elements of the therapy together, including suppliers, supplements, liver and vegetables and then:

"We'll really start!"

Before she left Sheila gave me Jones's number, a retired engineer who knew a great deal about the Gerson therapy as his mother had done it. He was now working in bio-energetics. As Sheila pointed out:

"You'll need all the help you can get".
Besides Sheila, Jones would provide another lifeline. Its curious how in one's hour of need "God provides," as they say.

As Sheila left, I apologised for having no funds with which to pay her.

"Ne're you mind, just get well".

After she had gone, for many days I still felt her enormous presence in my kitchen. She had the mystery of the Irish about her, a kind of magic that is the best of them. That night after putting the children to bed I rang Jones. Jones was incredibly knowledgeable on alternative therapies and medicine. He told me he had been a chief engineer with a company for many years and in the days of tough opposition and economic downturn of the 80's had managed to keep his job as a designer. Now he was retired and could devote himself to the field of bioenergetics. Jones glided through the subjects of geopathic stress, metal toxicity, bioenergetics, the industrial revolution and the hour and half slipped by almost unnoticed. This conversation led to a long list of topics for further research at some point, but would have to wait until as Sheila had suggested that I get everything ready to start the full therapy.

I contacted Mr Whitier a butcher in Croydon about the liver. Mr Whitier was a kindly large man who lost a daughter to cancer and claimed that she would have lived had she done the Gerson therapy, but had instead deteriorated very quickly from what he claimed was, "too many drugs". In her memory he now tried to help as many Gerson patients and he could, by sourcing and supplying the organic calf's liver. We arranged that I should collect the liver twice a week, but since I would not be relieved of the juicing schedule until the evening, he agreed to tie it to the back door of his shop and I would slip a cheque weekly through his letter box.

I located two brothers – the Pickles brothers as they were known from Yorkshire, who operated a wholesale organic fruit and vegetable business from the back of a budget rental truck at night, on the Nine Elms Road in London. They would arrive from Europe and literally sell the vegetables on arrival from the back of the truck. It seems incredible now that this is how the organic scene was in 1986. For once the gods were smiling I thought, it seemed too good to be true, I could drive to London twice a week at night, when the therapy was over for the day and pick up the liver and vegetables – I had not however accounted for the dreaded healing reactions.

By Christmas I was ready to go.

7 Battles and Dreams

Christmas lunch was a dismissal affair of the usual Hippocrates soup and baked potato and salad, eaten alone. In previous years I had always baked before Christmas. The table would be set with garlands and rosettes and a menu with the date. Exhausted after four months of almost constant "flare ups" and the awful healing reactions and caring for the children alone, along with the arduous therapy preparations, I felt it would be only fair to let the children spend Christmas with Max.

I mentioned finances, which had become an increasing distressing problem. He replied bitterly that I had set myself up against all the doctors all the experience and all the evidence of cancer and that he was heartily sick of talking about cancer. He pointed out that thousands of women develop breast cancer each year and "do not make the fuss you are making".

For the millionth time during our relationship the shutters came firmly down, recognising that not only were we driving in separate cars along separate roads, but we also existed on different planets, with different realities. Talking to him was exhausting and I just longed for him to take the children and leave. If there was a deep sense of regret, it was that we could not agree on the one topic I felt very strongly about – my life. There was a sense of disbelief that his character was so flawed. As I would go on to discover in regressive therapy, a past life we shared and possibly two lives, was at some level asking him to confront something he could or would not confront.

Over the holiday I started the full Gerson Therapy, trying to make a schedule before the children arrived back after the holidays. It was only just manageable without healing reactions. Sheila had made a wall chart with times for each part of the therapy, which resembled a daily battle plan – I felt exhausted just looking at it.

The first battle day after the children returned, I was pleased that things were running to schedule. I had washed all the vegetables for the juices the night before, which freed up time between juices every hour, for the children. I could just about get Rufus to school, before another juice was due. On returning I was busily preparing the liver juice when Barnes tired of playing with his toys on the carpet, crawled over to me and tugged at my jeans for his 11 o'clock bottle:

"Bott bott....bott bott!" he cried ever more loudly and insistently.

Hands full of pressing cloths, liver and carrots, I tried quickly to launch them into the grinder, but had left the shield off for the umpteenth time. Liver and carrots sprayed all around the kitchen. By this time Barnes had worked himself up into a screaming lather, not pleased at his bottle not being delivered. I sank to the floor, with Barney's bottle, cuddled him and as he stared up into my eyes searching them, I just thought: It can't be done, it can't be done they were all right.

Looking at Barney's face his big eyes staring up at me in complete peace and trust, his little fat cheeks sucking heavily on his teat, his eyes looking with enquiring interest all over my face, it was as if he was saying:

"Yes you can - do it for us".

Maybe, the cancer won't come back, maybe if I just go back to the hospital and take the drugs.... but then I remembered the woman whose cancer had returned - it wasn't an option. I realised at some level that the Gerson Therapy was a means to an end, there was something more I *had* to find out.

I looked at the schedule and the clock on the kitchen wall, with its hands ticking ever onward. The liver juice ruined all over the floor and walls and 20 minutes of preparation gone and now it was 12 o'clock and that meant a green juice. I knew Barney would not be happy, if I put him down, so how was it to be done? Suddenly a thought hit me. In some societies where mothers have to work and take their babies with them, they tie them to their backs. I made a papoose by tearing up a sheet from the airing cupboard and strapped Barnes on to my back. As his heavy little head rested on my shoulder and I could talk to him, a great sense of relief emerged, as I realised that he was happy and I could complete the juice schedule.

By the middle of January my health deteriorated badly, with one healing reaction after another. My hands had turned blackish grey, which I was told were toxins eliminating from the skin. I shuddered when I remembered the dream I had when first diagnosed with cancer, when I had seen Max standing with another faceless woman and I held out my hands to the children, only to look down and see they were black, as if in a fire. It was as though their eyes were pleading: "don't go, don't leave us." I would show them to Barry Luxton although I refrained from telling him about the dream. For some reason also my teeth and jaws ached, which although at the time I did not understand why, was a past trauma surfacing. As Gerson had pointed out old illnesses are recapitulated and come to the surface during the therapy. This was not a past illness however; it was a past trauma that was deeply hidden in my mind. It would take many years of research, to discover the mechanism by which the Gerson Therapy could do that. As it was, I stumbled on from one physical crisis to the next, barely hanging by a thread both mentally and physically.

I felt in a constant state of loss. A picture taken of me holding Rufus when he was just 10 weeks old sent me into floods of tears. There had been so much hope and promise then. The loss carried tremendous grief. In a long conversation with Sheila by phone, we agreed that the peculiarity of the therapy was that the emotions seemed to be in some way linked to what was happening in the body at the time of the past incident. Other patients on the Gerson Therapy were also undergoing emotional reactions. In some way and by some mechanism the therapy was able to bring these past traumas to the surface, with the emotions that were inherent in the trauma at the time. I remarked my eczema, had an emotion of intense anger with it. Again it would be some years later, when through regression I would discover why.

My mother, who was still trying to come to terms with the grief of my father's death from cancer, would come over occasionally, to tell me the reason I was exhausted was that I was not eating properly and juices were no substitute for a good steak and kidney pie. She brought some rubber gloves, insisting that I wear them to avoid spoiling my hands. On one occasion she brought over a picture of a girl in soap filled bath, drinking champagne under the usual red top banner headline of "I fought cancer and won!" Naturally she had gone down the orthodox route. Some years later I noted the young woman had died. I could not blame my mother for her total lack of reality about my condition, she was locked into her own world and cancer to her was just too frightening after witnessing my father's painful decline.

Occasionally, I would check the lump under my arm and was encouraged that although it had not gone, it had not got any bigger. By February however a small lump had appeared on my neck. As the lump got larger the fear turned to

52

a controlled panic. I was not to know then, that fear and terror are the major emotions that occur at around 4-5 months into the therapy and at which point, a number of patients I knew had thrown the rag in and run to the hospital and gratefully taken the drugs.

The unknown source of the depth of fear and terror was in itself terrifying. On one occasion when I was returning to the house, a blinding terror hit me as I saw the house emerge into view through the car windscreen. I was not to know that the house had become associated within my mind with loss and that feeling then precipitated or re-stimulated other losses, multiplying the fear and terror by degrees in summation. The terror at the sight of the house was like a huge enveloping wave, it just hit me like a wall. The devil himself could have been after me, as I put my foot hard on the gas, squealed past the house and headed down the A3 to London. I 'woke up' at the Robin Hood Roundabout, slowed down and stopped with my heart racing. I sat for a moment trying to regain my composure – "What did it mean?" I asked myself.

I would later ring Jones and tell him what had happened. As always he was practical and unflappable.

"I don't know whether I can carry on with this Jones", I told him truthfully.

"Look Renee you know that's *not* an option" he replied emphatically.

"Jones I think I'm going mad".

"Renee you're not mad, it's the therapy others are going through something similar. Steel your mind to it Renee don't give it any room, emotions are bad things, they dissipate energy, energy you can ill afford".

"I don't know Jones; perhaps I just feel that I'm driving myself to the edge here".

"You have to carry on Renee, What are you going to do if you stop? Take the drugs? You know that's not the answer".

In my heart I knew he was right.

"Put your blinkers on Renee, don't look right, don't look left, just keep plugging on and you'll make it. Look, other Gerson patients ring me and they have all got help, they get plenty of rest, they are not looking after two kids after being deserted... what do you expect Renee, you're a pioneer!"

"Well I guess it's tough for pioneers," I reflected never having thought of it that way.

"It takes guts to stand alone Renee. It takes guts to do what you are doing, don't ever forget that".

Over the next few weeks, I decided that Jones was right, if I was to survive the emotions that arise from the therapy and the healing reactions, I would have to as Jones put it "steel myself." I looked into warrior codes. The idea of a warrior in peacetime is unusual. The idea of life long training and self-development, are central tenets of all warrior codes. Under Bushido the Japanese Samurai spent long hours in mastery of martial skills, but also they had to practice such things as tea ceremony, painting and poetry composition. The ability to control emotions by will and the balance of such endeavour meant a man was not led, but rather could he lead and exhibit loyalty, honour, veracity and justice, or rectitude. The code was demanding and undeviating. Courage for the Samurai meant an integration of physical and moral bravery, based on moments of serenity balanced by moments of danger.

The warrior's life was shaped by his awareness of death. 'The idea most vital and essential to the Warrior,' wrote Daido Ji Yufan in the seventeenth century in his treatise 'Primer of Bushido': 'Is that of death which he ought to have before his mind day and night, night and day, from the dawn of the first day of the year until the last minute of the last day of it...think of what a frail thing life is, especially that of a warrior. This being so, you will come to consider every day of your life, your last and dedicate it to the fulfilment of your obligations'.

I remembered my father just before he died saying: "Some people do great things with their lives and others do nothing at all".

I remembered having felt loss when I looked in my wardrobe, to see the white lace dress I had worn, walking down from the Palais de Croisette in Cannes with Max. I had laid it on the bed and taken off the polythene wrapper and stroked the lace in my hands. The once lightly tanned hands, with cerise tipped

54

fingernails entwined in a pearl bracelet. The hands now grey. Now I felt that these things were not losses, but a parting of the ways. I had for a long time lost the true path and now that I had found it, it was useless to hold regrets for things that no longer mattered in the scheme of the Universe. Slowly I was re-discovering my true self, as if I had for some time taken the wrong road.

I read the books of Carlos Casteneda. In the late 1960s and early 70s, when America's young and privileged were avoiding being drafted into the Vietnam War –"draft dodgers", they were reading the Carlos Casteneda books. The central theme of the books was that life is meant to be lived at its best and every instance of it, should be lived as a warrior. In 1963 Casteneda an anthropology student became the apprentice of an old Yaqui Indian named Don Juan Matus who lived in the north Mexican desert. It is widely thought that the visions that Casteneda had were drug induced. Out of the five books the 'Journey to Ixtlan' was the most interesting. Casteneda through his Master becomes a 'man of knowledge' and in order to do so Don Juan tells Casteneda that he must adopt the Warrior's Code. Not a warrior that goes to war or kills people, but rather one who exhibits integrity in his actions and control over his life. The warrior's courage is unassailable, but even more important is his will and his patience. He lives every moment in full awareness of his own death and in light of this awareness, all complaint, regrets and moods of sadness, and melancholy are seen as foolish indulgences.

Don Juan's warrior pursues power and acts strategically in order to achieve self- mastery. The spirit of the warrior is not geared to indulging and complaining, nor is it geared to winning or losing, the spirit of the warrior is geared only to struggle and thus the outcome matters very little to him. The warrior aims to follow his heart, to choose consciously the items that make up his world, to be aware of everything around him, to attain total control, and then act with total abandon. He seeks in short to live an impeccable life in readiness for the afterlife.

Although I never took drugs, which was somewhat unusual for my generation and having passed through university in the early 70s, years later I would read 'Red Cocaine' by Dr Joseph Douglass [7]. 'The familiar, complacent view of the contemporary drugs scourge, which is ravaging the minds, bodies and souls of Western youth, is that it 'just happened.' The financial rewards, according to that argument, are so enormous that there will always be evil forces willing to distribute narcotics for money. *Red Cocaine: The Drugging of America and the West*, explodes this ill-informed opinion' (*Appendix 4*).

The young learnt that irresponsibility paid, that money and celebrity mattered more than knowledge, integrity and honour. Governments and politicians sought to jump on the 'freebie' bandwagon and the world became a grotesque parody of 'The Rake's Progress', an opera in three acts and an epilogue by Igor Stravinsky. The story concerns the decline and fall of one Tom Rakewell, who deserts Anne Truelove for the delights of London in the company of Nick Shadow, who turns out to be the Devil. After several misadventures, all initiated by the devious Shadow, Tom ends up in Bedlam, a psychiatric hospital south of London.

During this time I had two more strong vision-like dreams. In the first dream, I was on a boat or ship sailing on an ocean, when suddenly there was a storm and I was blown into the harbour of an island of great beauty. I had no idea what this dream meant, but it seemed highly significant. Astoundingly the dream came true seven years later.

In the second dream, I was sitting in a field where I seemed to be making food from the very flowers. A bee hummed and birds sang in a scene of utter peace. Suddenly I heard a deafening sound like cattle stampeding. As I turned and looked I could see an olive skin people, in their thousands running and jumping over a cliff edge. One man wandered over to me and asked what I was doing and I said:

"Come sit with me and I will tell you many things".

And so he sat and listened and then suddenly he jumped up and cried:

"You have spoilt my day!"

"Far better to spoil your day than your eternity", I replied.

And with that he ran and jumped over the cliff with the others. I was sad but just felt somehow it was inevitable. Years later I would wonder whether the vision referred to the Greeks as they lived in the 90s for today and not tomorrow and forgot their great history of Teachers. Or was it Islam? Or was it just a metaphor for mankind in the 90s, where he wished to party on and not think of the consequences? Was the dream my destiny? – To speak of many things?

8 Down and Out in Beverley Hills

I managed to find an alternative supplier of organic produce to the Pickles brothers, who for some reason failed to appear now on the Nine Elms Road. Martin and Clive ran an organic wholesale business in Covent Garden. Later sadly the market closed – another part of the heart of London removed. The first time I arrived and asked if I could buy my own vegetables from them Martin quipped:

"What do you think this is, frigging Tesco's?"

Laughing at my dismay he added: "Help yourself love".

As finances were critical and the money from the sale of furniture and jewellery had to last, together with a loan from a friend, then buying the vegetables wholesale was I considered a stroke of genius.

At 12 midnight, twice a week I would carry the sleeping boys to the car wrapped in blankets – a land rover type car, where with the seats removed I had placed a foam mattress, on which the boys would sleep through the journey. Once or twice they would wake up at the Market and find this as I did a vibrant busy and often humorous place. There was 'Ape Man' as I would call him, who wore a leopard Tarzan-like leotard and only ate organic fruit. Mostly there were the alternative fringe pioneers of organic food who used to be called the 'sandal brigade.'

On the way back from Covent Garden, I would drive to Croydon to pick up the liver from Mr Whittier, where I would rummage around with a torch for the plastic bag at the back of his shop. The outside world became an increasingly hostile place to me. I became an observer, where news only portrayed ideals and loyalties were fading. Selfishness, bigotry and most of all egos were becoming prevalent and children now were being led down the wrong path.

Jones was of the 'old school' and certainly not a lover of the mass of humanity whom he referred to as "quatermass": the term taken from an old movie 'Quatermass and the Pit', where mankind became zombies.

"The least I have to do with the outside world the better," he told me.

"Selfish, nasty load of individuals, look at you Renee you've been made to feel an outcast from society, but if you stand back and look at what this means, our society today is violent and totally devoted to greed and selfishness. It is degenerate in mind and body and soon two out of three will die from cancer and heart disease. Is this what you are an outcast from? It is a privilege I'm an outcast but by choice. When people condemn you for what you are doing, you should consider not only the spoken word but also the speaker, one learns in life to assess not only the advice, but also the quality of the person who gives that advice. Fools tend to be more generous with words than the wise. The way we are going now Renee, the holocaust will come and only those who live by God's laws will survive".

It wasn't that Jones hated humanity, otherwise he would not have helped Gerson patients, but in a fatalistic way he was no doubt right as greed would later precipitate the banking disaster in 2008, but then the bankers did survive to profit again, so what lesson lies there – perhaps 'survival of the fittest' and bankers inherit the earth; pity that everything else will be extinct, after all a predator cannot survive without prey in the food chain.

I told Jones that I had actually been turned down for help from the local Church of England in Esher with the words: "we don't get requests like this very often": probably not in the stockbroker belt of Esher and Oxshott.

Jones continued with his biblical analogies in response to this story:

"I suppose you have heard the excerpt from the Bible - The Good Samaritan, where a man from the church walks by a beggar in need, and also a rich man walks by, but a man from Samaria, which I think would have been the equivalent of a man from the East End of London, helps the beggar in need. You could learn a lesson there perhaps Renee. Perhaps if you had lived in the East End, you would have got more help- you know in my day people helped one another a great deal more, it's all different now. You live in Esher where I should think if you dropped dead it would take them a couple of days before they cleared you up".

I suggested that perhaps if children had been taught different values, they would not act the way they do, which further ignited Jones.

"That lot of quatermass out there, you still like to call humanity" he fumed. "The young of today a lot of selfish layabouts, walking around like a lot of zombies, filling themselves up with junk food and watching those junk programmes on TV. In my day we came from hard times, hard backgrounds, we had to fight to rise above it. We didn't sit around moaning, waiting for people to do things for us we had to get on with it in my day".

Sometimes I just listened and let Jones get it out of his system and there was no more igniting topic for his wrath than the state of the country and "quatermass".

I told Jones, that I would like to set up a cancer charity and undertake independent research in earnest when I finished the therapy. Jones however was not convinced.

"Look Renee, most of the populous is doomed, you can't help most of them simply because they don't want to be helped, and in fact they would probably get extremely aggressive if you tried to help them. Do you think I would make my research public, they would laugh me off the streets, like they laughed at Prince Charles when he tried to do something better for himself".

I had to agree with this point, when I remembered a brief conversation with the Chairman of an advertising agency whom I had once heard described as a "butcher's dog" whatever that meant. He told me about his daughter who at 15 was on two shots of insulin a day. When I had suggested the Gerson Therapy, which Gerson claimed had shown success in diabetes he rounded on me, his lips curving almost viciously as he virtually spat out the information that he had taken his daughter up and down Harley Street and spent thousands of pounds in trying to find a cure.

"What do you think you know about it," he retorted. "Do you think you know more than the experts?"

Startled and nervous by this extremely rude reaction I smiled nervously.

"Wipe that smile off your face!" he concluded as he 'politely' turned his chair at the table to face his back towards me.

As I recounted this story to Jones, he exclaimed:

"Well there you are, don't bother even saying hallo to that type of person!" and continuing:

"Renee you are living in the real world now, before you had some vague notion of it, because you surrounded yourself with lightweights, now you are a heavyweight".

"Hey watch it Jones, the upholstery is a sensitive issue," I teased having dragged Jones through numerous accounts on the state of my body, following healing reactions.

"Blooming upholstery, you never give up do you, I'll be glad when your hair falls out finally and perhaps you'll stop worrying about it, we deal in engines not upholstery," he teased back. "Well if you ask me, the sooner your upholstery gets a few holes in it the better, you might attract a better class of man then".

As usual Jones was right on the nail.

"Well if you saw me you would wonder what you had been talking to all this time. Poor old man, trench jacket and felt wide brimmed trilby, that's what I wear, the trilby is 30 years old now, it's been through a lot that hat," he joked: "You can't get hats like that now, I see the kids looking enviously at it".

"Ah ha" I laughed "Indiana Jones!"

"Who's that?" he asked innocently.

"Jones, you should really get out more", I teased.

Jones was soon back on his favourite topic: "quatermass".

"Well these days they make all sorts of excuses for kids, bad family backgrounds, poor education, no job, now they talk about food additives...oh it makes me sick, what they really mean, is that they've got no backbone, they don't know what it is to fight".

I could not entirely agree with Jones, considering the dire circumstances in which some children live. Poverty is something that can be overcome with difficulty; cruelty and emotional abuse and neglect however cripples a child for life.

After the conversation with Jones, I began to seriously think of what values I wanted my children to have. The children would return from Max's where cream cakes, sweets and meat were all allowed. Barney hated meat and would develop some food problems, from being forced to eat it by his father: one lawyer's letter later Barney now required the game of 'aeroplanes' to get him to eat. I would spend ages flying 'spitfire' spoons of pasta around in the air to again make eating a joyful experience, before asking him to "open the hanger!" and delivering the payload into his laughing mouth. It occurred to me then, that anyone who would try to control what another person eats is a seriously controlling person.

The boys had their own diet for breakfast and supper, but I shared the Hippocrates soup and baked potatoes at lunch with them, where they had cottage cheese or tuna and I was limited to the three tablespoons of linseed oil allowed on the diet. The troupes soon rebelled. I once told them a story of Jesus healing people with the soup, to try and get them to eat it. Thereafter if Hippocrates soup was ever served they would shout: "Oh no, not Jesus soup again mummy". Barnes would be more demonstrative spitting it into his plate with shouts of "Uck!" Hippocrates was removed from the menu.

During the intense healing reactions, Rufus who was still only 5 would offer to wash the carrots. He would pull a chair up to the sink and I would watch him with his little knobbly knees scrubbing away, with his favourite tunes on. Mainly however, the boys would hike down to the back garden, at the bottom of a long path. The garden was not observable from the house, but Rufus could always be relied upon for being totally responsible even at the age of 5, having been given responsibility from an early age. I never went to the back garden, as it was now a jungle, having no time to tend it. I had a bugle, which signalled them to come back to the house. It was a surprise when after a year on the therapy, I ventured down, to find the boys had built their own 'city' down there.

Rufus had once come into the kitchen with a plastic hammer and toy tools and asked me: "How do you expect me to build things with these?" He certainly had a point, but then he was only five years old and I had to consider whether it was responsible to give him a full set of tools: but there again was I destroying his male psyche by not allowing him to build? I decided there would be building and I brought him a proper set of tools and explained the seriousness of such tools and how to use them safely. Apart from a minor mishap no serious incident occurred and both boys became adept at building things.

In the evening the boys and I would play the pastry shop. After their bath I would roll them in a fluffy white towel and pretend I was making a sausage roll, with much kneading and prodding and tickling to squeals of delight. Then I would quickly fling them out of the towel and shout "And out of the pastry shop!" Monster across the bridge was another favourite. A story would follow and cocoa, before bed and then I would start the round of vegetable preparation for the next day and research any items on my list of 'to do'. I was back with my books in the library of my childhood. It was definitely a very healing time.

It was during the evenings with the boys, that I recognised how our lives despite the horror, was at least happy and balanced with importantly a rhythm. I reflected how different our lives would have been had I not developed cancer. I still wasn't grateful for the disease, but I could see that it had been a warning sign and I had heeded it. Years later I would see that it was a crossroads that would shape my life.

Max on one occasion turned up unexpectedly to collect something and we were having a vegetarian barbeque in the great hall. We had set up the barbeque outside, but it suddenly started to rain, so we dragged the umbrella, table and chairs and the barbeque into the hall. The enormous stone fireplace, which I had been told once belonged in Winston Churchill's home, whether true or not was a work of art, with its cupids and garlands. If it had seen grand days, then now it was stacked up with carrots and other organic vegetables. Max took one disbelieving and withering look around before exclaiming "The Beverly Hillbillies!"

"More like down and out in Beverley Hills", I replied.

The boys from an early age were very aware that there were two different life philosophies and roads one could take.

9 A Near Death Experience

I had always managed to retain a sense of humour, despite the battle like experience of completing the Gerson Therapy each day, alone with two children. The healing reactions were comparable to being wounded and yet still having to carry on.

Philosopher Glen Grey, a world war two combat veteran wrote in his book 'The Warriors': 'No human power could atone for the injustice, suffering and degradation of spirit of a single day of warfare.' So it was one Tuesday evening towards the end of February, I struggled into Barry's office, off the King's Road in Chelsea.

It was always so warm and cosy, so bright, but most of all safe in Barry's room. Even throughout the most appalling times I had managed to laugh. Barry would say: "Your sense of humour will see you through Renee". That night at the end of February, I wasn't laughing anymore and hadn't laughed for three weeks.

I looked at the familiar comfortable brown brogue shoes, the pipe lay on the desk, and if I had noticed, I would have realised that I had lost my sense of smell and could not detect the faint smell of tobacco in Barry's office. I felt desolate that evening.

Years later, I would recognise that after three to six months on the full therapy, Gerson patients encounter overwhelming emotions such as fear and terror. I would also recognise that the therapy, whilst causing the physical and emotional content of childhood traumas to surface, could also cause the memory to go back further to past life traumas and losses. If those traumas were experienced in an emotion of fear and terror, as in the case of a traumatic death, then this emotion would come forward in *present* time.

In Barry's office, I was left without explanation other than Barry's concern that I was exhausted physically and mentally. I listed my familiar catalogue of woes, the lump under my arm I was convinced was increasing in size, I thought the one in my neck was about the same, but could not be sure. The hearing had gone in my right ear altogether, which I considered just one more peculiar healing reaction. My speech was wrong and I could hear myself almost slurring my words. I felt disorientated as though I had cotton wool in my head and was in slow motion crawling through mud. Years later I would recognise the loss of the senses of hearing and smell, is a position close to death. To have survived that time, was as frightening as any front line battlefield, or Don Juan's visions in the Arizona desert.

Barry was asking me if I could remember what I had done that day. "Well it must have been the Gerson Therapy, but I can't remember". It neither dismayed nor surprised me; I accepted it and stared out of the window to the street below. Barry had always been against recommending that I go into the clinic for rest, because I was adamant that I had to continue with the therapy, but now he was gently trying to persuade me. I declined and in so doing had set the scene, for a life changing experience.

Barry had been ringing me every morning for a week, to check on me and said as I left that he would ring me the following morning, to see how I was. I left the safety of his room and walked down towards the King's Road, where my car was parked. It was as if I just about hung on until I got home. I paid the babysitter and I sunk to the kitchen floor, clasping the back of my head with my hands and curling into the foetal position. An emotion of such intense loss and desolation enveloped me that I had never felt before or since. A well of pain so great, that it would be difficult to describe in words but perhaps Elgar's concerto in E minor Opus 85 with Jacqueline Du Pre on cello, would partially describe the pain. A pain so deep and all enveloping that it seemed to be the pain and totality of all my existence.

Then an extra-ordinary thing happened. I was outside of my body in the region of the kitchen ceiling, looking down on myself. I could see myself quite clearly curled up on the kitchen floor. I noticed a green hair slide on the top of my head. I had a total enveloping feeling of pure serenity. I was surrounded by an intense ethereal bright white light, which was everywhere, but did not obscure the view of where I was.

A voice spoke to me: "You must go back" to which I replied mentally "No - I can't". The voice again said: "But you must go back," to which I again replied: "No, No, I can't" .The voice then used the only persuasive argument that would have forced me to return: "But who will teach the children?" In a flash, it was over and I was back on the kitchen floor. I pulled the slide out from the top of my head and looked at it. I had forgotten it was there. I looked around half expecting to see the Angel Gabrielle, but no just the vegetables waiting to be washed. I sat there not fully knowing what to make of it. Was it a religious experience? I felt an extra-ordinary peace, as though I knew now I was going to survive and there was a purpose in that survival.

Sometime later, I discovered I had gone through a 'Near Death Experience' (NDE). I became a member of IANDS (International Association of Near Death Survivors) and London Weekend Television, made a programme for the series '*Not on a Sunday*' which included my own experience and that of two others. All those who went through this experience, had either been very ill, or had experienced a life threatening situation such as a road accident, or had actually physically died when their heart stopped in an operation. If I had not returned, the inquest no doubt would have given 'Heart Attack' as the cause of death. Although science would like to put this experience down to lack of oxygen, or build-up of carbon dioxide etc., it is the experience when the Spirit leaves the body. Those who have not experienced it try to explain it away in Newtonian terms, those who have experienced it simply *know*.

Years later, I would discover that the incident was the night when the summation of all losses, including past lives, would cave in on me, causing a rapid exit of the Spirit from the body. I would remember the experience as the night the crab and I fought to the death! At some level that night, I did recognise that I had finally put my foot on the right path. It was not that I feared death for myself; it was that I had always felt some purpose, something I was supposed to do and had not. I would dwell on the reminder: "Who will teach the children?" Teach them what? There seemed something more that I was destined to do, where I had found the road, but a note had been left: "Gone on!" The journey was not over, the road stretched far to the horizon.

Barry rang met the next morning as promised. I was about to tell him, what had happened, but decided that it was probably wiser to keep the experience to myself. This was 1987 and you were considered insane if you took coffee enemas and ate organic food, without discussing Near Death Experiences.

After the crisis I was amazed that the therapy became easier and the emotional feelings began to be less frequent and intensive. There was of course the daunting schedule but it was more manageable. As with other unremitting practises, regular attention to it causes the technique to become internalised so that one is no longer conscious of executing it.

I felt increasingly more in control and began in any spare time, to research the role of the mind in illness. The black 'burnt' look of my hands subsided and the lump in my neck went down and the one under my arm disappeared altogether, much to Barry's surprise and proof it seemed to me that I had been right to do the Gerson Therapy. As I looked at the boys, who were fed only on organic food, they looked the picture of health, with boundless energy. I felt that whatever horror or 'Rite of Passage' I had survived had been worth it.

Always in my mind, was the NDE experience and what seemed a goal I should complete? I concluded that thinking and existence is not limited to a body. I could think and reason *out* of my body. I became interested in the belief of reincarnation and studied numerous texts and books. Rufus at one point when I was very ill had said: "Are you going to Jesus mummy?" I realised that I should talk to the boys and explain what had happened and share any fears.

On another occasion Rufus asked me: "What happens to you when you die mummy?"

"Well my lovely" I replied: "I believe in the philosophy of what they call reincarnation, that the real you leaves the body and goes off," I tried to think of an analogy, to help him understand. "Look think of it like this, you are the driver and the car is your body, when the car is so old and beaten up that you can't drive it anymore then you have to get another one".

Rufus looked puzzled: "What do you mean you can really leave your body?"

"Well I believe that you are not your body, any more than a driver is his car, *you* or the Spirit is *you*" I replied.

"Where do you get another body from?" He asked quite reasonably: "Is there a body shop?"

"Well its jolly difficult I think to pick up a new body, you might have to wait an awful long time in the queue to get one, so you have to make sure you use it well and wisely and for good purposes", I replied not wishing to be very specific.

"Why do you have to use it to do well?" he replied evidently pondering any misdeeds.

"Well, what would be the point of waiting all that time for a new body or like a car, if you intend to drive it badly and smash it up, or fill it with mucky petrol or use it to smash other drivers and their cars, it would all then have been a waste of time and a life wouldn't it?"

Pondering this 'sermon' in ethics and the need for healthy 'petrol' or food Rufus declared: "I'm going to look after my car!" And virtually in the same breath complained: "Mummy I don't like those muesli bars you brought, can we have some jammy dodgers again please?"

Later that week I noticed that mice had moved into the kitchen and begun to help themselves to the crates of organic food. We tried blocking all exterior pipes and humane traps, but the herd kept multiplying and I realised I would have to take more severe measures. As we surveyed the cull one doleful morning and prepared to make the necessary funeral arrangements Rufus asked:

"Mum is it a Buddhist mouse?"

"I don't know" I replied: "Why?"

"Well when it comes back again in the next life, I should like it as a pet".

Rufus would return from a visit to his father one weekend, and tell me that he had asked him what happens to you when you die. His father had told him: "That's it, you are gone so enjoy it while you can you only get one". I said to Rufus: "Well some people do think that and you are going to have to make up your own mind about it, when you get older". However in that moment I could see there were two philosophies in that marriage and thus it would never work. Little did I know then that a past life history was re-playing: another scene, another time, different faces, but the players were all there on the theatre stage once more.

10 A Bridge Too Far

At one point, near to the end of my two years on the therapy, Max had initiated a meeting towards reconciliation, but as Princess Diana would famously state: "well it was a bit crowded, there were three people in the marriage". He was however doing what men do, road testing the alternatives before deciding which, was the comfiest position for him to be in.

I noticed that his presence brought back the old feelings of exhaustion and by now we had two completely different points of view. Although I struggled to find it, I found I could find it in me to exercise the Christian value of forgiveness, for not having supported me on the therapy: however the betrayal was far too great to ever forget. His actions pointed to serious spiritual flaws. Any reconciliation would require not just a wallpaper job, but also a renovation from the foundations upwards.

Max's main obsession was the relentless pursuit of pleasure, money, cars, restaurants, and holidays – but mostly the relentless pursuit of power. Successful men everywhere show this condition. I quote from my diary of the time:

'For the son of ambition
He'll pay the full price
His success is his condition
A heart burnt to ice'.

In a philosophical note I had added the question: "Will greed exterminate our species?"

On January 2nd I walked into the offices of my solicitors and asked them to file for divorce; the decision had been a New Year's resolution. On returning home the babysitter told me the cellar had flooded, "Now what!" I exclaimed, exasperated that once again, something else needed fixing. After filing for divorce Max having lost control of me, decided to exercise it through the only method left to him – money.

I only had a couple of months left to do on the therapy and like the prisoner; I would then be released into the outside world. Knowing that if I resorted to yet more solicitors' letters that the pump would be leaking for the next year, whilst the solicitors circled at hundreds of pounds an hour, I fixed the pump myself.

Brown envelopes, now mounting were stuffed into the drawers of my desk. Even the word "money" could bring on palpitations. My car then hit the dust. I rang the insurance company to find out Max had only insured it third party - typical I thought, but of course his Aston Marten was fully insured. My lawyer's mind-set was typical of the time, where even a man earning £120,000 a year, in 1988 was seen as a benefactor and not under legal obligation. As I was on the phone explaining why a car was necessary, if not to get the children to school and back Rufus yelled from the top of the minstrel gallery.

"Mummy! Barnes has pulled the chain on the loo and water's coming up all over the floor!" Explaining the Children's Act and Equality to my solicitor would have to wait.

I was just about coping with the house, springing leaks in all directions, drawers full of brown envelopes and a dangerous car that Max's solicitor Mr Tooth thought was OK to drive with the front left side missing, when my solicitor rang me.

"The other side would like a medical report on your condition".

"Well I don't think that's necessary".

"Well I am afraid they are insisting on it".

On a Tuesday morning in July, I sat in the GP's waiting room; I had been there two years ago, when I was told I had a cyst and that it was nothing to worry about. This time however I felt the chair beneath me, this time I was real. The receptionist, a near neighbour, coloured up red and busied herself, so she would not have to acknowledge me. I thought of Jones's 'Good Samaritan'.

The doctor was uneasy in my presence, shuffling his papers, having assured me two years ago that I only had a cyst. I told him my husband's solicitor required a report on my health. As he examined me he said:

"Well you have two lumps in the right breast and I see that your left arm is highly swollen". His blunt statement, said in a matter of fact tone, conveyed his view, of what did I expect if I would not take orthodox therapy and follow chemotherapy and the doctors' orders.

"You must go back to your surgeon, you are showing signs that your cancer has spread and I must say that it is not unexpected".

My breath stopped somewhere between my lungs and mouth, as once again I was cruelly thrown back into the black abyss. On the way home, I was numb with disbelief. How could it be? Not now just as I was coming into the stadium after the marathon. Would I have to go back and run this race again – another two years on the Gerson therapy? I was crushed.

I rang Jones.

"Had the bone waived at you again?" he said matter-of-factly.

"Look Renee, the two lumps you did have, went didn't they, a year into the therapy, this is probably just some toxic pocket, nothing to get scared about. At any rate you know why your arm is swollen, the blooming doctors did it, when you had radiotherapy".

He was right about the arm it was caused by the radiation and was permanent damage. I felt less panicky and our conversation turned to the journey we take through life.

"You know Jones, I have been looking for myself, for a long time, and I even went to Marrakech in the 70's – the road to Marrakech and all that".

"Did you find yourself then?" teased Jones.

"No I found chronic diarrhoea" I laughed.

"You never cease to amaze me Renee, with your daft exploits, still you have seen a bit of life".

As I put the phone down I felt calmer, but shortly another incident would shake my faith. Sheila rang to say that Sylvia, one of the Gerson patients who had been doing the therapy for nearly a year had died. Sylvia had done well on the therapy and had even joined the darts team as she progressed. She had however encountered the dreaded 'wall' and had gone into the fear and abject terror emotions. She had experienced painful healing reactions and despite Sheila's encouragement and assurances that it would pass, and my own account of the horrific episodes I had endured, Sylvia had entered a downward spiral and died: they thought it was a heart attack, it wasn't the cancer. I thought of the episode in my kitchen and the NDE experience, where no doubt if I had not come back, the autopsy would have read 'heart attack'.

I forgot all about my lumps and bumps and went back to my research and the drawing board. Sylvia had died the same way as Mary, in abject terror. It had nearly polished me off on the kitchen floor. Mary had one healing reaction after another, until at about the critical 4 month period, she too had been overwhelmed by terror and finally had given herself into the hands of the doctors and orthodox medicine. She took chemotherapy and died at the end of it. I began to look carefully at the biochemical mechanisms, trying to tie this to a mechanism of the mind. I would write a definitive statement in my notes: 'LOSS IS THE KEY'. It was definitely a 'eureka' moment! Key links were then written in large words on sheets of A4 paper stuck to my office walls, where a mechanism for cancer was beginning to emerge, based on *loss*.

That week I felt in need of going to Barry's Thursday group session. As we all settled ourselves down, in the safety of the comfortable room, I felt exhausted. The familiar faces around the circle, with depressingly familiar human problems. Peter was the conscientious executive, too conscientious, too competent and too sensitive. It was part of the reason that forced him into a nervous breakdown. Peter, like me tried to develop a sense of humour to stave off the pain:

"Oh yes," he said: "when people know you've been in here, they think you are going to jump out on them with a knife and attack them, still it's useful if you want to get rid of people fast".

"Not as good as telling people you've got cancer," I contributed.

Burnt out company executives, army post traumatic stress burnouts, divorcees, burnt our rock producers; here we all sat with our own pain having: "seen a bit of life," with no wish to jump back into it. The walking wounded from the battle. Everyone I noted had suffered *losses*.

Terry a veteran survivor had lost his Directorship in a company and feared he would never get another one, but had fought his way back to Managing Director, but then had felt utterly exhausted by the ordeal.

"Life is full of opportunities as soon as one door shuts another slams in your face," Peter quipped.

It was through listening to these men that I realised men count their losses in terms of material advancement and women count their losses in terms of relationships. It seemed that evolutionary survival genetics and the roles of male and female were not as insignificant as one would like to dismiss.

Brian an auctioneer, a charming man, who had once told me that I should auction off, or sell to the Americans, Winston's fireplace in the hall and it would solve all my financial problems, asked what had been happening to me since the last time I attended. I spoke of my deep financial problems since filing for divorce. Brian reminded me of the fireplace and Peter quipped about the lawyers arguing over a gutted house. Terry who was astute when it came to money, advised me to pay good attention to financial matters, as he thought my soon to be ex-husband would: "play dirty" and told me the barrister and solicitor my husband were using, were well known expensive "Rottweiler's". He warned me to start looking for offshore accounts and scrutinise bank accounts. Perhaps I should have listened more carefully as his predictions later materialised: the prospect of being set upon by the "Rottweiler's" however seemed to be less pressing than the newly discovered lumps and the death of Sylvia.

After I mentioned this more pressing worry, there was a long silence in the group: "Just my luck," I laughed off the silence. Peter spoke first, mentioning something like "brave" and "fighting spirit". I could not feel anything, I just felt emotionally numb, tired and exhausted.

Over the next few weeks, I was catapulted back into the black abyss of despair once again. This time I felt I was too exhausted and numb to crawl out. Barry, concerned that I had suffered what he felt was a "cruel blow," asked me at my next meeting with him to come in the following morning to the clinic "for a rest". I did not know it then, but he feared I would 'top' myself. I told him: "I don't want to fight anymore, I am finished".

Even then I may not have succumbed, but one morning there was no hot water coming out of the tap. I went down to the cellar to find water gushing out of a large cylinder. The water stopcock, for such a large old house, resembled a wheel on the Titanic, as I tried to turn it off. The room started to spin and I collapsed.

I sat in the back of the cab and on arriving at the clinic I drew the curtains in my room and fell exhausted onto the bed. My body felt like a dead weight and there in the darkness I felt that I no longer wanted to live, it was far too painful. Someone came in and mentioned, "Doctor".

"No doctors, no drugs, otherwise I can't stay".

"All right Renee" a voice replied: "Just rest Renee".

They say "God will provide" in your hour of need and so it was Tomaz arrived.

11 Poems and Flowers

Dreams and faces faded in and out, as I lay in the dark stillness. The peace and quiet was only interrupted occasionally.

"Do you mind if I open the curtains a little?" A young man stood before me, looking like a younger version of John Cleese and with a comparable sense of humour.

"I can't read your notes very well, just a crack that's all I need," he said as he parted the curtains slightly.

He opened my notes and read for a few minutes and then looked at me. He suddenly got up from the chair and came over to my bed and folded his arms around me. Tears rolled constantly down my cheeks. He told me he was the nurse "John" in charge of the section I was in. After he left, the dreams and faces came and went in the half-light and John would occasionally appear with meals, which came and went without being touched.

Through the dimness, I opened my eyes to see a feint figure sat in the chair facing me. His hair was dark and fell in curls framing an exquisitely beautiful male face with eyes as dark and deep as pools, taking their time as they observed me. I had never seen eyes like that on a man, but it seemed as if I knew them. They say the eyes are the entry to the soul and here was a beautiful soul. He was dressed totally in black, and I supposed I had imagined the face until he spoke:

"Hallooo..." the word falling softly from gentle lips: "I am Tomaz".

He was young, probably no more than his mid-twenties. He was a recovering heroin addict. He asked me what had happened and I find myself telling him in the briefest of ways, because I didn't want to discuss it any more. Afterwards he says:

"I don't know what to say".

"Well don't say anything", I reply and tell him: "I am tired" and he apologises and leaves.

It bothers me that I seem to know him. I close my eyes, the Adonis face floats beside me, he is wearing an Egyptian white gown and so am I. His gown falls softly in long folds as he walks away from me, the eyes heavy and smiling, he holds out his hand, the fined boned hands of intelligence. The temples and pyramids loom high and we glide through large pillars covered in blue and gold scrollwork. My eyes follow him and I know him so well. But *who* is he?

I open my eyes. He sits curled in front of me, eyes watching, taking their time. We talk and I tell him of my Near Death Experience.

"I always knew it was so Renee" he replies thoughtfully.

As we continue to talk, he suddenly cries: "Renee! Renee! You have a strange orange glow all around you... I feel soooooo happy".

"What is it Renee?" he asks in wonder.

I felt it too. For a second suspended in time, we seem to spin around the room in ecstatic joy. I feel we have found each other, but *who* is he? I ask him what he feels and he tells me we are spinning together in joy. I am amazed that we have exactly the same experience. He asks me again:

"What has just happened Renee?"

"It was your appointment with fate, I am glad you could come," was all I could say.

He tells me that he will never take Heroin again and asks:

"How from that brief experience, do I know this?"

I remember my own NDE experience.

"It only takes one glimpse of who you really are Tomaz, change often comes suddenly and unexpectedly".

He tells me that he doesn't know how it came to be that he took heroin, but adds without recognising his pun:

"One day I woke up and decided to become a heroin addict and I gave it my best shot". He laughed feeling now the futility of it.

He tells me I am beautiful, but I laugh it off, pulling at my candyfloss hair.

"Actually" he says quietly "I like your hair" he pauses and then continues: "Actually I love everything about you, even the mascara that has run down your face, from crying".

His gentleness so contrasts, with my husband's brutally emotional world and the world of advertising, a world that had wrung me out like an old dishcloth, throwing me away when of no further use, whilst the lawyers circled to haggle over the remains of a marriage and family. The most precious possession that I had lost was naivety and trust; in its place there was now a core of acceptance of what man was capable of. I could no longer pretend and the rose coloured glasses I had worn in the 70s were now gone. I could no longer bear to watch anything that involved suffering, especially if that suffering involved innocent children. Betrayal takes lifetimes to emerge from.

"Significant, significant, significant," cried John as he placed a tray of fruit and salad beside me: "just a crack, just a chink of light coming through the curtains," he observed teasingly before heading for the door.

"John", I cried.

"Yes?" he answered popping his head back around the door.

"What day is it?"

"Saturday," he replied: "by the way there is a letter here under your door," which he placed on my bed.

Had I really been here nearly a week I wondered as I opened the letter, with: "Good Morning!" on the envelope. It was from Tomaz.

'You know how people talk about their dream come true, well you are my dream come true. I don't know how much this says or doesn't but it's all I can say. When Pam entered the room, I felt she was the only human soul in that room and that human soul disturbed a spiritual force, you and me. I'll never take drugs again thanks to you. You have given me so much'.

The note lifted my heart and I went to the bathroom. I looked terrible with five days of mascara that had run down my face. My thoughts ran to the children: 'I must leave and go back' I thought, but was overwhelmed by anxiety and a desperate panic of returning to that house where I had endured so much. There was a knock at the door it was Tomaz. As he came forward into the room he held out from behind his back a yellow bunch of freesias.

"For you!" he said smiling broadly.

This produced floods of tears: "I'm sorry...it...it's just such a long time, since anyone showed such gentle kindness," I said quietly.

"Do you ever feel great pain Tomaz - emotional pain?"

"Yes a lot Renee, perhaps this is the reason I take drugs".

"Where does the never ending well of pain and loss come from?"

"I have always been trying to get out of my body with drugs or whatever, perhaps to avoid the pain of living", he says quietly stroking my hand. "Pain" he continues "keeps you in the human way, it gives a bond between human and animal alike, pain bonds us in compassion for others. When people have an illness it is sad it is painful emotionally and we should listen and be aware of this sadness, for it binds us together, as does joy".

His words are very wise for one so young. I make a mental note that I must find out where the pain comes from, where the fear and panic comes from, I will find out where the crab is hiding in my mind.

It is Valentine's Day February 14th and Tomaz leaves a Bob Dylan poem 'My Love She Speaks like Silence', with a red rose on my pillow.

God provides in one's hour of need as they say and each day Tomaz leaves flowers and a poem on my pillow.

'Standing alone withdrawn
You feel the cold and long to hold
Someone who will run with you
Much faster than time
Your heart's confused, you're feeling used
You'll never plead, but still you need
Someone who will lay his love
Comfortably on the line
Swimming on the sea of thoughts
You drown in confusion
And realize the truths too far
You see through people with magic eyes
While remaining inscrutable yourself
You control your desire to dominate
This is no challenge to your strength
You are mine but I'm not yours
Is how you like to keep it with the boys
Love is missing from your eyes
But you'll never be won by lies
You probe the shadow when you can
To find the leisure that you seek
You play no games with happy talk
And patiently wait for what you need'.

I decide that I would try to go out again. The last attempt caused terrible anxiety, with people rushing at me, cold staring faces rushing at me, everywhere noise, traffic, people. Tomaz had left another note and flower.

'People are strange when you are a stranger
Faces look ugly when you are alone
Women seem wicked when you are unwanted
Streets look full when you feel down
A lonely dance in the crowd'.

Tomaz suggests that we walk together to Sloane Square on the King's Road and soon we are walking in the crisp watery sunshine of spring. We stop at

Blushes for a juice. There in the window seat we watch the street, the people rushing along and the traffic and I realise I have no anxiety. I tell Tomaz that I will be leaving the clinic. He suggests we drive down to his villa in the South of France.

"You know I want to be with you more than anything".

I gently tell him I have responsibilities, my children and that the age difference between us was a consideration.

"Perhaps it's not so great," he replies.

"Not now maybe" I reply "but it will be" I pause and add playfully: "I do not want to grow old counting every wrinkle!"

He chastises me for thinking him so shallow. Seeing his despondency I suggest we both have journeys to finish and that he must return to Egypt and detoxify his body from all the drugs; whereas I must continue with my journey as I felt it was far from finished. Tomaz asks me about the 60's.

"The English are peculiar; they have a long history of suppression, the British Empire and all that. People for the main in the 60's were recovering from the second world war and the young, just wanted some fun," I sipped my juice and continued: "There were a lot of police battles mainly in France. The young particularly the students were crying out for change. The student 'French Revolt' was really the equivalent of Vietnam for the Americans. It truly shocked the authorities and the police brutality shocked the students but apart from the American Embassy protest, there was not much else in Britain".

"Did you protest then?"

"I didn't like the violence .We felt the authorities were lying to us, but the students never pinned down the lies and perhaps like Dylan, I felt you could protest in words rather than with violence". I paused continuing: "protest can only occur when you have the lies pinned down. Looking back perhaps I was taking the long route round preparing myself with education to look at facts, the weapons if you like to win a much bigger battle".

"Perhaps you made your protest by doing the Gerson therapy" Tomaz suggested. "Perhaps this was part of your future battle?"

"Perhaps as you say it is part of it - do you know that the French students occupied the Sorbonne and established a commune also establishing a French Parliament, where free discussion sought to wrestle democracy, choice and freedom back into the universities. They wanted the universities to be a seat of development, other than what they are now at least in science as poodles to the Drug Companies and those who pay the research grants, that's why the Gerson therapy has never been fully researched, there's no drug money in it. New ideas now in British politics are seen as a nuisance to the order of things".

"But what was the point of the 60's?"

"A good question" I replied "I think the students recognised that there was little opportunity for control of their own lives; few ways in which to participate and little chance to contribute. There was deep dissatisfaction with the way things were" again I paused to reconsider the question: "Where did all the protests get us? - look at the force thrown at me just because I sought to do something different, you can't say that we are living in a democracy here in Britain".

"Is socialism a good thing?"

"Rich men or those who do not live in the real world, always promote socialism, whilst following completely different principles in their own lives, just another hypocritical lie to think about. They promote state schools and send their own to private schools, because they know the game is rigged that way from cradle to grave".

"Did you go to a private school?"

I laugh: "No, I guess I wheezed and scratched my way through childhood, with asthma and eczema and spent a lot of time in hospital. I failed the 11-plus and went to an all- girls' state school, where it was ceaselessly drummed into us, that since we would be poor when we married, we had to economise at every level. I remember my silent protest, when the nun in home economics explained pastry had to be made exactly to fit the dish with no wastage. I would secretly roll mine much bigger and drop the waste into the drainpipe

82

outside the window, until one day it rained and white sludge spread all over the playground".

Tomaz laughed: "Perhaps you were protesting, but how then did you go to university?"

"I was a very good artist and at one point I painted this picture of a white blossom tree in the middle of a slum. Perhaps my art teacher not only recognised talent, but the psychology of such a painting. She called my mother in for a meeting with her and the Headmistress, and suggested that I should aim for art school. I just said 'Oh, but I'm going to university to read science' – I just had that determination. I remember the Headmistress laughing".

"That's incredible Renee".

"Education I used to think was the key, but then how do you explain the wealth gap among equally-achieving African-American and white families? The key is evidently the accumulation of financial resources, the richest one per cent of western populations owns virtually half of a country's wealth and that mainly comes down to inheritance and tax avoidance".

"There is poverty in Egypt; the wealthiest people have many more chances".

"Did you know" I reflected: "A few hundred schools in Britain dominate entry into elite universities, and monopolise the production line of future leaders in professional and political life?"

"It is the same in many countries".

I remembered a quote from Oscar Wilde.

"In England, education produces no effect whatsoever. If it did, it would prove a serious danger to the upper classes".

Tomaz laughs: "And yet you Renee survived this system".

"Not really, education is not the great social leveller it was promised to be, it is still the protector of privilege and please don't get me started on *male* privilege and advantage!" I replied laughing.

"Yes, I suppose if you start with money, there are all sorts of advantages, like my own life I suppose".

"Why then Tomaz, did you become a heroin addict?"

"Yes there was money, but my parents were never there".

"Ah - the stalker again - *loss!*" I reflect.

We sit silently for a while before Tomaz remarks: "Total government does not like people who think, people like you, thinking people cause trouble, they spot lies they follow alternatives, but mostly you can't control them and they are afraid of that".

"Well no problem with that, because it seems there is no time to think now," I laugh and relate to Tomaz an anecdote about the Scientist Ernest Rutherford. One student in Rutherford's lab was very hard working. Rutherford had noticed this and asked one evening if he worked mornings too. The student proudly answered that he did, expecting to be commended, whereupon Rutherford replied amazed: "But when do you think?" We both laugh and I am glad to see that my sense of humour has returned.

Later that evening Tomaz passes another of Dylan's poems under my door.

'People tell me it's a sin
To know and feel too much within
I still believe she was my twin, but I lost the ring
She was born in spring but I was born too late
Blame it on a simple twist of fate'.

As I am leaving the clinic, I bump into Pam sitting in the lounge, where there is a terrible commotion. I ask what the commotion is about and placing the wool over her knitting needles, without pausing she explains: "Oh that's Jan she's been out on the bottle - blind drunk": her needles clicking she continued: "terrible waste".

I thought about the waste, it seemed the bottle subdued Jo's pain and I wonder about Max's pain and whether the bottle achieved that for him or whether it was just a reckless indulgence. As we watched Jo running around naked jumping up and down and singing, Pam complained about the drug and alcohol addiction programme she was on. "I mean Renee, it was truth day today, you had to admit the worst thing you have ever done whilst under the influence," she paused adding without recognising the hilarity of the remark or the purpose of her stay at the clinic: "I mean you come in here to forget all that" and finishing her line of stitches, she reversed the needles and started another line.

Barry had agreed that I could leave saying: "You just needed time to get some skin on you again". Was I raw? Yes I had been but now there was a resolution to discover the cause of the pain. Did it come from this life or many lives? Barry had kept me from sinking to the bottom and had undoubtedly kept me afloat, but over a year I still was capable of roller coasting down a huge terror filled dip only to go up the other side and then down again. I resolved to find a regressive therapist who would find the root of the pain.

Tomaz left another poem and red rose on my pillow.

'And now from where I stand
Upon this Hill I planted from Nepal
I look around I search the skies
I shade my eyes, so nearly blind
And I see signs of half remembered days
I hear bells that chime in strange familiar ways
I recognise
The hope you kindled
It's off, so easy now
As we lie here in the dark
Nothing interferes it's obvious
How to beat the tears
That threatened to snuff out
The spark of our love

Then the moment of clarity
Faded sometimes
Just like charity does
Sometimes
I opened one eye

85

And I put out my hand just to touch your soft hair
To make sure in the darkness that you were still there
And I have to admit I was just a little afraid
But then
I had a little bit of luck
You were there
I couldn't take another moment alone'

I recognised instantly the *loss*.

I am elated to be back with the children, determined to resolve the pain once and for all, the final month of the therapy passes and the prisoner is free after two years of incarceration. Two lumps have disappeared but the two new lumps are still there. I tell myself "two down, two to go".

Three letters arrive. One is from BUPA, the private health insurer informing me that they have paid the considerable costs of my stay at the clinic. The second is a poem posted from Cairo from Tomaz entitled 'Farewell Until Now'. It ends with:

'We'll feel separation
Yet know it's pretend
For the moment between us
Is one without end'

The third is from Max, who informs me he is deducting £60 for telephone calls to the boys, during my stay at the clinic.

11 A Pilgrims Progress

Like Christian in Bunyan's 'Pilgrims Progress', where he arrives after much difficulty and many vicissitudes at the house of the Interpreter, I was able to go over all my research and the biochemistry of cancer in relation to the mind.

Whilst the biochemical mechanism I had formulated seemed very clear, the mechanism by which it could be manifested at the physical level by the mind and vice versa, eluded me. I looked at numerous theories of how the mind works: Otto Kernberg, Brenner, Freud, Bowlby, Fairbairn, Kohut, Jeung and numerous others.

None of the theories seemed absolutely right and certainly provided little explanation of how a mind actually worked or could cause illnesses such as cancer. Arthur Janov's work was interesting where accidentally in 1968, during a regular group therapy session, he witnessed a strange occurrence. A shy student called Danny Wilson, which I believe is a pseudonym, described a theatre performance with a man, who had paraded around in a nappy on stage shouting for his mummy and daddy. Noting Danny's fascination with the act, Janov asked Danny to call out for his mummy and daddy. After a hesitant beginning, Danny was suddenly writhing around on the floor in agony and finally let out a 'piercing death like scream'. Neither Janov nor Danny understood what had happened, but afterwards Danny seemed transformed. Danny had said he'd "made it" and he "could feel".

Later Janov who treated John Lennon and Yoko Ono, came up with the word 'primal scream' to describe the intense experience. Janov then observed another patient, who in addition to the scream had been 'flooded with insights' thus 'making his whole life fall into place.' Janov published his findings in his first book '*The Primal Scream*' in 1973. His basic theory was that the frustrations of the child's needs, creates psychological pain, which if repressed will accumulate and lead to neurosis. The technique of the removal of psychological pain was to re-experience the suffering of the unmet need, to express one's need as fully as possible and thereby 'drain the primal pool of pain'. The basic concept was that traumas or unmet needs create emotional pain, which must be discharged. Although Janov did not describe emotional pain in terms of loss, it was evident to me that loss was the key.

Janov maintained that the traumatic process did not need to arise from obvious dramatic events like rape or parental loss through death or divorce, they could result and often did, from these experiences but could also result from general aggressive family atmosphere or parents whose emotions stifled children's natural joyful expressions and under these conditions the child could become neurotic. Janov also saw the needs of the child hierarchically arranged, where development of each new level of need depends upon the fulfilment of an earlier need.

I wondered if I rolled around the floor screaming, whether it might discharge the pain, but decided that more research into this was required. Janov saw repression as the basic defence for making us unconscious of pain and cited secondary defences for surviving pain as isolation. I recognised the isolation I had been forced to enter, whilst completing the Gerson therapy and yet the boys and I despite this had turned the house into a regular hive of activity, where they were constantly making things and completing craft projects, I set for them. In some ways, it was fortunate that they were so young and still happy within their home and garden. Beata Bishop in her book spoke of '*A Time to Heal*', which necessarily isolates one.

Janov spoke of first line traumas, gained from trauma in the uterus up to the age of one year. I had developed eczema and asthma at around that time and wondered what trauma created it, and kept it active throughout my childhood. Janov confirmed that first line traumas, give rise to such symptoms, 'due to the lack of psychological structures' and further claimed that if the traumas were large, such as a bad birth, then they caused psychosis: further claiming that birth traumas were responsible for half the neurotic suffering.

Second line traumas Janov maintained were related to feelings of not being loved or accepted which he also maintained gave rise to specific psychological symptoms and certain body 'somatic' problems, such as muscle tension. Third line traumas or those attained at the age of cognitive development or understanding, mainly in the teen years, such as divorce, separations, death etc., would not have lasting effects, *unless* compounded by earlier pain.

Recognising that my own children had gone through my cancer and the break-up of the family, then I was aware that I would have to try and bring the boys to a level of cognitive understanding before their time and allow them to discuss the effects of these events upon them. The boys by now had a non-stop agenda with outside activities and it was surprising that they had come through it so well. The fact that I made the house into a playground full of bikes, skateboards, rock climbing gear a billiards table and table tennis table, was a stroke of genius that seemed to counterbalance the losses including the necessary auction of virtually all the furniture to help pay for the Gerson therapy.

Janov's work tied with the work of Laurence Le-Shann, Levenson and the Simmonton's and a picture of how the mind worked and its role in illness started to emerge. Janov saw defences organised into a personality system called the unreal self, which represses the suffering and the real self. He also noted that unless the differences became very rigid, unresolved problems are usually acted out. A current event may be over reacted to, or a present relationship simply because an earlier similar unresolved trauma dominated the solution to the present one. One might see this as a current event, re-stimulating an earlier traumatic event, which is similar to the transference concept in conventional psychoanalysis.

Janov claimed that neurotics, which most of the population are to a degree, are constantly seeking situations or persons reminiscent of earlier traumas, in an attempt to resolve them: repeating one's parent's actions or marrying someone who reminds you of their most annoying traits.

So I pondered, if neurosis is an attempt to resolve an earlier conflict, then what did or *who* did Max represent to me and what earlier conflict was there? Had I married Max to re-create something I needed to resolve in this life and/or something that hadn't been resolved in a past life? Further did I have a first line eczema and asthma trauma?

The questions of my existence were answered by regression therapy, which also revealed the source of the well of pain. I will only cover briefly a few regressions to assist understanding of my journey and will only recount one past life in some detail.

One regression saw me at around two years old in this life spread-eagled and tied down to a cot, by my arms and legs in hospital. During the regression I was able to enter my conscious stream at the time of receipt of the trauma – including thoughts, feelings, smells etc. I am angry and itching, but I can't scratch as I am tied down. I turn my head and to each side there are other children tied down to their cots. I feel I am not loved or wanted and this is a punishment – there is a feeling of abandonment and rejection. I must not cry, or they will never take me home and love me. I learn to internalise my loss and grief and the anger of the constant itching. If I cry I have learnt that no one comes and all grief and anger is internalised and self-contained. I stop crying – I realise no one comes and there is no help.

As I ran through this incident time and time again in regression, the feelings of great distress and grief, anger etc., slowly dissipate as the charge and mental anguish associated with the incident is released with each recounting. Finally, in the session I was able to use my cognitive mind, to reflect upon this trauma. I had chronic eczema and that is the way it was treated in the 1950's at The Royal Free Hospital and the National Hospital for Skin Diseases in London. I reflect that the treatment was inhumane and akin to torture of a young child. That experience had led me throughout my life to be passive and internalise any upset particularly grief and anger, as I felt that if I 'made waves', I would be rejected. At some deep level this incident had taught me to become a victim and place others needs above my own. The sense of self was lost, the self that I had fought to find again through my illness. I reflected that this incident together with the damage done to my arm through radiation was in part responsible for my insistence of not creating any more damage to mind or body, by undergoing orthodox treatment. Subconsciously by seeking an alternative treatment for cancer, I had sought a total healing and desire to know exactly why I had cancer. It seemed amazing to me that at some deep level I had known from the start that there was a psychology at work.

In the session, I was able to 'see' or become that small child and connect with that black abyss of pain, loss, desertion and abandonment. The months of mind numbing 'nothingness' staring at a hospital ceiling were re-experienced along with that overpowering smell of carbolic and stark brown desolate emptiness of the hospital ward. When I was untied for meals and baths, there was the fear, panic and terror of then being tied up again.

I had no outward memory of this incident and had to ask my mother about it, who confirmed that this had happened, explaining that she and my father could only visit on Sunday's because of my father's work and the hospital was in central London. I had asked my mother about the first conscious memory I had at around 2 years old, when I remembered being dressed in a 1950s style pink wool bonnet, leggings and a coat – I had stood with my mother watching

90

the trains at Kew Gardens station. My mother confirmed this was the day I was brought home from hospital. It must have been a momentous day and I can remember nothing before or immediately after.

The Gerson Therapy brought the eczema; *physically* forward to be healed, together with the *emotions* of anger, grief and panic but the actual incident was not recognised until I underwent regressive therapy. The abandonment by Max only turned the trauma full on or re-stimulated it, without my conscious recognition of content. This is the peculiarity of the Gerson Therapy, in that it will cause earlier illnesses even very early childhood illnesses to the surface and past life emotions and phrases. For quite some time and throughout the Gerson Therapy I also found myself hunching my shoulders and bowing my chest. There was a constant desire to push my shoulders up and forward. There also seemed to be a chronic tension in the area and in the groins, where there was again an overwhelming desire, to push the sides inwards and curl my torso.

I had read the works of Wilhelm Reich and the Ida Rolfe and was aware that old conflicts are held as memories in the body cells and organs including muscles, but did not resolve this re-stimulated trauma until I underwent regressive therapy.

The regression saw me fighting for breath during a chronic asthma attack, on my mother's knee as a young child of three years old. In the session I curled up as I was at the time and even felt the fear and terror of not being able to breathe. My father who had to get up for work in the morning got out of bed and stated, "I'm leaving". I had taken it literally believing he was leaving the family altogether, when in fact he was going to sleep on the sofa. My mother replied "she can't help it" and so another defence mechanism against people leaving was born. Every time I felt loss, the asthma and eczema would be re-stimulated as a way of gaining sympathy, ensuring no one left me. The thought of leaving Max, was to lead to fear and subconsciously it was better to tolerate it than face the torture and abandonment of myself as a baby or the terror of not being able to breathe. Inhalers were not available and chronic asthma was a frightening condition for a child in the 1950s.

Of course the incidents were hidden in the irrational mind and so, leaving and loss was accompanied by fear and terror, strung together in memory on what was a line of similar events involving asthma, loss, eczema, people leaving and a fight for life and breath and significantly and more importantly - betrayal. The last experience of betrayal was contacted and recounted in a number of past lives.

It has taken some degree of thought as to whether or not to include the following incident as a deeply personal trauma. I do so in the hope that paedophiles recognise the immense spiritual anguish they cause to their victims and families and in the hope they recognise they are digging their own karmic grave, not just for this life but eternally.

There was an immense evil betrayal as a young girl when under anaesthetic (gas) I was sexually assaulted by a dentist and his assistant. On reflection of the incident I could only wonder how many more girls this man and woman had inflicted their broken minds on – children with the enormity of the incident locked in as a Level 1 trauma inaccessible unless they underwent regression. The incident then re-stimulated a whole line of past life betrayals. Further, it seems that the early incidents which had an element of betrayal of trust (by the medical profession) and to a certain extent by my parents in assenting to such treatment, then re-stimulated a whole string of past lives with similar content i.e. betrayal of trust and these lives had to be regressed into in order to relieve the entire charge of betrayal.

I was also able to contact the past life betrayal and the incident that surfaced in a dream in 1986, when I was first diagnosed with cancer. In my dream Max had stood with a faceless blonde woman. The extra-ordinary thing was that the past life involved the same woman he had left me for this lifetime. I could not be sure at the time it was her but later another extra-ordinary incident would seem to confirm it. In the past life regression I had called the woman "Lady Susan". I accessed this incident in regression in 1990 before my divorce hearing in 1991. I was sitting in the Holborn (London) law courts corridors with my barrister at a table and he was going through the bank accounts of the co-respondent that he had subpoenaed, when he casually observed that the Christian name we had all known her as, was in fact her middle name.

"Did you know she is called Susan?" my barrister casually commented.

I sat astonished and remembering the content of the past life replied: "No, but let me predict she has attained a lot of money from my husband, correct?" My mind turned to the dream I had 5 years previously and it seems that I had predicted her appearance. The same scene would play out as the players did not recognise each other's faces in this lifetime. I concluded that Spiritual awareness is far greater than we recognise. It seems as though the betrayals as a child, had pulled in past memories and even personnel who were part of those betrayals – as in karma I was being given a chance to heal and disentangle myself from past events.

Even more extra-ordinary was the fact that events which finally saw Max and I part ways in this life, were virtually identical to the past life, but of course different scenes, as though we had sleepwalked an act in a play that we had played before in a different time. Predictably Max had not changed a bit, but I had changed considerably, where I had chosen another path and found the personality I had been in many former lives.

Shortly after undergoing regressive therapy, the two lumps vanished. A nice happy ending you might think, but this was a journey that had only just started. Max not knowing the past life (or lives) that we shared and the events in those lives, was like a dog with a bone, he just could not leave it alone. At some level he was trying to solve his case, but that irrationally meant controlling me, so I could not leave. How could he do that? Well get yourself a "Rottweiler" solicitor such as the "fearsome" Raymond Tooth and barrister and use the law or what passes for so called "justice" to help you play out the rest of the past life and your psychological case.

The past life scene was played out in court in 1991 and as I watched Counsel Nicholas Mostyn in a disgusting theatrical snorting mucous down his nose into the back of his throat and spitting it out into his handkerchief a foot from my face, ranting "you're a religious zealot aren't you" many times, I could easily have been in an ecclesiastical tribunal of the inquisitional courts of the Middle Ages with the Grand Catholic Inquisitor, trying a heretic. I had to remind myself this was a divorce hearing case for finances to settle my children's secure future – but then you are not there for that of course in the British courts of Alice in Wonderland. This scene would be re-enacted many times – and 'stuff' the Declaration of Rights and Human Rights so say the judges and barristers!

Although it is considered bad form to relate one's past lives there was one incident that made me realise my true nature and recognise that I had unfinished business in this life as the NDE reminded me: "Who will teach the children?" It was the beginning of the fourteenth century and I was a young French nobleman, very learned and one of the highest members of a religious-philosophical sect. There had been a siege of our castle and it was expected that we would all be slaughtered. Four of us had been chosen, to get important documents out, so that they would not fall into the hands of the Catholics. These documents were so important, that they would threaten the Catholic Church should they be known. We were each given certain documents and we would travel to the four points of the compass to agreed destinations where the documents would be kept for safekeeping. Firstly we had to scale down the most precipitous and dangerous freezing mountainside, which I would later reflect had put me off mountain climbing altogether in this life.

It was very early spring and as I rode across France at top neck speed on my horse, I re-experienced in the regression the intense cold, as my hands were frozen to the reigns, despite my leather gloves. I seemed to be very young and as I rode I constantly looked over my shoulder, for the black hooded figures. I gave my last bread loaf to the horse and spoke kindly to it, stopping to water it by a river: "a little longer, we must travel my friend, we cannot let this fall into their hands". The horse was a beautiful white breed, with some markings and I seemed to love it dearly and felt bad that I had to ride it so hard.

Exhausted I arrived in England, but did not trust the Prior (?) of the Priory (?) where I had been told to leave the document. He was not the Prior that I had expected. I left not mentioning the document, but then they were closing in and I must hide it somewhere, I followed a river until I came to Alfriston a small hamlet in East Sussex, where I saw a large church. I entered what seemed to be a small room at night and took out the fourth brick up and along and placed the document behind it and made a sign of the circle on the brick on the outside of the church: the Circle of Eternal Return. In the regression I saw that a window was on the right side of the small room where cloaks were hanging and through the window, I could see a slope down a grassy hill. In the dawn light, I stared hard at the scene, imprinting the memory of it into my immortal Spirit, so that one day I could return and pick up the document and trail.

The life ended badly by being horribly tortured (once again) after being caught on a ferry to what I thought was the Netherlands. However I never revealed the whereabouts of the document to my torturers. On reflection I seemed to have spent many lives hiding secret documents so "they" would not get hold of them. I seemed to have in each life access to some deeper vein of knowledge. I had evidently been on a secret communication line of some knowledge for many lives. I reflected how when I was young I had set up a 'Secret Club of Nature' and fully expected high membership, but ended up with just one member – myself. Sometimes I would dress as a nun and a film that fascinated me was the 'Inn of the Sixth Happiness', where children are lead to safety over mountain terrain in China during the Boxer rebellion. Past life memories often play out in early childhood, but then submerge as the child grows up. I was also fascinated by the story of a disinherited princess, who led a life of poverty after being betrayed and having her inheritance stolen. In pottery class as a young child I had made a figurine of what looked like a very old and wise woman holding a baby and talking to it – was she teaching it something ?

I would relate this life and the story of Alfriston to the boys and they suggested we should go to Alfriston and see if there was a church there with the small room. The boys and I arrived at Alfriston never having seen the scene before and it was exactly identical to the way I had described it in my past life, there was even a sign on the brick of the doorway where I had left the document four bricks up, although it may have been added to and was described now as an "unusual sun dial". There was more to this incident, but I will return to it later.

At the end of each regressive session, I was asked to find a pleasurable memory. When this request arose after the first heavy session as a child in hospital, I retorted:

"Well if I could remember the happy times, I wouldn't be sitting here with you would I!"

It took a little time, to find a pleasure moment early in my life. It was 1966 the year England won the world football cup. A young group had brought a London Transport red double-decker bus, a number 7 to Clapham Junction and called the group the double-decker club. That year we had taken the bus to France and Cliff Richard's film *Summer Holiday* released in 1963 was the inspiration. Everywhere we went, we attracted attention and virtually brought the whole of Paris to a standstill, as we busked off the back platform wearing top hat and tails. I was sixteen and full of life.

World cup fever was everywhere in France and the bistros and cafes were full of Frenchmen gathered around blaring TV's drinking pastis or with emerald bottles of aniseed 51 on the tables. My standard order would be the delicious: "jambon beurre baguette", or egg mayonnaise baguette wolfed down whilst playing table football and joking with the locals: "Aren't you interested in your team they are in the final?" asked one astonished Frenchmen.

The truth was, I was there to experience the social fabric of France and there was always some interesting person to speak to in the cafes and bistros. There was a feeling that you existed amongst the midst of humanity, something I had not experienced in Britain. The bistros were like the "parliament of the people" where one could sit for hours and debate any issue: how different from England, where people went to work and then went home, never meeting their neighbours for a chat. In one conversation with a Frenchman, I discussed the decline of this social dimension in Britain and the loss of communal spirit, where people have less time for one another. The bistro was a "lieu de vie" – a place of life, which I remembered fondly.

I laughed when I remembered how we had met an unexpectedly low bridge and the broom we held out of the top deck front window, indicated not enough room to pass. The road was too narrow and on a mountainous incline, to let the mile or so of backed up traffic to pass. We were in the process of backing up the traffic jam, with no hostility as I remembered it, but good-humoured acceptance by the French drivers at this young group of eccentric English teenagers, when the French police arrived on motorbikes, scratched their heads and laughed loudly. Political correctness and Health and Safety had not yet been born, as a policeman told me to hop on his motorbike and we reversed the traffic jam. The following year on another trip, a London Transport Official spotted us; we later received a letter stating that we could not legally travel abroad in a red bus, as it might be mistaken for an official bus from London. I wondered how many French people would hail a bus going to Clapham Junction! Political correctness insanity had emerged. We were told to repaint it, but the whole point would have been lost, so we sold it.

That strange beguiling song 'A Whiter Shade of Pale' by Procol Harem accompanied our last holiday again to France. I remembered too that on Bastille Day, I was overcome by a sense of nervousness, without knowing why, which would only be explained by a recalled past life. I remembered also how I had been walking on a long French road, which led to Paris, when I felt very sick and had a flash vision of carriages and soldiers. Only years later would the incident be identified, as being part of the French Revolution, at the time it was just an inexplicable incident that I dismissed. The French Revolution and the immense betrayal would become part of what I would "teach the children", in the *Theatre Earth* series.

I came to realise that a man or woman's difficulties arise from cowardice. To have difficulties in life means to run away from the business of living. The less one confronts the more problems one has. Inevitably a total confront will mean having to decide who you actually are and in the event that one discovers unpleasant memories, then one might have to confront those or even the past lives one has lived, where one made wrong decisions that affected others.

Confronting ones actions then inevitably means that some degree of emotional pain occurs and some degree of courage is required, to go back and try to reverse those actions. I have heard people say: "I have enough problems in this life, without worrying about past lives". It seems that some people will never get it and as Jones was apt to lecture: "Look after yourself and your own".

Objects and people become less real the closer a person moves towards apathy. A person in sub-apathy sees a very watery, thin, dreamy, misty and unreal world. The more real a person becomes, the more real the colour and solidity of things around them become. If two people agree this tends to make the other more real. Two people who argue constantly have little reality. There is a definite link between agreement and reality. A marriage is supposed to bring agreement and affinity or love, but fails when two people have little reality upon which they can agree. Those things are real which we agree are real.

I tried to honestly look back at my time with Max - why could I find few pleasure moments that had endured? I alighted in therapy upon the time when I had walked down the avenue from the beautiful Napoleon III, Hotel du Cap, Eden Roc in Antibes, set in a private hectare park; towards the Eden Roc Pavilion. Kirk Douglas was playing tennis on the courts, much more diminutive than I had remembered him from his role as 'Spartacus'. The Pavilion stood on a terrace looking out to sea and one could swim in the spectacular overflowing swimming pool. Max and I were sat in the Eden Roc restaurant, overlooking the ocean watching the water skiers. Had I been happy? Even then, it was as though an uncomfortable truth was being presented, that my destiny did not lie with this world, I was being asked at some deep level, to reject this path and find my true purpose, along another path. The lives I had spent fighting a cause for truth particularly in religion and social justice, sat uncomfortably on the terrace of the Eden Roc; everyone else there had escaped from reality then why couldn't I? It seems that destiny had another path in mind.

13 A Cycle of Eternal Return to Greece

It was during such sessions, that I realised that I had a purpose; a purpose I had carried for many lifetimes, but found it difficult to identify that purpose exactly. Perhaps it was to cover my cancer research. I had by 1989 published a scientific paper outlining a mechanism for cancer (*Appendix 1*), which explained the psychology and biochemistry as linked. I had set up the Karmak Trust and with Sheila hoped as a charity to gain enough funds to open a centre for application of the therapy and to further research. The legal Wardship proceedings undertaken by Max along with traumatic events at Michael Hall School – a Rudolf Steiner School in Forest Row, East Grinstead; had exterminated all hope for the project. The thought of having to confront the likes of Nicholas Mostyn again in court was enough to force me to follow Jones's advice of not attempting to help cancer sufferers. Nicholas Mostyn had also ensured that I would not be able to cut loose from Max and I would be tethered to his chaos.

The boys agreed to board at a school in Sussex, when they realised I was right and that Max would go on interfering at great detriment in my life unless I left the country. I would go to Greece with the goal of setting up a homeopathic business, under Greece's more relaxed rules, following union with Europe. The boys would stay with me for all holidays and half terms for 26 weeks a year and board for the remainder until after a year they would join me and attend the Tassis Hellenic School in Athens.

There were always two sides to my personality, one the deeply rational scientist, who likes facts and figures and most of all proof: the other side was intuitive instinctive and visionary. As a child I was talented in both the arts and sciences, which was unusual. In today's terminology I might be considered left and right brained. In a world especially in science, where right brain thinking or rational argument is valued and left-brain or intuitive thinking is dismissed, then perhaps the idea of gaining proof for past lives, was another objective on my mind.

I had been impressed by how accurate my memory of the scene at Alfriston had been. Later I had studied Alfriston Church and its history and found that it was a large church and called 'The Cathedral of the South Downs.' It appeared to have no additions to when it was first built in the 13th Century. The Church had unusually been built on the sign of a Greek cross. Good Heavens I had thought, why a *Greek* cross? At that time in England, it would have been considered very unusual if not unheard of, to have a church built on the sign of a Greek cross. There were also stories surrounding a supernatural event at the Church. The stones for the foundations of the Church had been placed in one area, only to be mysteriously moved overnight to another, on the mounded hill, which was where the church was eventually built. It was deemed that it was God's wish to have the Church built there and so it was.

In my memory of the past life, I had remembered being in a "small room" when I had been seeking to hide the document. I could clearly see the view from a window to my right, in the room. However when I visited the Church with the boys, we could find no evidence at first for a small room. The boys and I searched everywhere. When asking a woman at the Church who was arranging flowers, whether there was a small room, or had it been removed, she thought for a while and then replied, "Well there is the porch". As I turned excitedly she added: "Don't forget to look at the unusual sun-dial on the wall". I had run excitedly from the church to see a sign, altered slightly from the one I left, but not much. There was also a window in the porch, just as I remembered it. I had recounted in my past life regression that the document was left four bricks up and four along, from the base of the wall, there at exactly four bricks up was the sign, where I had left the document behind the brick. When I covered this life in regression a phrase in connection with the document arose 'Help Me'. Help whom? I wondered at the time. If this referred to humanity, then they could help themselves, because by now through my experiences, I no longer cared to help.

Apparently a man had moved into the area at one time and had collected important documents and one night a spark flew from the fire and burned everything. I wondered whether he had found the document. A toothpick object and tongue-scraper had been found in the churchyard, in the 19th Century, with the unusual inscription of 'Help me – Adio Hurst'. I wondered whether the parchment had been found, perhaps by now burnt in the fire. I also considered whether 'Adio Hurst' was an anagram for 'Taro Hid Us' and made a mental note to look into the Taro, which figured in the *Theatre Earth* series and which did indeed hide a secret – Hermes the Charioteer who looked left and right.

Unusually too for the area, no important family had come to live in Alfriston. There had been no manor house, certainly unusual in that period of English village life. It was as if sleepy little Alfriston had been protected until my return. There were trips to Michelham priory, where the boys and I signed the visitor's book in the autumn of 1993. Had this been the priory, where I had been told to leave the document? It did have an octagonal room as in my past life memory.

I pondered for a long time on the document and past life. Perhaps the document related to some unknown religious truth concerning Greece and Christianity that mostly threatened the Catholic Church and male priesthood. I tried to recall what was written in the document, it was written in some form of code from right to left. Years later, I discovered this type of code was used by the secret group of the Rosicrucian's. Although I could not remember the exact contents of the document, it was a condemnation of humanity of some sort, for falling away from the truth. It seemed to be connected with the Apocalypse – 'the end of things', written by John the Apostle (Evangelist) and yet it seemed to be a different secret version.

The scientist in me began to seek proof of past lives and I reasoned that past life memories if they could be recalled, were comparable to holograms. In hologram theory, if one part of the hologram or 3-D picture is re-produced it can cause all other elements of the hologram to manifest. I wondered what would happen if I had a parchment made, written in a code, which replicated the original document *tone* of condemnation. Perhaps it would re-create the original hologram and being a part of that picture from the past, I would discover more. It was an interesting theory but even my intuitive self could not have imagined what would occur next.

On the day I left England on the 17th September in 1993, I left a parchment at Alfriston and posted one with the story of the sundial to the Archaeological Society in Sussex. No doubt it was tossed into the bin, or just archived away as another case of 'oiled pots' and the hiding of parchments, which tell a different truth, to the one we are led to believe in. Perhaps my experience would have to be locked away for a future enlightened time.

After driving from Milan to Ancona and taking a ship to Patras and from there driving to Piraeus to catch the ferry to Crete, I had forlornly travelled across three oceans with only the thoughts of my children in my mind. There was it seemed an intuitive fantastic urgency and yet that was coupled with the scientist's mind and question "is this is a crazy theory?" This was counter-acted by the question in the Near Death Experience: "Who will teach the children?"

If there were doubts, then the experience of being stranded during my journey to Crete on the island of Patmos for three days, after a large storm stopped all ferryboats in the Aegean, made me realise that some larger science of existence was at work. I was truly amazed and dumbfounded that a dream I had some six years previously of being stranded on an island of immense beauty after a large storm, had now materialised! Had I really foreseen all this and how could I have possibly known that a storm would materialise – even weather forecasters can't predict storms 6 years ahead! Further had not John the Apostle been blown into Patmos on a storm? Had the *tone* of the document in some way pulled down an entire hologram from the past? The ship I was on was destined for Crete, but had to run for cover in the port of the island of Patmos as the storm worsened and all ferryboats in the Aegean were cancelled for three days. How could I possibly have predicted that event six years before? The only alternative was to consider the power of the hologram of the past and my *intention*. Did I really make that storm happen? "Oops" I thought, I certainly did not want a bill from the Greek ferry companies for lost revenue! I decided that the document was probably an alternative version of John's Apocalypse, a version that the church did not want known.

Even more extra-ordinary, in a past life I had been an eyewitness to the events of the crucifixion and my account bore no resemblance to the official story. I have recounted this in the *Theatre Earth* series, so there is no need to recount it again here, but suffice it to say that the events hardly corresponded to the orthodox version. The information was unusual and I was inclined to dismiss it at the time. How could that be proved or disproved, was all I thought. It never occurred to me at that time that I would prove it at least to myself, through the *Theatre Earth* books and my research in Greece.

I had been in Greece three months when I literally bumped into 'the Mazarin'. Greece had once been the crossroads of the world for information and yet it seemed impossible at that time, to even get a phone line in Crete. I had spent

102

virtually every day for a month queuing at the government office, which dealt with phone lines, where I am sure an imprint of the frustration and complete exaggeration of an Englishwoman still exists. Queuing would occur from 8am onwards and infuriatingly just as I got to the top of the queue, the office would close for lunch and siesta. The Mazarin suggested I buy a phone number on the "black market" and at £500 it seemed cheap compared with one more day of queuing in the stifling heat.

As soon as I arrived in Greece I felt I was home and had returned. There were many hilarious things I liked about the Greeks. One day I was in a busy office and the phone kept ringing and the woman dealing with another large queue would have to answer it, to the frustration of the queue until a man, quietly stepped forward opened her draw and put the phone in it and closed it. The woman just gave him a quiet look, accepted it and the queue diminished quickly. I could not begin to imagine how some British government official would have responded to that, but then in Crete, they told me they kept guns, to make sure Athens kept their distance. The first New Year's Eve the boys and I spent in Crete, was celebrated with a release of gunfire all over the island, including machine gun fire as the clock struck midnight and the Cretans ran out and fired their weapons into the air. I would have given anything to watch the face of a health and safety inspector in England, confronted with that experience. There was a certain defiance and independence about the Cretans, who in World War II took to the mountains and fought a guerrilla resistance war.

The nickname Mazarin derived from the chief of police that Maria Antoinette hired -too late, to act as a spy and find out who was behind the French Revolution. She had suspected the Freemasons, but was fooled because; "they have God on their lips". A pity she did not find out which God. My Mazarin was hugely knowledgeable and held a large library of nearly three thousand books, many of which covered the occult "necessary in order to understand politics," the Mazarin assured me: as the Mazarin pointed out, "If you read that lot you will go mad". I was amused to think that the spirit of Greece with its independent intellectualism and wit was still surviving, most importantly with its own library. It was incredibly annoying that a lot of the documents were in Greek and the Mazarin tried earnestly to teach me the written language, but when I found out there were three 'e's I descended into exasperation: "There's not enough time in the Universe!" I wailed. It was at times like that I resented the sub-standard education received in State British schools, where Latin and Greek are not taught, compared to public schools. I made a mental note of taking some time later to learn Greek in the interim the Mazarin would interpret.

I explained a little of my experience and particularly the events surrounding the Crucifixion and Alfriston to the Mazarin and he walked over to his library and fingered the books with a sense of pride, "which?" he pondered might explain some of my experience. He chose 'The Holy Blood and the Holy Grail' by the authors Baigent, Lincoln and Henry. It was factually well researched, but unfortunately was followed years later by Dan Brown's books, which gave people the impression that The Holy Grail quest was fictional, perhaps not altogether a coincidence. One of the most important claims of Baigent, Lincoln and Henry's book, was that a mysterious group – the Ordre du Sion, a secret group currently called the Prieuré de Sion, hoped to reinstate the Merovingian dynasty on the thrones of Europe: a dynasty or bloodline descended from a child of a proposed liaison between Jesus and the Mary Magdalene. It did at least hold some support for my own (past life) witness evidence of the events surrounding the crucifixion, but did not identify what I felt was a secret communication line and branch of knowledge not known outside of the highest echelon of Christianity as it emerged. Neither did the book reveal my own memories of the facts surrounding the crucifixion.

I spent much of the time I was in Greece, studying and visiting archaeological sites and museums and going through their stored collections, putting together the hidden story and knowledge not only of events surrounding the crucifixion, but many world events. Connections started to appear between the secret groups, past wars and revolutions. A thread started to form, a golden thread, which Ariadne had laid for Theseus to follow in order to find and kill the Man-bull Minotaur in his labyrinth.

The Mazarin and I would curl up on his "thinking couch" discussing the various texts and if any new books or papers arrived from England or France, the Mazarin would tear them open immediately; he liked to be fully briefed. Once when we discussed European Union, he commented: "they won't let it last, it will be broken up soon". "Ah! I replied I knew you worked for intelligence". The Mazarin denied all of course.

The Mazarin once asked me why I had married my husband, to which I replied laughing: "Well you know what Plato said that love is a mental disease". The

Mazarin who had served in the military, reminded me of Jones when he commented, "emotions are dangerous things, romantic love is the most dangerous because it casts you from the heights of ecstasy to the abyss of despair". He wandered over to his Greek dictionaries to look up the definitions and derivations. The Mazarin was a patriot and was convinced everything derived from the Greek.

"Why?" I would ask him, "can't men be like gerbils and stick with their partners for life? I explained my research on gerbils back in the 70s and the intense bonding that occurs.

"A man does not like to be reminded of his own mortality, he likes to be Zeus!" was the Mazarin's reply.

The Mazarin would laugh heartily in such moments when I fumed about inequality particularly in science. I reminded him that Jocelyn Bell a physicist graduate PhD student under Anthony Hewish was not recognised or included for the Nobel Prize after she first noticed the stellar radio source that was later recognised as a pulsar. "Hewish and Martin Ryle picked up the prize in 1974", I told him: "And then what about Rosalind Franklin who was not acknowledged for her important work on DNA x-ray crystallography, which was absolutely key to working out the double helix in DNA, but Watson and Crick and Wilkins picked up the Nobel Prize in 1962". Science at least in Britain has always been sexist.

The Mazarin reminded me it was a two way street: "Well didn't Marconi get the Nobel Prize for work on radio even though Nikola Tesla was awarded the patent first?"

"Mm.... yes your right and I seem to remember that Tesla could have done with the money, as he went bankrupt shortly afterwards. That's what they do they don't give you a penny in research costs and then the vultures descend and pick it over for themselves".

On reflection I added: "There was Henry Eyring who did not receive the Nobel Prize for chemistry because of his religion, he was a member of the Church of Jesus Christ Latter Day Saints".

"So" remarked the Mazarin: "Perhaps it is the origination and genius of that, which they cannot acknowledge...maybe because for example Tesla's research was too important to the American military and Dr Gerson's work was as you say too threatening to the medical orthodoxy".

"Like poor old Wilhelm Reich, who they imprisoned and he lost the will to live," I retorted adding: "Well, non- acknowledgement is one thing, but what about betrayal?"

"Whose betrayal?" asked the Mazarin.

"Well the Mary Magdalene betrayed by Jesus and then there was Maria Antoinette who was betrayed by the Freemasons and the Duc D'Orleons who I might add was paid in Britain! And poor old Jeanne D'Arc betrayed by Duke Henry D'Anjou used like Mary Magdalene for her visions and when of no use thrown out and killed".

The Mazarin would leave to make tea during such rants and return, wearing a World War II helmet and a rifle (part of his collection), shouting: "Wake up, World War III has just started!" His humour and eccentricity was quite close to my own.

I would discuss with the Mazarin the effect of past lives on the present. I had accessed an even more astounding past existence, which involved a live crab. The scientist in me once again, refused to accept the data, finding it too beyond what I could confront, or perhaps what I wished to confront. Even so it sat there and bothered me, I mean what if it *was* true – everything else had checked out so why would this be wrong? I decided to check the data by the same method I had used before. I argued that if I returned to the exact location or place where the incident had occurred then my presence would cause all parts of the hologram to manifest in present time repeating at least elements of the past life. If it were not true then those elements would not manifest. So I wrote down my predictions of what would happen based upon the past life and then posted them to myself in a sealed envelope, such that I could not elaborate.

I predicted that a live crab would appear, I would be treated in a hostile fashion by someone, who did not want to hear what I had to say or who would reject my message. In fact I had chatted to a cafe owner, who was very interested in my philosophy and said that I should meet an old man from the mountains, who was incredibly versed in such matters and asked me to return the following day. As I sat at the exact spot in the past life, and waited, the hermit philosopher arrived and not long after got up angrily and walked off. The cafe owner apologised profusely, saying he had no idea of what had gotten into him. At that point a man walked up carrying a crab. I laughed and said, "Do you mind if I break its *left* claw?" The cafe owner replied, "that would be cruel", to which I said, "Yes it would, I was only joking". Virtually the whole incident from the past life had just manifested and even I was left jaw-hung with the thought reverberating in my head: "My God it's all true!"

I was attempting to note in the light of my past life experience, which objects or scenarios, were repeated. Much of this might seem rather irrelevant to western thinking, but in eastern beliefs, it would be a perfectly plausible hypothesis. The idea of a repeated pattern, or scenario played out time and time again, until as in Buddhist (or Hindu belief), the pattern is recognised and the individual releases himself from it, to reach a state of Nirvana, described under the laws of karma.

The Dalai Lama of Tibet was chosen as a child, as the living incarnation of the previous Dalai Lama. Recognition of objects used by the previous Dalai Lama was seen as some proof. Where then does intuition cross with reincarnation? My research in Greece became more than academic; in a cycle of return I was *remembering* things I had forgotten.

I had intuitively purchased the book '*The White Goddess*' by Robert Graves and without any logical reason that I could give, applied the Ogham finger alphabet – Beth Luis Nion alphabet, to decode 'The Shepherd's Monument' inscription at Shugborough Hall in Staffordshire England. This monument and its inscription had been mentioned in the book *The Holy Blood and the Holy Grail* and yet no one had ever been able to decipher it. I seemed to know the codes as if in a past life I had learnt them.

Staffordshire was a centre of Masonic activity in the mid-seventeenth Century, when Charles Radclyffe was the alleged Grand Master of the Prieuré du Sion: a secret group mentioned in Grail history as defenders of the Merovingian bloodline – an alleged bloodline from a union between the Mary Magdalene and Jesus. My research, not only was bringing me closer to providing proof, for my own past life memory of events surrounding the crucifixion, but I seemed to be retracing a hidden underground knowledge, once known to me.

Again I might question whether it was intuition, or experience and memory from past lives, that made me return to England from Greece, to visit the Summer Smoking Room at Cardiff Castle, Wales. I had wanted to view the coded concentric circular floor, which to a degree is mirrored by the pavement floor at Westminster Abbey. It was the boys' half term and they loved my "expeditions" and were pretty excited to visit the Castle.

We took the normal tourist route around the castle, with a guided tour. At the end of the tour, I asked the guide if we could see the Summer Smoking Room, which was closed to the public. Eventually a gracious man, Peter Erikson agreed to take us to the top tower, where I could view the floor, with its coded concentric circles. It was there to my astonishment, that my son found a crab mural on one wall, where Celestial Hercules is clubbing the crab, with a cut to the *left* claw. I was again left with the reverberating thought in my head: "My God it's all true!" Far from my research discounting my past life memories, time and time again my research confirmed them.

The boys loved our time in Greece, where they would excitedly come on my "expeditions" to the various archaeological sites and museums and where I would explain the significances of the objects, which were not listed in the tour guide. My goal was to teach the boys to always look beneath the superficial explanation, for a deeper hidden meaning. On one occasion in Heraklion museum near the site of Knossos, I was explaining the hidden knowledge behind some Cretan seals, when I noticed that a small group of tourists having left the main tour group were following and listening. One American man who had been listening intently to my explanation of the seals turned to me and said, "Jeeez, you should be running the tour here". The boys later suggested that I write a book on my findings, but the depth of knowledge and the nature of my findings, meant that it would be an almost impossible book to write.

I did roughly and I do mean roughly, publish an initial book '*The Battle of the Trees*' in Greece. Money was again tight, having paid the boarding costs for the boys and in travelling to and from Greece at half terms. Max predictably was causing numerous problems back in England, which meant almost certainly I would have to return to sort out the mess. The book was briefly placed in a bookshop 'Free Thought' in Athens. The Mazarin shortly afterwards told me the bookshop had been blown up. Shortly after that I knew I had hit some bare nerve with the research, when the Star of David was carved on my front door and my car badly damaged. Evidently someone thought I was Jewish. It at least confirmed to me that the Masonic research pointed to a Jewish underground vein of knowledge I had tapped into and certainly it started to explain the hidden account of the crucifixion. If it was a warning, then it seemed sensible to take it and return with the boys to Britain.

Greece had indeed been a healing experience for the boys and me. They still claim that our "expeditions" gave them a spirit of adventure and made them see that they had not lost from their bad experiences in childhood, but gained something instead. I remembered the Near Death Experience and the question: "Who will teach the children?" I had opened their eyes to something more about this world than one hears on the nightly news bulletins, or reads in newspapers.

One of their fondest memories was the time we spent naked, living on a beach in a remote part of the island. We pitched our tent on the pebble beach, overhung by steep cliffs, upon which wild goats grazed. We dug out a large hole in the pebbles, which was filled by pure mountain spring water, filtering down through the cliffs – it was our 'bath'. Another hole was dug for our 'refrigerator' and our provisions sunk in a container into the cold mountain water. This was pure boys own stuff! My goal was to teach the boys they could experience true happiness without material trappings.

Our days consisted of rising at 6am to walk (clothed) 10 miles over the mountains to the nearest village. The views were breathtakingly spectacular and the smell of wild thyme heavenly. At the village we would buy our bread and any provisions for the day. We ate breakfast at the small taverna, usually Greek yoghurt with honey and fresh-baked bread and orange juice. We would then catch the small daily boat back to 'the beach' arriving in time for our swim and snorkelling in the crystal clear emerald waters of the bay. As the sun reached its mid-day climax, we would while away our time in the shade, at a small taverna eating cheese pitas and reading, until by mid- afternoon, we would take out the canoe and paddle around the cave inlets fishing for our supper, whilst singing 'The Owl and the Pussycat.'

After the Germans arrived, they organised the suppers for everyone, pooling the day's fishing catch and making the most delicious fish stew. One could always rely on the Germans for organisation; they even had a small cooler fridge hitched up in a cave. After supper there were songs and guitars around a campfire or the boys and I would skim pebbles across a moonlit ocean. It must have been like that in the beginning, before man 'evolved' and swapped the beach for the stock market.

The boys discovered one could live on very little and be happy and years later Rufus would tell this story to a man in hospital who had suffered a stroke brought on by financial worries. The boys mostly remember the simplicity of life and the "old men": two brothers from Athens, who must have been well into their eighties, who lived on the beach. They would spend the whole summer on the beach and return to Athens for the winter. They were life- long naturalists, brown as berries and as fit as men half their age. They would often flash past us on the walk over the mountains, wearing their retro circa 1930's buttoned short cardigans and shorts. Whilst we took the boat back, on my insistence that ten miles was enough, the "old men" would hike back carrying their provisions. Their routine consisted of sunbathing on the hot stones with no towel or sunscreen, with evidently no concern for skin cancer, followed by a swim and then an hour lying under a plastic sheet that acted as a sauna. Through a Greek interpreter, they told me the secret was to remove toxins, which through the Gerson Therapy I was familiar with.

After the boys returned to boarding school in the Autumn, I received a letter from the Headmaster, informing me that the boys usual compulsory first English essay, 'What I did over the summer holidays,' was the most engaging and interesting he had ever read!

Care of Max the chaos was now mounting back in England, it would be necessary to return and go back to the dreaded lawyers. I was sad to leave the Mazarin, but the life I had sought in Greece had to be left, along with the homeopathic centre and the hope of extending that into an alternative cancer centre; and with a sense of impending doom, I returned to Britain.

Doom, because I was plagued by the question: "Who will teach the children?" As if I was constantly being urged to write down what I knew and to make that public. Perhaps the sense of doom emerged from memories of past existences where I had been forever taking responsibility for some precious knowledge, hiding documents for safe keeping less they fall into the wrong hands: documents which I hoped to retrieve in another incarnation. There was also, the memory of the constant flight and fear of those who sought the documents and the loss of any comfort and security that most people expect in a life. If it was the Inquisition and Freemasonry in past lives, it became judges and barristers in this life together with the usual assortment of flotsam and jetsam – those who had done nothing in their lives but sought to wreck yours, through some miniscule allotment of perceived power they had achieved for themselves.

At a time when I was writing the original manuscript for this book in 1989, Sheila and I were belting up Goodge Street near the University of London, on our way to Cranks vegetarian restaurant. The sun was shining down gloriously for once. Furiously running alongside the diminutive figure of Sheila, her red hair flowing, there was an enormous expectation that one could achieve something in this world of broken dreams.

"Whatever have you got on now?" I laughed looking down at Sheila's black boots with orange laces and nearly colliding with a newspaper stand.

"Aye never quite up ter the minute!" she laughed.
We sat on Crank's doorstep taking in the sun, when Sheila commented, "You know you used to pretend that you were not able".

I laughed, "Well perhaps I was hiding away this lifetime, not wishing to be burnt at the stake again, or hunted down by the Inquisition and subjected to their insane trials!"

I felt a great energy, I could feel it pulsating down my spine, it had been a long time since I felt exhilaration. I leaned back on my elbows and lifted my face to the sun. I had my blue jeans and 'bikers' sunglasses on and '*Tango in The Night*' by Fleetwood Mac was playing.

"Well that's it then Sheila", the end of that journey – cancer".

"Aye it looks like it Renee," she replied in a bored way, squeezing a small carton of apple juice trying to hit a tree opposite with the juice from the straw. It missed and nearly hit a smartly suited gentleman who looked at Sheila with an obvious stare and his trousers for any signs of juice.

111

"Will you stop that Sheila MacLean, I bring you to all the best places and look what you do," I laughed "you ought to be locked up!"

"Aye, well when you've written that book that's what they'll be doing to ye".

Perhaps she was right and the research would have to be hidden away once more, until a more enlightened age. Significantly '*Go your own way*' was playing by Fleetwood Mac. I boxed up the manuscript and research and left for Greece to find my *own* way.

14 "Off with her head!" Alice in Wonderland

The book '*The Battle of the Trees*' researched and published in Greece seemed to pull in a wide range of what seemed to be the 'old crew'. 'The Shepherds Monument' inscription had remained enciphered for twenty years, since its mention by the authors of '*The Holy Blood and The Holy Grail*'. My decoding of the inscription together with the decoding of the paintings '*La Fontaine de Fortune*' by René d'Anjou (Jeanne D'Arc's mentor from the secret groups); '*Et in Arcadia Ego*' and '*Les Bergers d'Arcadia*' by Poussin; and '*Et in Arcadia Ego*' by Guercino, along with Salvador Dali's ' *Persistance de la Mémoire*', certainly created a wave of interest and invitations to lecture on my research.

A doctor who had come across my cancer research encouraged me to pursue it telling me, "It's brilliant, and you really must make this research known". I had already been through Wardship proceedings due to the cancer research and been virtually burnt at the stake in my divorce proceedings by Counsel Nicholas Mostyn (whom I later learnt ironically was a Catholic), because of it and had with the boys suffered horrendous events in two schools including the Rudolf Steiner School of Michael Hall in East Grinstead. I had left England because of the upset and really had no wish to put myself, or importantly the boys through any further trauma. However, against my better judgement I was persuaded in 1997 to give it a last shot.

I spent a month in the library, researching the ancient Right of Petition and having approached nearly every Member of Parliament finally gained the consent of the MP for Lewes, Tim Rathbone to table the Petition in the House of Commons. My mother helped me stick on the postage stamps at more personal cost, but with one stamp short for envelopes to about 300 MPs I put two in one envelope and asked Alan Johnson MP if he would kindly pass it on to the colleague MP. He took the bother to write back telling me: 'I am not the postman'. The Petition was predictably and inevitably 'scuttled' by the Conservative Government and the research neatly channelled off down the dark, non-transparent labyrinthine corridors of power (*Appendix 2*). I felt I could do no more and certainly there was the pressing goal of putting together the research of twenty years into book form for publication, which would become the *Theatre Earth* series, in addition to holding down a job and caring for the boys.

'*The Battle of the Trees*' had been cobbled together with 'Prit Stick' in a T-Shirt factory on Crete. Power cuts, problems with computers affected by power cuts, printers, staff and a myriad of other problems, had caused me to think that this research was being fought at every level. It was as though the message was being fought and was facing an enormous barrier of lies, which defeated truth at every turn. The '*Theatre Earth*' series turned into four volumes. The books contained knowledge yes, research yes, but they also contained *a message* I had carried through many lifetimes. It was with some predictability that the knowledge would be taken and used and the message deleted – that is the story of the Holy Grail: the golden cup more important than its contents.

It would be no surprise that by the time I gave up entirely, my research had been used against me no less than nine times in various court hearings and incidents including employment. I had sent my books to Stephen Hawking at Cambridge, but received the reply that his disability and shortage of time prevented him from reading them. I had hoped he would take up my research and explanation to Einstein's singularity as a geometric universe, built on the foundation of the 3-D tetrahedron geometric of the Hydrogen atom: space-*time* being merely the product of implants as described in *volume 3* of *Theatre Earth*. I guess my problem is that I have always been ahead of my time and there was never a time when anyone could duplicate the data.

One minor suggestion I did put forward in the books, was that aliens had 'planet hopped' and devastated the resources of any planet they landed on. In one court hearing my books were ridiculed along with 'aliens' and the barrister for the other side, managed to violate nine points of the Code of Conduct for a barrister along with nine violations of Human Rights. This rather mirrored the Wardship proceedings and matrimonial hearing, where another barrister used my research in order to win points for his client and influence the judge's decision. In all court cases my research was put on trial and not the case before the court.

In one court case, another judge, who unknown to me at the time was a Grand Master of Freemasonry, suddenly replaced the judge who was due to hear the case. Even without knowledge of that membership he was found to be so bias,

I had to have him removed. As my books are anti-Masonic then one might reasonably ask how un-bias a Grand Master could be.

'*So where is the justice in judges being allowed to keep their wrongdoings secret?*' asked a journalist in *The Daily Mail* (*March 17th 2009*). Despite volumes of letters about these cases to the various legal complaints departments and bodies, no remedy was ever forthcoming in violation of Article 13 of The Human Rights Act 1998 – the right to remedy. The tape recording of the hearing involving the Masonic Judge was eventually 'wiped' with 'apologies' by the Court, when I was due to use it in a court case I intended to bring on my own; despite evidence must by law be retained for six years and the Court had agreed by letter to save the recordings. In fact this case was before The Right Honourable Jack Straw then Justice Minister, when he announced that as no serious conflicts had ever been reported, Masons do not have to disclose membership as that membership would have no bearing on the outcome of proceedings. In my case I had clearly shown that the judge was removed for bias comment and pre-determination to judge the case in a particular way, thus determining *outcome* of the proceedings.

A barrister may use your research in a court of law, to adversely influence the judge, even though you are there to settle another matter entirely. Barristers constantly flaunt their Code of Conduct using what they consider 'bad points' (in my experience usually violating Article 9 & 10) in order to influence a judge and as a result I have been robbed and traumatised by Courts in Britain, all over my research and this does not count loss of employment, where hundreds of thousands of pounds were lost.

I may have been ridiculed in Court for my views on aliens, where I had to remind myself that this was a trading standards case and not an Inquisitional trial, but when Stephen Hawking repeated those views he obtained coverage in '*The Sunday Times*' newspaper. He would not find his disability ridiculed, or ideas on alien life ridiculed in a Court of law as I did and here you have another violation of Human Rights in Britain – equality before law. No doubt if Stephen Hawking had written to Jack Straw he would not have been fobbed off with some ridiculous reply. Britain is an unequal society. As Snoopy once observed sitting in cattle class with a polystyrene cup, 'you have to pay for respect'. The only time they pay attention is when they fear they will be publicly exposed – the nature of the coward.

The ideas, the knowledge, when stripped of the message of the Grail becomes a power base and in such form is acceptable, because the lies of history do not require answers from politicians, who have their sound bites to rely upon: "we value the individual who takes responsibility" (John Major circa 1996 at the time I was presenting the cancer research by Petition and the government was refusing that Petition); "a more transparent society"; or "taking politics to the people"; or "the big society". The best jokes however are the mission statements by the various departments that I applied to and lists of values they claim to uphold. If it were not so sick, one might laugh at the replies from some of these departments, such as the Bar Council, The Office of Judicial Affairs, the Parliamentary Ombudsman or Jack Straw's Office of Justice, which I use in the very loosest way. One recognises to use Simon Carr's term what: 'prodigious waffle monkeys' these people are. If the parliamentary system was found in the expenses scandal to be institutionally corrupt, then from my own experience the legal system is questionable, since they are bound by law to maintain law and yet I have sat in courts since the passing of The Human Rights Act in 1998, where I counted at least nine human rights violations in one case by a barrister; and I can assure you that not even the justice minister was vaguely concerned, or the fact that the Bar Council offices were broken into and my data amongst others stolen. One must assume that even an idiot burglar would not attempt to burgle the central office of barristers and so it must have been an inside affair, with a motive, but apparently even the police have yet to come up with that conclusion.

Whilst child slave labour was occurring in Britain during the 18th and 19th centuries, where children as young as four were forced down tunnels in the coal mining business, dressed in rags suffering from starvation; or mutilated by the cotton mills machinery being forced to scramble under working machines picking up cotton; the upper classes and aristocracy were more concerned with the morals of slave trading abroad. Britain has a history of ignoring the rights of its own citizens, whilst portraying itself as a moralist nation abroad. 'All fur coat and no knickers' as the saying went. The Dickensian mentality still exists in so far as despite my numerous complaints and one to William Hague, who is now foreign secretary, it was reported (*The Guardian 15.09.2010*): 'The foreign secretary will today pledge to strengthen the role of human rights in British foreign policy and will announce the creation of an independent advisory body to help identify abuses abroad'. I raised my eyebrows when I noted that Hague in a speech at Lincoln's Inn - London, the heart of Britain's legal establishment, Hague was quoted as saying, 'our standing is directly linked to the belief of others that we will do what we say and that we will not apply double standards'. Hypocrisy is a term that constantly applied to my story.

In 2005 I forwarded some of my research (*Volume III Theatre Earth*) to *New Scientist* and *Scientific American* magazines, with a view to covering my research on the geometric universe and Einstein's singularity and the emergence of four-dimensional space-time from the tetrahedron (3D) or triangle (2D) as the basic geometric. I also sent my research to the Niels Bohr Institute. The magazines did not cover it and I received no reply from the Institute, but some years later I noted a comparable if not identical theory, was laid out in both magazines ('*Quantum Universe*' *Scientific American July 2008; 'Grand Designs' New Scientist 14.06.2008*). The authorship was male orthodox professorial - naturally.

New Scientist had in fact previously rejected my work on the Minoans ('*Who Killed the Minoans?*'), but in the next issue ran a standard orthodox theory of the demise of the Minoan civilization, by male orthodox scientists - naturally. The standard orthodox theory for the Minoan's demise on the island of Crete is a volcanic eruption on the neighbouring island of Santorini, which caused a tsunami, travelling to Crete and which then wiped out Knossos and the Minoans, one and a half thousand years before the birth of Christ. The researchers produced smart wave action diagrams generated by computers in their laboratory – well naturally they received research grants. As I pointed out the following week in a letter to the Editor, had the researchers ever left their laboratory and visited the archaeological site, they would have discovered the whole site is covered in gypsum, which dissolves in running water as I stated: 'Oops!' The article even produced a picture of the icon I had used in my own proposed article – a man holding his hand to the third eye in the middle of the forehead, with deep religious meaning. I am afraid I could not resist asking the Editor: 'If the icon was meant to convey the thought woe is me, here comes a tsunami!' Needless to say my teasing letter was not printed or the research on the Minoan civilization, which was actually important to the history of science as the Minoans it seems from my own research, may have grasped the science of the re-cycling universe, which they incorporated into their religion of a Cycle of Eternal Return: but at least it seems they probably held beliefs on reincarnation, which powered their creativity and fabulous art.

Certainly one should question whether the original Apocalypse version and perhaps the document I hid in the 14th Century, conveyed this cycle of eternal return, which was then edited out of *Revelations* in *The Bible* to hide the trap for humanity. So you see despite scientists can't prove how the Minoans were actually wiped out, only one view – the tsunami view is accepted and all other views or evidence is barred. That's how science *actually* works. In my own research, in *Theatre Earth,* I proposed that the Late Minoans wiped out the Early Minoans in a religious revolution, which eradicated the belief in a Cycle of Eternal Return. That belief was at base I claimed behind the secrets shared between Jesus and the Mary Magdalene, whose close relationship is evident in the *Lost Gospels.* Further just because the eminent archaeologist Arthur Evans decided Knossos was a palace (and not a burial place as my own research shows) and published many papers on it – then no one may now question that: As Peter would have said at the Charter Clinic and to misquote: "science is full of opportunities as soon as one door shuts another one slams in your face".

Recently Richard Dawkings and Professor Hawking have both strongly rejected any spiritual dimension in the universe. As Dawkings famously remarked in his book '*The Selfish Gene*': 'we are survival *machines – robot vehicles* blindly *programmed* to preserve the selfish molecules known as genes' (*author's emphasis*). Although Dawkings did not realise the depth and significance of his words, there is more than an element of truth concerning the trap in them, as I covered in '*volume 3 Theatre Earth*'. Science in its rejection of religion prefers such a view and it may be pointless to explain that every person who attacked my research, in holding a belief only in *bodies* (derived from genes) with no spiritual dimension would indeed have sought to protect the *material* universe and hide the *spiritual* trap man finds himself in. Such people do not consider that they will be here at the end, when the sun becomes a red giant and their whole being and identity will be re-cycled in the *universe of matter*, which they sought to protect. Everyone is entitled to his or her view and if they want to go down with the ship, it's their choice. Stephen Hawking remarked in his documentary televised in 2010 that the purpose of the universe and our being here is not known. It's a tough universe and no one promised it would be easy – *staying ahead of the game and surviving as a spiritual being and evolving upwards on the spiritual ladder* (to?) **is the purpose**. Some people will entirely 'get it' but I am afraid the majority as 'programmed' 'robot' 'vehicles' won't.

The first lesson here on earth appears to be 'find out who you are' – recognise you are a spiritual being and leave this doomed cycle on earth. If you don't learn the lesson then of course you will go down with the ship you cling to and be re-cycled as stardust.

I had bribed the boys as Rufus now approached the awkward teenage years, to go with me on one last expedition, by promising them three days at Disney Paris, if afterwards we went to the birthplace of Jeanne D'Arc at Domremy and lit three candles in the small church: followed by a visit to The Temple de l'Amour at Petit Trianon built by Maria Antoinette and to see once again the little Austrian village she built. The boys asked me why I wanted to go there and I just replied: "I want to say, I know what happened, I know your betrayal".

After looking at Petit Trianon the boys and I visited Versailles and as I wandered down the Hall of Mirrors, I caught a glimpse of myself, I looked tired and old - battle weary. I remembered in history how Maria Antoinette's hair at the age of thirty-three had turned white with shock, supporting her husband Louis through a serious mental breakdown and watching her young son the Dauphin, who could have been no more than eight years old, being battered by his jailor Simon, filled with alcohol and smeared with VD and made to claim in court he caught it from intercourse with his mother. Maria whilst battling the Freemasons through the French Revolution and watching her family and friends murdered also witnessed her closest friend's head waved on a pole in front of her. Before she went to the guillotine she bumped her head on a low beam and when asked if she had hurt herself she replied: "Oh no, there is nothing more you can do now to hurt me".

There does come a point, when after spending thousands on your research, continually thwarted in trying to set up a clinic and having your research picked over by vultures without due consideration as to the costs of that research, then you just wake up one day and you simply don't want to carry it anymore: and so the research and my biography went into a box in the attic and there it has stayed for 20 years.

Today in Britain expressing an opinion is a dangerous activity and a scientific opinion more so; as pharmaceutical companies and the Medical Council, silence you with threats of excommunication from your profession. Britons believe that they live in a democratic country, where their opinions count.

They don't. Your request for an inquiry that is completely independent from the powers that be; your Petitions presented to The House of Commons will be ignored. Your complaints and protests will go ignored and your letters will go unanswered. They will do whatever they want to and will not be accountable. Most of all they do not want thinkers, because thinkers ask too many awkward questions.

A Russian scientist colleague once told me that what had happened to me would not even happen in Russia and is more reminiscent of the Gulag days. Whilst I was walking in Holborn in 1989 a barrister said to me: "just remember from now on Big Brother is watching you". I thought it a joke, but he wasn't joking.

So many freedoms in Britain have just disappeared. One used to be able to stand on Hyde Park Corner in London, traditionally the place of free speech and give forth on any topic to anyone who would stop to listen. The police started harassing speakers under Tony Blair and Jack Straw, once Political Correctness came into force. European Union ironically whilst enforcing liberties and equality has in other ways reduced them. It's got to the point where no one dare open his or her mouths anymore and freedom of expression (Article 10) in my case was shown not to exist.

A measure of a democratic society is access to law. In my own journey, I approached ten legal firms who practise in Human Rights legislation including top firms like Bindmans, Leigh and Day and Public Interest lawyers. One solicitor in declining to uphold my rights under Articles 6, 9 & 10 said, "if you were a terrorist or a member of a penal institution we would be able to help you". I thought he was joking but he wasn't. Legal Aid or government funding is not it would seem available to protect a British scientist under Article 10 (Free Expression) or redress (Article 13). Another told me, "You are just too controversial in your views". I thought he was joking but he wasn't and the irony of Article 10 lost on him.

I also found out that judges couldn't be questioned. A *'Daily Mail'* newspaper article on this topic stated: 'It is an almost unbelievable fact that when judges do get into trouble, their misdemeanours are very likely to be swept under the carpet'. Well indeed when I wrote to the Office of Judicial Affairs concerning the bias of a Judge who was a Grand Master of Freemasonry, I was fobbed off. Later the tape recording would be 'wiped' with apologies of course, despite

120

the evidence was supposed to be retained for six years and was needed in a private case I wished to bring against the barrister, for nine violations of Human Rights and as many violations of the Code of Conduct. It is only when you challenge the system that you find out Britain is not *actually* a democracy and Article 13 (the right to an effective remedy) is simply ignored. It always looks fine until you get to the small print and how it *actually* works where you inevitably find catch 22.

"The Big Society" was David Cameron's (Conservative Prime Minister2010) mantra; and: "We value the individual who takes responsibility", was John Major's (former Conservative Prime Minister) mantra at the time my Petition as a democratic right was being swept under the carpet in 1997, before the 'triksy' Tony Blair came to power. If you do take responsibility in the "Big Society" let me forewarn you that you will end up like me. On March 30th 2010, I opened a newspaper to see Lady Levene wife of Lord Levene of Portsoken, Chairman of Lloyd's of London, sitting in front of one of my treasured possessions I had to give up for auction, when yet another barrister had used my research to influence the judge. It was an oriental lamp, with a cream silk shade I had especially designed and made. Ironically it was Lloyd's of London which reneged on my insurance policy, which in clear black and white statement, had promised to cover all violations of 'Rights': apparently not Articles 6, 9 or 10 rights. If you find the energy, you could send your complaints around the various Ombudsmen, only to find that they evidently cannot read black and white print either. No - don't take responsibility, unless you wish to be driven mad and bankrupted.

Even if you do survive the legal battles, Article 10 (free speech) is fought in Europa wonderland at the level of publishing. As George Orwell discovered when he wrote '*Animal Farm*', one of the greatest satires of the 20th Century: 'It is so not ok politically that I don't feel certain in advance that anyone will publish it'. This may be the first reference to the term 'political correctness' that we know. Orwell also astutely said, 'what sickens me about Left-wing people, especially the intellectuals, is their utter ignorance of the way things actually happen'. But if the "Big Society" is anything to go by, then the right-wing hasn't got a clue either. It seems some intellectual rediscovered the 18th century philosophy of Edmund Burke and repackaged it as "the big society". The way it *actually* works is that the Establishment will always erect barriers to guard against the undeceived; in order to maintain a compliant deceived populous – the 'selfish gene' will always protect itself.

To hear the Conservative government talking of citizens "collective" control over their lives, is to realise such rhetoric has no reality, but is merely a clever political branding exercise. If you are prevented from access to justice and continually experience violation of the most fundamental right of fair trial (Article 6) then you do not have control over your life. To quote from the Conservative Party manifesto (2010):

'...Our alternative to big government is the big society: a society with much higher levels of personal, professional, civic and corporate responsibility...'

Evidently they need to emerge from their private clubs and schools and run the wheel of life in the *real world* as hamster, as I have done to find out how it *actually* works. Let us take the view that the Human Rights Act applies to all citizens and Article 10 – Freedom of Expression is protected along with Article 6 (fair trial). Not so. If ministers now view the Human Rights Act as a, 'Charter for undeserving criminals,' it is because the legal system is run by greedy solicitors and barristers, who won't pick up a pen, for less than £5,000. No solicitor or barrister in the UK will pick up a pen for a point of principle. The price of legal representation is too high to take action against violations of Human Rights and Article 10, so you will have to go it alone and if you do, you will experience violations of Human Rights in a Court of Law. Represent yourself as litigant in person and you can throw the law out of the window. Nearly 90% of litigants in person fail to win their case according to the Department for Constitutional Affairs – a figure, which illustrates the failure of Human Rights in British courts.

And yet we condemn China where the jailed human rights campaigner Liu Xiaobo, who was nominated for the Nobel Peace Prize, is being actively prevented from receiving it. Whilst the west quotes article 35 of the Chinese Constitution, which says that, 'Citizens of the People's Republic of China enjoy freedom of speech, of the press, of assembly, of association of procession and of demonstration': the west or at least Britain actively bars that in more devious ways in that Article 6 (unfair trial) in Britain is only applied to convicts and terrorists and I am told courts do not like to apply Article 6 and unfair trial to ordinary citizens, because 'bias of a judge is published'. This surely means that Britain at least is hiding its violations of human rights and bias in court proceedings to ordinary citizens, whilst publishing only figures in relation to a prison population and terrorists.

Despite a ruling in Scotland Meerabux v A-G of Belize [2005] 2 AC 513: where it was pointed out that there was no difference between the common law test of bias and the requirement for impartiality in Article 6 of the Convention, which was also a decision in Lawal v Northern Spirit [2003] ICR 856: the law courts in England will not grant you Article 6 violations in a case of judicial bias. It seems that British courts are not willing to confront the fact that they are bias towards certain citizens who hold views contrary to e.g. Freemasonry or religious beliefs that have been designated as a "cult"; or who hold political views contrary to the policy of the government or even those who challenge the legal system on fairness.

Before Mr Liu's last trial, the United States government called on Beijing to release him 'immediately and to respect the rights of all Chinese citizens to peacefully express their political views'. Once again the word hypocrisy arises, when American citizens are not allowed to determine the fate of their lives and treatment for cancer, when they have to cross the border with Mexico, because they hold a different philosophical view of cancer, which contradicts political policy.

In 1913 in Scott v Scott, which is the closest Britain came to a constitutional case, the Law Lords declared that, 'every court in the land is open to every subject of the King'. Today that should be amended to: 'if you have the means to pay' which contravenes Article 6 and access to justice. As former judge Lord Darling dryly observed a hundred years ago or so: 'like the doors of the Ritz Hotel, the courts are open to rich and poor alike'. Even if you take out insurance as I did, by the time you find out where eventually your insurance has been bundled to, much as in the banking crisis of sub- prime mortgages, you will find out that suddenly they can't read the black and white print of your insurance contract, as was the case with Lloyd's. It's all very well for the government in Britain to cut back on public legal aid funding, telling people to take out legal insurance; but in the *real world* as I found, squabbling with your insurance company over default is more likely to result with another year squabbling with the Ombudsman, none of whom can read black and white print.

How can one experience nine Human Rights violated in a court of law? As Gavin Phillipson told the British Academy forum, attempts by Parliament to instruct the judges on how to interpret rights have not achieved much: 'Judges do not like being told how to interpret things because they see that as their job'. It must be then, in the court case in 2003 that The Human Rights Act of 1998 and the Code of Conduct for a barrister had entirely slipped the judges memory.

You would think that organisations like *Liberty* would have been helpful. Shami Chakrabarti however refused the 2003 case, explaining that with limited funds, there were more important cases abroad or immigrant issues in the UK. Then why have the organisation in *Britain* if it applies only to immigrants or foreign nationals?

Even if you do manage to persuade a higher Appeal Court of justifiable doubts or grounds for a judge's bias and lack of impartiality in a lower court using a list of legal cases, you will find that even though *you* were not responsible for the bias, *you* are expected to pay high legal costs if you go ahead with a full hearing which on past experience in all probability will fail. The innocent party as litigant in person who had expected an impartial hearing is then forced up the legal case ladder of increasing legal complexity, where barristers have spent years in training into the courts of high costs, which acts as the final barrier to justice. It then becomes just too prohibitive to fight for principles of justice before the law in courts of justice (the two are not the same).

Whilst environmental campaigners have won a significant victory under the Aarhus Convention which came into force in 2001 and was ratified by the U.K in 2005 where the government is obliged to give rights and remove financial barriers for citizens to mount legal challenges to cases of environmental damage; no such right exists for author's and scientists like myself who continually suffer bias which in at least 3 cases was based on their research and books in courts of law. Whilst at least environmental campaigners it seems have won a battle to remedy gross unfairness in the U.K legal system that does not apply to scientists like myself. Like the case of cancer once they admit that one dissenter through – they fear the agreed upon system will come under attack.

Surprisingly (since Geoffrey Robertson QC, was a recipient of one of my letters), in arguing for a British Bill of Rights he stated: "There is no liberty in Britain that is safe from the meddling of politicians", presumably misquoting Thomas Jefferson.

If my case illustrates anything it is a reflection on the hypocritical words of Geoffrey Robertson QC in his article in *The Independent* (*1.06.2010*) where he argued for 'The case for a Bill of Rights':

'We teach our children nothing about Lilburne and Milton and Wilkes, or about the Petition of Right or the 1689 Bill, or about Tom Paine and the brave booksellers who died in prison for selling *The Age of Reason*, or about Erskine and Bentham and the Tolpudle Martyres'.

Well indeed, 'brave booksellers' or publishers like myself are still being 'zipped up' in law and in my case it has been on-going for 20 years, where my family have been traumatised by courts, schools and employers. Jack Straw's Green Paper in 2009 concerning a "British Bill of Rights and Responsibilities", seems to me to be hypocritical since he had before him my case at the time – but did nothing. Subsequently Straw ruled that Freemasons did not have to reveal that membership in Court, even though I had to have a judge removed for bias - a frightening ordeal if you are acting alone as litigant in person.

The irony is that The Human Rights Act of 1998 already allows for the Right to Democracy, where everyone has the right to take part in the government of his country either directly or through their Member of Parliament. But try exercising that Right (Article 21) as I did and feel the wrath descend upon you. Article 29 also covers responsibility, but try exercising that responsibility and you will wish that you had never stuck your head above the radar screen!

In my case a judge was removed from a case in 2003 after my complaint of astounding bias, when it is virtually impossible to achieve that especially as litigant in person unless the court felt there was incontrovertible proof of bias. Subsequently the evidence and tape-recording was 'wiped' by the court despite the fact it was needed in evidence in a private court case I wished to bring. I later found out the judge was a Grand Master of Freemasonry and as I write anti-Masonic books then how could there be no "real danger" of bias?

The House of Lords unanimously upheld that in cases where no actual bias and no direct pecuniary interest give rise to a presumption of bias, where there is a <u>real danger</u> it is the *possibilities* and not the probabilities, which matter. (<u>Taylor R (on the application of) v. Stipendiary Magistrate for Norfolk</u> [1997] EWHC Admin 611 (1st July 1997).

According to the maxim 'nemo judex insua' 'nobody should be a judge in his own case' – or you can't judge a case in whose outcome you have an interest'.

After that case in 2003 in a further case in 2010, to avoid 'real danger' I requested a non-Masonic judge, but was never assured that I would not be given one.

The Rights of Freemasons not to disclose (privacy) fought and won by the 'Brotherhood' as a legal case in The European Court and to which Jack Straw then Justice Minister for Labour bowed to, do not override the rights of litigant in person to assure that no direct conflict of interest is present in a hearing by those in a decision making position where 'impartiality' under Article 6 is an absolute right, which cannot be infringed under *any* circumstances. It *guarantees* the right to an 'impartial' hearing in 'determination' of the case and also *guarantees* procedural fairness.

The problem is that as the Labour M.P Chris Mullin said in the late '90s, 'you cannot have at the centre of your criminal justice system an organization...which swears oaths in secrecy to each other'. Mullin led two parliamentary inquiries into allegations that Masonic corruption pervades Britain's police forces and judiciary. Mullin brought a Bill in 1992 which through the Hansard Debates, required members of secret groups, principally Freemasons to declare their membership before taking up a public office or a position in public service. Mullin stated:

'For some years I have taken a particular interest in miscarriages of justice. That intent has brought me into contact with people at all levels of public life in the police and legal professions, particularly in the west midlands. I make no allegations of impropriety, but one would have to be blind not to notice that many of those with whom I have dealt are freemasons'.

In 1997 shortly before 'New Labour' came to power Jack Straw said that freemasonry should be a 'declarable and registered interest' for members of the judiciary. Labour won and a rule was introduced declaring that anyone who was made a judge or magistrate had to declare membership of freemasonry. Many resigned rather than declare membership, which is in itself curious if there is nothing to hide, although it has long been questioned what rites in Freemasonry are required that exclude women from the 'Brotherhood'? However just as an election loomed in 2009 and it was clear that Labour would not win it, Straw suddenly issued a statement saying that he was as Minister for Justice scrapping the rule over freemasonry declaration that he played a role in introducing. In fact the freemasons had threatened to sue the government, based upon a ruling by the European Court (2006) in the case of freemasons (Grand Lodge) in Italy, who objected to the rule of disclosure on the basis that it violated *their* human rights. As I say individual Human Rights do not matter and *your* right to an unbiased hearing under Article 6 of the Human rights Act. So you end up fighting a case of bias through the appeal courts, or formal complaints procedures that run you around until you expire in the wheel. That's how it *actually* works. Even then, the best you can hope for if you prove bias is a retrial, with no compensation for the year or two getting to that point or the legal homework you have to do as litigant in person. Even then the court will ignore Article 6, which guarantees your case will be heard within a reasonable time. You might wait a year or so for the first case, then when bias pops up you then spend another year going through appeals and if and when you win that you then get to go back to the beginning, this time with the threat of costs hanging over you! 'Access to justice'?

History has enough quotes and evidence, as illustrated in *Theatre Earth*, to prove that freemasonry and the secret groups historically at least, fomented some if not the majority of the world's revolutions and wars. I have continually warned of the danger of secret societies and where members are elected to public office. In my own books, I show that the French Revolution and the eradication of Europe's monarchies was essential to paving the way for European Union and thus in the event that my case was brought to the European Court, it is debatable whether impartiality would exist, where an author is opposed to a Federal State, with un-elected powers. How could one be assured that a judge there was not bias against my books or a freemason? The more fascist (or Communist it makes no difference) a state becomes, then the less freedom there is to question that State and my experience reflects that.

In 2001, Charles Wardle independent MP for Bexhill and Battle brought the Secret Societies (Registration of Membership) Bill in the UK, requiring registration of membership to a secret society, principally freemasonry: 'To set an example to other public officials, members of the Committee on standards in Public Life have established their own code of practise, requiring them to register *any private interest which might influence their judgment* or which' and this is the crucial part '*could be perceived (by a reasonable*

127

member of the public) to do so. The inevitable conclusion must be that, sooner or later, the need for openness and accountability in public life...will lead to legislation embracing that principle' (*author's emphasis*). The question becomes whether '*a reasonable and informed member of the public*' would feel that a Grand Master of Freemasonry could sit without bias on a case where the author is anti-Masonic and seeks to reveal freemasonry's political and religious skeletons? That is the question in law I put to Jack Straw, then Justice Minister, who dismissed it.

In fact there is already legislation that would require this openness and lack of bias. The European Convention of Human Rights in Article 6(1) provides: 'In the determination of his civil rights and obligations...everyone is entitled to a fair and public hearing within a reasonable time by an independent and impartial Tribunal established by law'. Further, The House of Lords held the overriding consideration to be taken into account is '...whether the fair minded and informed observer, having considered the facts, would conclude there was a real possibility that the tribunal was biased' (Lord Hope in Porter v, Magill [2001] UKHL 67, [2002] 2AC 357, HL (E) at par. 103).

The reality is, as I found out by not enforcing declaration of membership, then in the event of bias, one is left to fall back on legal cases such as Porter v Magill, which are then ignored as the 'waffle monkeys' go to work and unless you can pay a Counsel, your rights simply don't count. As a woman too, in my experience you suffer appalling sexist behaviour by courts.

Wardle stated that in 2001 the Grand Master of Sussex Freemasonry wrote to him asking if he knew of any cases of wrongdoing. As Wardle stated, 'If the Grand Master of the society in Sussex doesn't know about his own membership, or flock, what price self-regulation?'

Whilst the sole religious component of freemasonry is a requirement at least outwardly of belief in a single God, I have questioned in The *Theatre Earth* books, whether that God is Pan, the God of Nature and whether Nature is the 'Grand '(Geometric) 'Architect'. Maria Antoinette who too late tried to find out who was behind the French Revolution, was fooled because she stated of the freemasons, "they have God on their lips", but which God? The God of Nature works to protect the 'selfish gene'.

128

I have recounted in the '*Theatre Earth*' books, the great ferocity of the French Revolution, where man gave way to beast and the reign of terror. Thomas Paine wrote the French *Declaration of Rights of Man*, a book that Maria Antoinette constantly referred to in her trial. Those rights however did not apparently refer to Maria and her family and she went to the guillotine with her husband Louis, on the basis of the position of their birth: whether or not your rights matter, depends upon policy of the government at the time.

Despite in 2009 Jack Straw then Justice Minister was aware of my case and had done nothing to fully investigate it or call upon me for the evidence and the tape recordings, or even organise a meeting over such a serious matter, he declared:

'...The review of the policy operating since 1998 has shown no evidence of impropriety or malpractice within the judiciary as a result of a judge being a freemason and in my judgement therefore, it would be disproportionate to continue the collection or retention of this information'.

Certainly the fact that the crucial tape recording involving the judge was then co-incidentally 'wiped' and evidence destroyed despite the six year rule of retaining evidence did nothing to provide confidence in the process of complaint or Article 13 and remedy. Thus by rebuffing casually such a serious complaint, without any due process of thorough investigation, it does nothing to convince one of transparency, impartiality or any workable system of complaint or redress. Straw stated in 2009 that the availability of a complaints procedure was enough support in: 'the proper performance of judicial functions'.

Gordon Prentice Labour MP in 2009, asked: 'How many judges have stood down as a result of a breach of standards of conduct in court in the last five years?' To which Jack Straw answered: 'Between 2004 and 2009, 95 magistrates, 14 Tribunal members and two judges were removed for misconduct. It is not known how many of these cases involved breaches of conduct within a courtroom. In addition, last year five tribunal members, 12 magistrates and two judges resigned during the course of conduct proceedings'. Again it is inconceivable and outrageous even, that Straw did not know whether these cases, which are numerous, involved conduct in a courtroom. He had a duty to the public to ensure that Article 6 (Fair Hearing) was not being violated in the UK. Even so, the sheer numbers of misconduct warrant a full public investigation. Court cases as I can attest to *affect lives*, often irreparably and it is not good enough to let this matter of misconduct or bias pass.

Mr Prentice replied: 'In this age of transparency is it not a disgrace that he has decided to allow judges no longer to declare whether they are freemasons, as we know that one in twenty judges is a freemason? Why on earth the cloak of secrecy?'

One woman took a case to the European Court claiming that judges' brief one another. I certainly had suspicions this might be the case and it would explain a great deal of my own experience.

Mr Alan Michael, The Minister of State for the Home Office stated in a Hansard Debate on 6th May 1998:

'It is worth underlining the fact, that it is the criminal justice system we are talking about, which is one of the bastions of a free society and of our democratic processes. It is extremely important that it should be free *from bias and for that to be seen to be the case*' (*author's emphasis*).

And just as pertinent to my case Mr Prentice observed:

'...The Government are concerned solely with dealing fairly and effectively with the legitimate expectation that the rights and freedoms of *all* are properly observed and safeguarded in any dealings with the various parts of the criminal justice system'(*Author's emphasis*).

The declaration rule followed a Report in 1997, by the Commons Home Affairs Committee that said: 'nothing so much undermines public confidence in public institutions as the knowledge that some public servants are members of a secret society, one of whose aims is mutual self-advancement'. However I would say that mutual *self-protection* also needs to be considered.

The Judiciary have assumed like the bankers, 'god-like' powers, where judges may not be questioned. There seems to be no accountability or transparency. As I write this update, I noted an article in *The Guardian* (*09.09.2010*) '*Vote trading leading to unqualified ICC judges*'. '*A 'toxic' system for appointing the world's most senior judges is fundamentally undermining the legitimacy of international courts, a new study claims'.* The article went on to say that: 'Unqualified judges, in some cases with no expertise on international law and in one case no legal qualifications, have been appointed to key positions because of highly politicised voting systems and a lack of transparency'. The ICC or International Criminal Court deals with cases of war crimes and crimes against humanity, and the international court of justice, the UN court, which deals with disputes between nation states' courts. It merely represents another case where standards no longer exist and where one could project a scenario of a defence lawyer appealing a case on the basis that the judge was not qualified. If law becomes ruled by politics, or 'mutual self-advancement' or self-protection, then one may as well turn off the lights and leave. How on earth can one have a judge with no legal qualifications sitting in serious cases?

So if you wish to take responsibility and trust the government's word that, "the big society" will replace, "big government" then you like I, will tiptoe naively into a mined battlefield where vested interests supported by government, will lay in wait. You will find that Human Rights do not apply to you, because you have sought to use those rights against excessive state power and secret groups who wish their activities to be hidden. But my case will send a terrible signal around the world, because countries like China, Russia, Burma and even Greece, will justify their own violations of free expression: it will be seen as a green light for undemocratic countries to justify and pursue their own abuses of power. Hypocrisy is one word I came to understand in my journey very well.

Britain has relatively few academics roaming the corridors of power compared with America. The political class has a profound distrust of intellectuals, a distrust that is often returned. In universities, academics are put under pressure to limit their research interests to those of 'policy relevance' and to undertake 'knowledge transfer' and consulting work, and to abandon the kind of critical perspectives that would result in asking awkward questions of those in power. The government's 'Experts' in academia are expected to toe the policy line and disregard any evidence to the contrary – the one-sided government policy argument.

As Professor Cohen remarked in his letter to *The Independent* newspaper (*2nd May 2009*):

131

'As a result, we have the worst of both worlds. We produce too many experts who are denied a hands-on role in policy making, and too few intellectuals who might produce and communicate radical new ideas'.

The problem is that 'radical new ideas' in science as the history of science shows even in my theory for cancer here, are likely to end in tears for the scientist - poor old Galileo, poor old Harvey, and poor old Gerson. New ideas rarely come out of the institutions, because of the politically correct constraints applied through the grant system and funding in addition to the peer review system. A new idea is only announced as an 'innovation' or 'breakthrough' provided that it does not conflict with government policy or vested interests and profits; and does not dethrone any prior orthodox theory set in stone. That is how it *actually* works.

In 2003 I forwarded my research on the geometric universe, with an explanation of Einstein's singularity (*volume 3 of Theatre Earth*) to Lord May then President of the Royal Society of Science. Apart from thanking me and commenting upon my "unique" research, that was it.

The case of cancer, started out like the debate on global warming, before it became a massive industry: after 1940 true research into cancer died out, when the big pharmaceutical giants took over. How it *actually* works, is that someone like myself, who cannot gain a grant from any of the funding bodies (I tried around 30) then has to fund their research themselves. Because they are not beholden to anyone, they are free to search for the truth no matter how incorrect politically the answer may be. L. Ron Hubbard (who founded the Church of Scientology) in his thesis: '*Dianetics: The Modern Science of Mental Health*', published in 1950 developed a workable method of erasing mind traumas or 'engrams' as he termed them. Now it would have been a whole lot easier for me had a regressive therapy for the mind, come from elsewhere – a politically correct orthodox source, but it didn't and so I am not about to change that fact for the sake of political correctness.

Dianetics is basically very similar to Freudian theory without the libido and dreams: except in the use of Dianetics dating from the 1950s people were running past lives. I suspect I could have passed a therapy of the mind (regressive counselling) off, without stating source using some of the psychological theories that have derived from Dianetics, I could also have omitted past lives; but my books have been aimed at *truth* and the correct and truthful facts of history. By bypassing what *actually* happened, I would be committing the same sin as those I condemn in *Theatre Earth* - using the Holy Grail cup of power and not the message. I used Dianetics as a regressive therapy, simply because it was reliable and worked and made sense in much the same way as the Gerson Therapy made sense. It's an individual choice as to what type of regressive method one uses and there are different methods, it just happens that I personally felt Dianetics was the most reliable method *for me*. I think it would be fair to say that many psychologists have adapted Hubbard's original work, without revealing source, just as many dietary therapies used Gerson's work without acknowledging source.

Personally my view (from my own experience) is that Scientology has its overts on money, with its casualties through that and it has its sycophantic pandering to 'celebrities,' whilst it tramples the 'little people' placing fame and money above *spiritual power*. Unfortunately the woman as source was erased from Hubbard's work, in much the same way as The Mary Magdalene was virtually erased from Christianity as a source. Hubbard never knew or did not say, where origination came from in the case of *what to audit* for his Operating Thetan Levels (OT) grades. The OT levels deal with whole Time Track History of the Planet. Hubbard famously left virtually no references as to his sources: but because Hubbard did not originate the 'OT rituals' giving access to past time track data, which he used on his 'Operating Thetan' courses – therefore knowing what to Audit, he did not understand the data at least not in scientific terms. He did not have a science degree either. The ridicule that Scientology has withstood lies in this basic fact, that Hubbard did not have the science background and did not originate methods to obtain whole track data – which he probably acquired in his connection with the secret OTO (Ordre Templis Orientis) group – an offshoot Masonic group connected to Aleister Crowley through Jack Parsons a rocket propulsion scientist, who was head of the OTO Lodge in Pasadena California.

Hubbard's interpretation of whole Time Track Earth Event data was not voiced with an understanding of science and the geometric universe. His was an *interior* viewpoint, whilst the message came from the *exterior*. Evidently however the Mary Magdalene's research including *'The Book of Nature,'* which was stolen, ended up in the Masonic groups and principally the secret group of the OTO (Order Templis Orientis) and Rose Croix, with which in the case of the former, Hubbard was associated with at one time. As I have covered this in the *Theatre Earth* books, there is no need to expand here.

Hubbard of course given the chance to introduce an Anglo Saxon religion of reincarnation, indelibly stamped his character all over it and no-one who has read the Russell Miller book '*The Bare Faced Messiah*' or Jon Atack's book '*A piece of Blue Sky',* could have thought otherwise. Hubbard however like so many men who set up religions could not keep to a line of truth and 'dusted the tracks' for fear his omnipotence might be questioned, and without any sense of repercussion for his followers he omitted his sources, particularly the OT rituals and the origins in the secret groups and constantly made false statements. This does not alter the fact that Scientology now holds very valuable if not extremely important knowledge or what is referred to by Scientologists as "the tech"(technology).

Hubbard stated in 1972, 'The actual barrier in the society is the failure to practise truth...Scientology is the road to truth and he who would follow it must take true steps'.

Those who inherit a religion as it forms a Church try to sanitise and alter the past and in the case of Christianity, the belief in reincarnation was erased along with the role of the Mary Magdalene. Her association with Jesus and the secret knowledge they shared, was not known or revealed to the disciples and for which reason the '*Lost Gospels*' never became part of *The Bible* even though they were of comparable antiquity and yet told a different story. The Church hierarchy then decides what was the truth based upon retaining vested interests. In removing the background to the Mary Magdalene and the Cycle of Eternal Return – reincarnation, the belief in the resurrection of Jesus, was retained and the idea that He had 'come back' or returned in his own lifetime a fete only possible as the 'Son of God'. Of course such a notion would have passed in antiquity before atomic physics would question that. Jesus' body could not have dematerialised without causing an atomic explosion to wipe out the entire Middle East. Lies or creative editing, have a horrible habit of catching up. The *Cycle* of Eternal Return was also edited out of *Revelations* (*the end*) and *Genesis* (*the beginning*) – again this has been covered in *Theatre Earth*. Revelations was written with knowledge of the cycles, but its connection to the beginning of a new cycle (*Genesis*) has been glossed over except for the curious referral to 'giants in those days'.

'The Nephilim were on the earth in those days, and also afterward, when the sons of God came in to the daughters of man and they bore children to them.

These were the mighty men who were of old, the men of renown.' (*Genesis 6:4 English Standard Version*) or in other translations:

Gen 6:4 'There were giants in the earth in those days; and also after that, when the sons of God came in unto the daughters of men, and they bear children to them, the same became mighty men which were of old, men of renown'.

'Then they said, "Come, let us build ourselves a city, with a tower that reaches to the heavens, so that we may make a name for ourselves and not be scattered over the face of the whole Earth".' (*Genesis 11:4*)

'We saw the Nephilim there (the descendants of Anak come from the Nephilim). We seemed like grasshoppers in our own eyes, and we looked the same to them.' (*Numbers 13:33 New International Version*).

As I proposed in the '*Theatre Earth*' series, it seems that a particular group and genetic line survived the demise of the last cycle, which must have been the wipe out of species 65 million years ago when giant dinosaurs roamed the earth. I pointed to either and/or a magnetic reversal or what seemed more likely an atomic war between two racially different types. The evidence was given in '*Theatre Earth*' and so I will not continue with it here.

Whatever the chronology here it seems a group evidently survived in this cycle a cataclysm that wiped out giant dinosaurs and presumably giant men in the last cycle, but not it seems a particular giant genetic line of important men or 'men of renown'. It was my proposal in '*Theatre Earth*' that this genetic line had survived through many cycles and had a *method* of doing so: which may account for the Noah's Ark story that occurs in many religions not just Christianity. Ultimately the 'men of renown' - the ultimate secret group on this planet, get a ticket out – the '*names*' as I have referred to in '*Theatre Earth*', which arise in secret documents. So this Earth will always at the start of any new cycle have those 'men of renown' to completely control the cycle from the beginning and throughout. It's rather like Groundhog Day as the same pattern is set in each cycle by a controlling group, who are completely cold, mechanical and compassionless. I referred in my books to the 'magnetically reversed case', with psychotic (anti-social) psychology.

Often in ancient texts these 'men of renown' are described with reptilian features and recorded as such in Palaeolithic cave drawings I suggested (*Plate*

135

11b p.572 Theatre Earth Vol.II). That genetic line catastrophically would have populated earth as it had done in previous cycles, creating an inferior species – effectively slaves, unless spiritual intervention had not succeeded in spiritualising the ape line, which gave spiritual man a chance to incarnate into a free genetic line. The evidence for that is produced n *'Theatre Earth'* and so there is no need to elaborate here. I consider those in this cycle who are obsessed with tinkering with genetics carry some memory of this and the 'giants' and are dramatizing the past.

I suspect that the document I carried and hid in the 14th Century retained secret information of the Cycles and survivors including the Nephilim or the old Adam (Y-chromosome) Eve (Lileth X-chromosome) line and the Anak. I also believe that the document or the secret version of Revelations I hid, connected the end to the beginning, which the orthodox version of *Revelations* in *The Bible* fails to do. The danger to the Catholic Church was that the document revealed 'paradise' as a cycle of construction and destruction on earth and man remains trapped by ultimately the 'men of renown' or the genetic line that is salvaged in every cycle. Mary Magdalene tried to reveal this cycle and was murdered for it.

The Catholics of course, have tried to sanitise the Inquisition and their role in stamping out those who tried to retain truer events, considered heretical. They also struggle today to contain and sanitise paedophilia in the church. As with other churches (and governments) the notion that truth should be advertised and not hidden is still seen as a PR disaster rather than an honest admission that man has advanced as a child advances to adulthood in order to assume responsibility. Humility lies in realising we make mistakes and making amends for them, but the ultimate secret group or genetic line is not capable of that humility. The psychotic has a computation that runs 'I must be right or I die' – if you managed to get a psychotic to agree he was wrong, you would probably kill him. Lies are merely a child's way of dealing with things he is not proud of, or which he feels he may be punished for. Notably Tony Blair claimed his biggest mistake was the introduction of the Freedom of Information law, presumably regretting not allowing governments and public organisations to act in secrecy. Neither he nor George Bush could accept they were wrong.

In the case of Scientology it has become a constant case of trying to sanitise 'Ron' (Ron Hubbard). Robert Kaufman who wrote *'Inside Scientology'* said

Kenneth Urquhart who was a senior executive in the Church saw a change in Hubbard after he researched and wrote OT3 (Operating Thetan Level 3) during his time with the Sea Org (Organisation). Hubbard became a transformed man who could suddenly and often would, scream with rage. Whether that change came about because he was using the rituals or channelling and/or using drugs to access whole Time Track data, on Earth, so he knew what to audit, is debatable but witness accounts do mention that Hubbard did use drugs and descriptive accounts during his time in the Sea Org (related in '*Theatre Earth*') do suggest to me that he was channelling information from the Akashic Record and using automatic writing. This practise of accessing past Time Track data has however been going on in the name of religion for thousands of years and in fact the Shaman used such practises to access the past event data of earth. I am not sure why people get so worked up about it – the idea of magick (with a k) should have been placed into the modern context of physics and energy fields and the electromagnetic grid, which I discussed in '*Theatre Earth*'. People however always fear what they don't understand and vested interests can always be relied upon to whip up adverse opinion, by playing their tune to the ignorant and deceived and of course they will inevitably go down with the ship. Ooh, don't look over there its dangerous, its occult, its witch-craft; it's a cult, its...Sly old magnetically reversed case that does not want you to find out what *actually* is going on.

On a personal level Hubbard's research never phased me, as I was quite capable of analysing it in terms of science and I always had the feeling I had seen it all before on the track of time. Oddly enough as I show in the '*Theatre Earth*' series Hubbard's research stands up to scientific scrutiny, although I have explained it in my terms of science rather than going with Hubbard's interpretations of the data. The great problem then with Hubbard's work, was his interpretation of data and his lack of science. In '*What to Audit*' Hubbard lists a series of 'incarnations' or a 'time-track' history in the evolution of man: the evolution, or 'genetic line', of the human body. Again I don't think that Hubbard made it clear enough to his followers that he was talking about the evolution of a *genetic lines* and *not spiritual memory* as such.

According to Hubbard the 'time-track' runs back to a point where the individual seemed to be 'an atom complete with electronic rings'. I think Hubbard should have emphasised here that this was a genetic line and *not a spiritual line*, which has created confusion. This would throw the reality of those with no science background. It is shocking how little science the average individual knows. This 'revelation' by Hubbard would then invite ridicule. However even on the very basic G.C.S.E course in science in the UK it states: 'sooner or later a star (our sun) runs out of small nuclei. None of them last forever. Stars like people, frogs and trees, have life cycles. The mass of a star determines how long it lives and how it dies'. Further, 'the most common element in the Universe is hydrogen. In stars, fusion continues to make bigger and bigger elements. When fusion stops, big stars explode as supernovae. Their debris, containing all the 92 elements (atoms) is scattered through space. When our Solar System formed, it gathered debris from dead stars. Except for Hydrogen and Helium, the chemical elements that make up everything on earth (including our bodies) come from stars; we are made of stardust (elements and atoms)'. So Hubbard writing in 1952 was really encountering the intelligent universe and the beginnings of our **bodies** from atoms and elements of a previous solar system - stardust. The Universe simply *re-cycles* – A Cycle of Eternal Return. Of course trapped into this cycle of *matter* is the spirit of man who then re-incarnates in a Cycle of Eternal Return – until he disentangles himself from his karma relating to matter and the 'selfish gene'. Everything in this universe is about cycles of construction and destruction.

There is a start, change and completion of any cycle – even the cycle of a cell or planet and star or perhaps even the 'great cycle' of the universe, which then on completion of the geometric pattern, returns to start and as I have proposed the simplest geometric origination or 'singularity' which is the 3-D tetrahedron of Hydrogen, which becomes space time, only when an implant is attached, which I have discussed in prior works as Hubbard's 'Incident One'. *Revelations* in *The Bible* simply failed to convey this cycle and the fact that the end (*Revelations*) returns to the beginning (*Genesis*) and of course with the controlling genetic line of 'men of renown'. With control exerted through a specific genetic line or 'men of renown' in each cycle there is *no change*. As I have proposed in *'Theatre Earth'*, the cycle of hopelessness simply repeats itself, a sort of Groundhog Day. Man will never achieve a cycle of hope unless he confronts this fact. Of course it now seems so beyond what anyone can grasp or wishes to confront and so much has been hidden that many will simply not make it out, because of karmic entanglement.

Sometimes I like to pull out the question papers for G.C.S.E science in physics and chemistry dating from the 60's - 70's in the UK, just to remind myself how dumbed down a science education has become. Some of those questions even A-level students today would be incapable of answering.

138

Returning to the *Lost Gospels*, which were never incorporated into *The Bible*: In the *Gospel of The Mary Magdalene*, Jesus and Mary appear to discuss this cycle (Pages 1 to 6 of the manuscript, containing chapters 1 – 3, are lost). The extant text infuriatingly only starts on page 7 unfortunately! Significantly over half of the Gospel of Mary is lost whilst the other Gospels found in the same ancient texts are complete. I hardly think this is coincidental and whoever removed those pages knew their importance. Mary Magdalene described as a 'prostitute' in translations, was likely to have been a priestess or female Pope (in Tarot). Certainly she would not, if she was just a mere 'prostitute' have been discussing with the 'Son of God' the fate of matter.

'...Will matter then be destroyed or not?
22) The Saviour said, All nature, all formations, all creatures exist in and with one another, and they will be resolved again into their own roots.
23) For the nature of matter is resolved into the roots of its own nature alone'. (*Chapter 4*)

This appears to state the now known fact that the cycle ends with saving only of the "roots" of matter i.e. the 92 elements.

It is clear that Mary and Jesus did share a secret communication line and knowledge, which was not imparted to the other disciples.

'5) Peter said to Mary, Sister we know that the Saviour loved you more than the rest of woman.
6) Tell us the words of the Saviour, which you remember which you know, but we do not, nor have we heard them.
7) Mary answered and said, what is hidden from you I will proclaim to you'. (*Chapter 5*)

It is also clear that the male disciples were quite jealous of the secret communication line between Jesus and Mary Magdalene:

'(4) He (Peter) questioned them about the Saviour: Did He really speak privately with a woman and not openly to us? Are we to turn about and all listen to her? Did He prefer her to us?' (*Chapter 9*)

Given my own experience of visions it is interesting that Mary questioned Jesus on this, asking whether it was the soul (genetic line) or Spirit, which sees the visions.

'(10) I said to Him, Lord, how does he who sees the vision see it, through the soul or through the Spirit?
(11) The Saviour answered and said, He does not see through the soul or through the spirit, but the mind that is between the two that is what sees the vision and it is [...]' (*Chapter 5*)
(*And again infuriatingly pages 11-14 are missing from the manuscript*).

This seems to imply the mind makes sense of the 'visions' which I agree with and have used as explanation of how Hubbard used his mind and experience to make sense of data from the Akashic Record or whole Earth Track history, which he interpreted in terms of what some saw as a science fiction epic. In '*Theatre Earth*' however I give a more scientific explanation, in terms of the geometric universe using my scientifically trained mind. The point here is obviously that the Mary Magdalene was speaking of 'visions' and those 'visions' I maintain came from usage of the secret OT rituals, which Hubbard probably eventually sequestered through the secret group of the OTO. Clearly here the secret knowledge that Jesus and Mary shared, which was not made available to the other disciples, was the knowledge of the history of earth, the cycles and that knowledge or the 'visions' were obtained through the Mary Magdalene and written down in Her 'Book of Nature', sequestered upon her murder in France, just north of Marseilles along with a child who would provide a bloodline – The Merovingian's and the Rose Line.

In the *Gospel of Thomas* Jesus once again appears to refer to the cycle:

'(18) The disciples said to Jesus, "Tell us how our end will be."
Jesus said, "Have you discovered then, the beginning that you look for the end? For where the beginning is, there will the end be. Blessed is he who will take his place in the beginning; he will know the end and will not experience death.'

Again this appears to refer as I suggested in '*Theatre Earth*', to a genetic group who survived the cataclysms on Earth and the end cycles of *Revelations*, to appear presumably from a 'Noah's Ark' at the beginning in *Genesis*, where a genetic line of 'giants' or 'Gods' appeared to repopulate the earth as Nephilim in order to control the genetic line, where the 'selfish gene' or X and Y chromosomes protect themselves. Hubbard was to claim that the arch controller was X̲enu but I gave the X̲-chromosome (female) which contains a full record of the genetic past and therefore the Akashic past; and L. Kin mentioned another line or Yatrus, which I gave as the Y-chromosome (which does not contain a full genetic record, but is composed mainly of so-called 'junk DNA'). Hubbard wrote science fiction and his interpretation of this complex data was in terms of *his experience* as a writer. Had he qualified in science his interpretation would have been different. The real vitriol against women by the priesthood is because women have full access to the Akashic record and are used in secret rituals for such.

Again in the *Gospel of Thomas*:

'(20) The disciples said to Jesus, "Tell us what the kingdom of heaven is like." He said to them, "It is like a mustard seed. It is the smallest of all seeds. But when it falls on tilled soil, it produces a great plant and becomes a shelter for birds of the sky.'

The opening and closing flower, the sprouting of the seed and the manifestation of a geometric grand design from the dot in the circle ('seed') are archetypes of ancient wisdom discussed in '*Theatre Earth*' and denote cycles of the Grand Design. The reference to 'seed' by Jesus is a sure indication He was referring to the cycles of Earth and these ancient archetypes.

However I can't think being reduced to stardust in the final cycle on Earth in this solar system, is exactly "blessed": even if a few as I have suggested in '*Theatre Earth*' survived the intermediate geological cycles here on earth, perhaps accounting for the 'giants' in *Genesis* of this cycle; there is no probability they will survive the end cycle of this solar system, after being buttered all over the universe as star dust and atoms.

And given ancient Indian texts and how at least one man-induced cycle ended in what appeared to be atomic war between two racial types, which could equally be Christians and Muslims in this cycle or even East (China) versus West, then another tract from *The Gospel of Thomas* is informative:

141

'(16) Jesus said, "Men think, perhaps, that it is peace which I have come to cast upon the world. They do not know that it is dissension, which I have come to cast upon the earth: fire, sword, and war. For there will be five in a house: three will be against two, and two against three, the father against the son, and the son against the father. And they will stand solitary".'

Whether Jesus is referring to karma in this tract from *The Gospel of Thomas* is unclear:

'(59) Jesus said, "Take heed of the living one while you are alive, lest you die and seek to see him and be unable to do so".'

This principle is well known in the East that one must seek the person one has harmed in the current life and make amends; otherwise one may seek him or her for all eternity and never find them in order to make amends.

Hubbard in his Time Track data described genetic evolution through 'seaweed' and 'jellyfish' and would describe the 'clam' incident. Jon Atack pointed out: 'The description of the 'clam' makes particularly fine reading. Hubbard was quite right when he warned that the reader might think that he the author had "slipped a cable or two in his wits'. Hubbard however had warned his followers of the dangers inherent in any discussion of the clam. Atack evidently did not possess a science background. The data never fazed me as I recognised it must have a deeper explanation in science. The incidents merely relate the evolution of a *body or genetic line* and I see no strangeness in that unless you have no science background; however that never stops the ignorant from voicing their 'scientific' opinions. Why shouldn't a genetic line in its evolution possess a sentience – how do they think a brain and cephalisation evolved!

There seems little point in referring to the Fatima miracle on 13th October 1917- an event watched by some 70,000 witnesses. During the event the sun appeared to   career towards the earth in a zigzag pattern, which frightened witnesses thought signified the end of the world. It was I maintained in my own research, a warning that one day the sun will run out of fuel, become a red giant and swallow the earth and if reincarnation is true, then it will take anyone on the planet at the time with it and all intelligence will end up in the atoms. Hubbard at one point described, 'a hole ahead of the atom', which can be explained by science perhaps as a black hole. However man is not interested in the fate of the planet or this solar system, or the fact that this universe recycles matter, because he does not think he will be here to witness the end, but has been led to believe he will end up in 'paradise'. I certainly have no intention of staying here, ending up supplying *my experience* to an intelligent universe or having that *experience which is my spiritual identity* buttered all over the universe as 'star dust'.

Whilst Hubbard designated Xenu as the arch controller and that threw the reality of many, in *'Theatre Earth'* I have given Xenu as the X-chromosome, the female chromosome, which carries a full history of evolution unlike the male Y chromosome, which carries a lot of so-called 'junk' DNA (seriously guys!). Women are often used in rituals like the psycho sexual ones described by Aleister Crowely and Jack Parsons because they carry the X chromosome and can access full earth event history. Women are more likely to be clairvoyant and were in antiquity oracles and temple priestesses (translated as prostitutes) for this purpose. L. Kin (a pseudonym) in his book *'The Pied Pipers of Heaven: who calls the tune?'* also identified a group, which I identified as the 13th tribe (male chromosome) and Hubbard made many cryptic comments eluding to this and the number 13, which must designate as I state in *'Theatre Earth'*, Hubbard's secret background. It is a complex story and it was a miracle that I could sort any of it out and I suspect that I could not have done so, if I had not followed the story in many lives.

'What to Audit' first published in 1952 claimed to be a: 'cold-blooded and factual account of your last sixty trillion years.' It is still in print minus one chapter under the title *'A History of Man.'* Jon Atack stated that the research was: 'A slim pretence at scientific method (and) is blended with a strange amalgam of psychotherapy, mysticism and pure science fiction; mainly the latter. What to Audit is among the most bizarre of Hubbard's work, and deserves the cult status some dreadful science fiction movies have achieved'. Again Atack was not a scientist and if he had studied science particularly physics, he might find a lot of it *is* like science fiction. Most people can barely get their heads around dinosaurs roaming the Earth, let alone the archaeological find of giant 'man' footprints in the Paluxy riverbed in Arizona, which show that giant 'men' roamed the earth *with* the dinosaurs. Of course orthodox evolutionary theory dismisses such evidence and gives no credence to the *Genesis* account of 'giants in those days'. Certainly no orthodox scientist would consider the theory I proposed in *'Theatre Earth'*, that those 'giants' survived a magnetic reversal that killed off the dinosaurs, or

the fact that their appearance is engraved in Palaeolithic caves (*Plate 11b p.572 Theatre Earth Vol. II*).

Hubbard famously wrote science fiction and thus *his interpretation* of data followed that aspect of his character and experience. I have tried to take Hubbard's data and that of L. Kin in his book '*The Pied Pipers of Heaven – Who Calls the Tune?*'(*1994*) as a basis for my own scientific research into the Time Track given in '*Theatre Earth*' volumes, but particularly the science in *Volume III*. Despite the fact that I was able to place Hubbard's work in the context of science, I am afraid once a religion is set in stone adherents cannot look anymore at the obvious or the more human traits of the founders.

Hubbard's former publicist, John Campbell put it very succinctly: 'In a healthy and growing science, there are many men who are recognised as being competent in the field and no one dominates the work...to the extent Dianetics is dependent on one man it is a cult. To the extent it is built on many minds and many workers, it is a science'. There is the pity of it, scientists should have evaluated Dianetics, but what has happened is that psychologists have merely adapted Hubbard's theory of how the mind works and erased Hubbard from the picture so they don't experience the witch-hunt I have. One can see the path of the Grail again, the power taken and the message and history omitted.

The Church of Scientology made their views quite clear to me when I suggested that they provide funds for a cancer centre using Dianetics in conjunction with the Gerson Therapy. I was told to: "Help the more able first". They do not take people who are ill, or those under psychiatric supervision, or those taking drugs (apart from the Narcanon project in the latter). Although this seemed callous to me at the time, on reflection given my own experience and the suppression I have experienced, then evidently the Scientologists don't want that suppression on their lines. They have always claimed that since they offer an alternative therapy of the mind avoiding psychotropic drugs that their main attacks have come through big Pharma and the psychiatrists. That is obviously a part of the attacks upon them, given that alternative cancer therapists went through the same mill, but I think that the Masonic connections of Hubbard and the fact he ran off with the OTO rituals and made publicly available, knowledge that was once only viewed in the secret groups, particularly freemasonry, may be more relevant: even so as I have pointed out in the history of alternative approaches to cancer, big Pharma and the orthodoxy only strike when an approach shows success. If Dianetics didn't work, there would be no need to attack it: when you see that much force thrown, you know that there must be a truth there.

Hubbard as far as I can see brought a lot of the attacks against the Church on himself by his own actions. If King Kong had used the elevator, instead of drawing attention to himself by thundering up the outside of the Empire State, he would probably have made it and found the woman. When John Mc Master and other senior Scientologists left the Church in the late 60s and others in the 80s including Captain Bill Robertson, to set up an independent organisation, they all felt the technology was of tremendous value, but questioned the motives of those managing the Church following Hubbard's death.

On a personal level, it never really worried me that Hubbard made money from the Church. As far as I could see he made no more than any chief executive of a company and certainly nowhere near bankers' bonuses. It seems that what defectors felt was unforgivable, was that Hubbard had lied to them, on his own personal history and motives. This did not detract from the knowledge, which is valuable. There lies the pity, in so far as although Hubbard wanted the knowledge widely disseminated, it seems his own actions would always prevent that. However once you release a method of running past lives, I should imagine it was always going to meet the resistance of those who inherited this earth in each cycle – the 'giants' and presumably the DNA, which is now probably inter-dispersed and accounts for Hubbard's psychological profile of the "Anti-Social Personality". This personality represents a small minority of men and women but causes the majority of upset and wars on this planet either directly or through contact with others.

In my own case, I was quite unaware of the background to the Church and Hubbard, when I took a look at its technology. After the Wardship proceedings taken out by my husband in 1989 to secure custody of the boys, the Church told me that all other similar cases of custody had failed, where Scientology was an issue. I was quite literally dropped like a 'hot potato' and the hypocrisy at least for me started to show up. If the Church of Scientology had never won a custody case this was not my intention, since it was certainly outrageous to me than anyone should be able to dictate what books one may or may not read or knowledge one may or may not look at, reminiscent of some Kafkaesque state. I won the case and it became a precedent in law, used I believe by the Jehovah's witnesses. Today of course there is the Human

Rights Act, which passed into law in 1998, but as I found out if you mention Scientology you will have that used against you and lose your case no matter what evidence you have got. It's tough for pioneers, as Jones would say. The judiciary is relentlessly opposed to Scientology and thus your case is open to bias before you present your evidence and that is before you mention freemasonry. Certainly in my own experience British Courts still violate Articles 6, 8, 9 and 10 in this respect. No doubt however if you are John Travolta or Tom Cruise with an expensive barrister, courts would watch their Articles – To misquote Snoopy sitting in cattle class with his polystyrene cup: "you have to pay for human rights".

In 1992 following terrible and traumatic events at the children's school – Michael Hall a Rudolf Steiner School I wrote to my then MP for assistance, which was refused. The MP Geoffrey Johnson Smith for East Grinstead never mentioned in his curt refusal that in 1970 he was involved in a libel case with the Church of Scientology. The events at my children's school were a very serious matter and the police protection unit were involved and yet as a constituent I was merely rebuffed by my MP, because he believed I was a Scientologist. In 1992 The Human Rights Act was not in place, but the position has not changed even after the Human Rights Act was passed in 1998.

Some years later I watched with disdain as Johnson Smith gave a Sports Day speech at my children's international school of Buckswood Grange, where he hypocritically praised the peaceful association of various nationalities and religions at the school. Hypocrisy was never far from my story.

Interestingly a Justice Browne adjudicated in the Geoffrey Johnson Smith case, which went against Scientology and a judge of that name was to adjudicate in my matrimonial proceedings where the 'Scientology card' was disgracefully and cunningly played by barrister Nicholas Mostyn, which was disastrous to the outcome: and where judge simply sat on, whilst the court violated rulings of the Law Lords and the Declaration of Human Rights of which Britain was a signatory at the time. I can't imagine John Travolta or Tom Cruise having to witness Nicholas Mostyn snorting mucous into his handkerchief a foot from their face, whilst ranting and calling them a "religious Scientology zealot," but then equality before law is a myth and certainly Mostyn could remember the law and his manners, in high profile cases for well-heeled and famous clients. Today of course there is Article 14, but courts in my experience still regularly violate this Article:

'The enjoyment of the rights and freedoms set forth in this convention shall be secured without discrimination on any ground such as sex, race, colour, language, religion, political or other opinion, national or social origin, association with a national minority, property, birth or other status'.

In the Geoffrey Johnson Smith trial the retired Governor of Western Nigeria, said of his involvement in Scientology. "I thought at first there might be something in it. I ended up convinced there was everything in it". The most startling witness was the former parliamentary private secretary to the Health Minister Kenneth Robinson – William Hamling who was the Member of Parliament for Woolwich West. He had decided to find out about Scientology for himself. I took much the same view and checked it out. He used the most direct method by going to Saint Hill, Scientology's U.K Headquarters and taking the communication course. In the witness box Hamling called the course "first rate". I thought so too when I did it. He said the Scientologists he had met were normal, decent, intelligent people and after the trial he continued with them. I thought so too, but then after an incident, which I considered the utmost betrayal I left abruptly. No doubt Mr Hamling, would not have had his employment threatened and been subjected to inquisitional courts.

The first time I came across Scientology, I knew I had seen it before on the track of time, it was just a case of remembering where and when. The Mary Magdalene had wanted to introduce the religion of a Cycle of Eternal Return, and the basis of the (Greek) Early Minoan Cycle of Eternal Return: Jesus however had other views and betrayed her. According to the *Lost Gospels* he "fooled them". That is presumably the reason the Church has so assiduously covered her story up and labelled her a "prostitute" – no doubt based upon use of her '*Book of Nature*' which included the rituals (she developed). Interestingly the secret rituals of the OTO are no longer available anywhere – unless of course the Vatican has a copy.

Unfortunately followers rarely question the true origins of their religions or the deeper meanings of the teachings. Christianity and I came adrift when they could provide no answer as to why if the body of Jesus had dematerialised in the resurrection, it did not cause an explosion to wipe out the entire Middle East: a pint size mug of material that dematerialised wiped out Hiroshima.

Even Jesus in the Gospel of The Mary Magdalene seems to accept that matter returns to its "roots" by which he may have meant atoms. The Archbishop of Canterbury in the UK - Dr George Carey in August of 1999, voiced his own doubts by saying: "we cannot know" that Jesus was raised from the dead. The Church at around the 6th Century AD wiped out the early Christian belief in reincarnation and led people to believe the resurrection was in Jesus' own lifetime. Dr Carey was nearly right however to point out that Jesus was an anti-Establishment rebel saying that organised religion and Jesus "do not mix happily". Only partially right because Jesus *was* an establishment figure at least in the end when it seems he sold out to the Egyptians (*The Lost Gospels*) and "fooled them", it was the Mary Magdalene who was not. The belief and message of a Cycle of Eternal Return, or reincarnation and knowledge of the cycles that Mary Magdalene hoped to bring back as a healing and ultimately salvation message to the people, practised by the Early Minoans, was betrayed as Jesus chose the status of power as a Sun King – the truer version at least in part portrayed in the *Lost Gospels* not included in The Bible, despite the fact they are of comparable antiquity to biblical gospels. The central mystery of the absence of Jesus body in the tomb at Golgotha was covered in *Theatre Earth* and so there is no need to repeat it here.

Religion always had a problem with science – and there lies the entrapment 'clause' in religions. It seems a sensible idea to leave this planet, given reincarnation and the fact that the sun is an ageing star, which will eventually expand to form a red giant and swallow the earth. Personally I see no future as a spirit, being re-cycled as stardust or being sucked into a black hole to be spewed out in another solar system, so that an intelligent universe of matter can evolve: the personality, the *essence* of who you are and your time track history of *experience*, which really defines '*you*' as a spirit, would not survive such an event. I often think what a terrible life on reincarnation suicide bombers and their victims must have, having fragmented themselves and the effects of that upon spiritual memory.

I look to the Jesuits and Catholic Church and see unforgivable paedophilia, so I guess it is a case of you 'pay your money you take your pick.' Personally I have never liked groups, because they have a habit of self- organising as a power pyramid, with a central all controlling apex, which will not tolerate questioning or new data, which results in stuck viewpoints and what is worse causes a loss of viewpoint and awareness. There is also a presumption that Messiah's and angels come in male form only - I can't think of one religion set up by a woman, discounting the true basis of Christianity, even though that story was well hidden by the Church. Further man does not consider that religions have throughout the ages been concerned to adjust their doctrines to ensure that the true spiritual purpose of man here on earth is veiled.

Polly Toynbee (*The Gruardian14.09.2010*) accurately observed: 'Women's bodies are the common battleground, symbols of all religions' authority and identity. Cover them up with veil or burka, keep them from the altar, shave their heads, give them ritual baths, church them, make them walk a step behind, subject them to men's authority, keep priests celibately free of women, unclean and unworthy.' She could have included forced marriage, ritual circumcision and marital violence, bullying and stoning: the Jews also "thank God" in their prayers that "thou have not made me a woman", as Tonybee observed: 'Wherever male cultural leaders hold absolute and un-scrutinised power, women and children will be abused'. That I might add even from my own experience includes courts of law and it is curious how in the UK under austerity measures of the conservative government, that it has been discovered women and children will bear the brunt of cuts.

To quote *The Gospel of Thomas*:

'(114) Simon Peter said to him, "Let Mary leave us, for women are not worthy of life." Jesus said, "I myself shall lead her in order to make her male, so that she too may become a living spirit resembling you males. For every woman who will make herself male will enter the kingdom of heaven".'

I suspected that the Y-chromosome genetic line which is saved, or the 'men of renown' is a *male* genetic line *and secret group*, which in past cycles was forced to mate with the genetically engineered old Lileth line ("haunch-ass"-"rib of Adam") covered more fully in 'Theatre Earth'. That was the case up to Spiritual intervention, when a new aesthetic non-engineered line appeared.

It also seems that in some countries there is no longer any right to decide how a woman wishes to give birth to her child. Dr Agnes Gereb a highly experienced gynaecologist, midwife and internationally recognised home birth expert, successfully delivering 3,500 babies at home faces a five-year prison sentence. As *The Guardian* reported (*23.10.2010*), this woman was *handcuffed and shackled* in leg chains in a court in Europe (Hungary) on 12th October 2010. When one gets to the bottom of this story one finds once again, choice

149

restricted by a medical male hierarchy of lucrative medicine and a monopoly. 'The state's campaign against home births has lasted nearly 20 years and is rooted in the determination of a clique of obstetricians to maintain their own power and earning potential from hospital births. Obstetrics is one of the most lucrative branches of Hungary's supposedly free healthcare system.... in which parents expect to pay up to a month's salary to the doctor, who is legally obliged to be present at each birth'. Apparently there is no choice where inductions and episiotomies are standard, despite the trauma they cause.

'When in The Gospel according to the Egyptians, Shelom asked the Lord: "How long shall death prevail?" He answered: "So long as you women bear children..." And when she asked again: "I have done well then in not bearing children?" He answered: "Eat every plant but that which is bitter..." And when she inquired at what time the things concerning which she had questioned Him should be known, He answered: "When you women have trampled on the garment of shame and when the two become one, and when the male with the female is neither male nor female." And the Saviour said in the same Gospel: "I have come to destroy the works of the Female".' (*Clement of Alexandria – Stromata, iii*).

Personally it never surprised me to discover Hubbard's history, having long experience of the secret groups inclusive of past lives. Jesus was accused of deceit and lies in a number of alternative texts omitted from *The Bible* (e.g. *The Apocryphon of John*) and interestingly like Hubbard His background up until he started his mission was obscured, as were his sources, which Jesus claimed originality on, as did Hubbard. Both Jesus (in biblical texts) and Hubbard have been accused of madness and there are many more comparisons. Perhaps their unknown similarity is that they both utilised the research of the Mary Magdalene (her "visions") which she recorded as rituals in the 'Book of Nature' and which it appears Hubbard used to develop his OT (Operating Thetan) levels having sequestered the secret rituals of the OTO, which he then claimed originality on. Hubbard however did not claim divinity, but he did claim membership of an elite council way back on the track of time, which may indicate an elite. Buddha never claimed to be God. Moses never claimed to be Jehovah. Mohammed never claimed to be Allah. Yet Jesus Christ claimed to be the true and living God. Buddha simply said, "I am a teacher in search of the truth." Jesus said, "I am the Truth." Confucius said, "I never claimed to be holy." Jesus said, "Who convicts me of sin?" Mohammed said, "Unless God throws his cloak of mercy over me, I have no hope".

I don't see the need to attack any religion, provided they don't try and force their edited teachings on me. In my experience any knowledge worth having was always withheld in the secret groups and in the past it was a matter of finding out what they had got and getting out in one piece. Scientology contains valuable knowledge and I don't see the point of attacking knowledge, despite my experience with them means that I could not recommend them. My experience was about par for the course and I certainly expected the blade in the back: after all, Hubbard himself stated at low tones help is seen as betrayal. Jon Atack after finding out the facts for his book *A Piece of Blue Sky* said: 'My idea of Hubbard as a compassionate philosopher Scientist, a man of great honesty and integrity, was shaken to the core'. For myself there was no big core shaking, I had seen it all before as a past life witness of the events of Golgotha. However one should remember if you get involved in big games, one can't whinge when it's not all apple pie and picket fence. It's my view that one learns from big games and so I am not about to stop anyone playing them. If you come a cropper, then better luck next time around, but at least you have learnt something!

15 Closed Minds

The Royal Society of Science under the presidency of Lord May had a closed viewpoint on global warming, just as there is a closed viewpoint on cancer. Lord May was once quoted as saying: 'The debate on climate change is over'. The society now appears to have conceded that it needs to correct previous statements by stating: 'Any public perception that the science is somehow fully settled is wholly incorrect – there is always room for new observations, theories, and measurements'. Sir Alan Rudge, a Society Fellow and former member of the Government's Scientific Advisory Committee, is one of the leaders of the rebellion who gathered signatures on a petition sent to Lord Rees, the society president. He told *The Times* (*May 29th 2010*) that the society had adopted an: 'unnecessarily alarmist position' on climate change. Sir Alan, an electrical engineer, is a member of the advisory council of the climate sceptic think-tank, the Global Warming Policy Foundation. He said: 'I think the Royal Society should be more neutral and welcome credible contributions from both sceptics and alarmists alike. There is a lot of science to be done before we can be certain about climate change and before we impose upon ourselves the huge economic burden of cutting emissions'.

Nobody, least of all government seems to notice or feel concerned that the indisputable idea of *man- made* global warming was written into the national school curriculum for science years ago (!) and is presented as a 'commandment of faith' in all examining boards at G.C.S.E. level. Ah yes brain washing starts early 'catch them before they can think' and preferably stop them thinking thereafter. This bias then breeds a new generation of witless sheep, who cannot evaluate scientific evidence, or set out a scientific two-sided argument; but they can protest. Generally however lack of scientific knowledge does not prevent everyone voicing his or her 'informed' opinion.

Interestingly Sir Alan remarked on his stance: 'One of the reasons people like myself are willing to put our heads above the parapet is that our careers are not at risk from being labelled a denier or flat-Earther because we say the science is not settled. The bullying of people into silence has unfortunately been effective'.

As I was to find out, when my career was threatened and I was dragged through legal proceedings by the witless politically correct sheep of *Animal Farm*; bullying, victimisation discrimination, lies, and violation of Rights are all par for the course if you put your head above the parapet. Scientists like the Army hierarchy generally don't speak out until their pensions are in the pot and no one can affect their careers. Ah yes governments and vested interests can rely on the fact that responsibility and courage are a rarity in the citizen whose livelihood is still open to attack. David Kelley the government scientist in the Iraq war case and the "forty five minutes" claim was an example of scientific courage and integrity and he paid dearly for that, with every possibility that he may have been murdered. The scientific community should have risen up in vociferous numbers, but quietly sat and dismissed it until five doctors and lawyers took up the case. Whistle blowing is actually a dangerous activity, for scientists.

A Drugs industry insider turned whistle-blower, who claimed to have proof that the multinational companies are 'bribing' thousands of doctors to prescribe their products narrowly escaped an apparent attempt on his life. Alfredo Pequito, a former employee of the German pharmaceuticals giant Bayer, needed 70 stitches after being stabbed by a man who scaled the back wall of the house in Lisbon in September 2000 where he was under armed police guard [8]. The attack came just days after Pequito told a newspaper in Portugal, where he worked for the German firm, that he had the names of 2,500 Portuguese doctors who had been induced with gifts to prescribe Bayer drugs. The Portuguese authorities were investigating 300 cases of suspected corruption. Investigators believed that as many as 17 major drugs companies could have been involved. The knife attack occurred just hours before Pequito was due to testify against his former employers. In another incident a car was alleged to have tried to run Pequito's wife off the road. Critics said that corruption of doctors by the pharmaceutical industry was becoming increasingly widespread but companies were taking greater care to cover their tracks. 'Written documentation (of abuses) is now hard to come by. It is done verbally now, and there is no written proof,' Alvaro Rana, a leading trade unionist and himself a former drugs rep, told *O Publico* newspaper.

Just as one comes to expect courts to avoid the evidence, so science operates. Lord Rees admitted that there were differing views among Fellows at the Royal Society over global warming but said the new guide would be: 'based on expert views backed up by sound scientific evidence'. I can assure you

153

evidence is not what vested interests or government 'experts' require and nowhere is this truer than in the case of cancer.

The case of Iraq was a clear example of lack of scientific evidence on WMD. How many members of George Bush's circle objected to the daily briefings about the progress of the Iraq war that Mr Rumsfeld gave to President George W. Bush, which contained quotes from the Bible? How many, if not the President himself or our very own 'Angel of Death' Tony Blair, objected to an F-14 Tomcat fighter jet roaring off from the deck of an aircraft carrier, with the words of Psalm 139-9-10 on the side? Who objected to a photo of Saddam Hussein with the annotated quotation by Rumsfeld taken from the First Epistle of Peter: 'It is God's will that by doing good you should silence the ignorant talk of foolish men'. The irony if not insanity seems to have by-passed him. It seems that a collective madness often overtakes leaders and the Iraq war was one example. Usually, when you nail these things down, you will find just one Anti-Social Personality hovering in the background smiling, as no one suspects *him* of the chaos.

One would like to think that sane men run the world, but evidence shows otherwise and history repeats itself. The problem now is that younger politicians are given high office and they are subject to testosterone, which appears to have a destabilising effect on sanity. It is frightening that the religious theme for the briefings prepared for the President and his war cabinet was the brainchild of Major General Glen Shaffer, a committed Christian and director for intelligence serving Mr Rumsfeld and the Joint Chiefs of Staff. This side of the 'pond' the British had their own lunatics to deal with, who avoided talking about oil supplies to Europe and pipelines or deposits in Iraq, whilst the government or Tony Blair lied to the people. The decision had been made to go to war it only remained for Tony Blair to present a case for why the British had to take part, and Saddam's weapons of mass destruction appeared the most persuasive. From then on any evidence no matter the source was leapt upon and evidence that did not suit the case for a policy of war was ignored.

So 'evidence' that Saddam had bought uranium from Africa, was based upon some obscure notice on the Internet. Then there was 'evidence' that came from an Iraqi taxi driver who claimed he overheard ministers discussing their weapons (third party gossip). This was all cobbled together with a plagiarised PhD thesis from the Internet. One would have thought that Hans Blix the

United Nations weapons inspector's evidence which stated that he'd found no conclusive evidence of weapons might have been faintly relevant as was David Kelley's intervention: but of course 'The Angel of Death' preferred to take counsel from the 'expert' source of Alastair Campbell and others. And so it came to pass in those days that 'The Angel of Death' declared: "I have no doubt Saddam has weapons of mass destruction, no doubt, absolutely no doubt at all". No one appears to have looked carefully and impartially at the evidence, or there would clearly have been doubts. Part of the government's later defence for going to war was that "everybody" believed Saddam had these weapons, so how were they to know any different? As if the public had access to Hans Blix and intelligence services: but what two million people in the UK did have was common sense, when they protested. As I stated nobody listens when you protest, your views don't matter if policy is decided.

My point in raising the case of global warming and Iraq is that evidence is only collected to support policy decisions *already made*. That is how it *actually* works. In the case of cancer there is a policy that cancer treatment must involve radiation, surgery and chemotherapy – that's the policy and so no other evidence of success or mechanism using any alternative is required or sought.

The IPCC (Independent Panel on Climate Change) made an enormous error in the case of the Himalayan glaciers. Many scientists are still at a loss to explain how the expert panel could have made such a mistake: the prediction that the glaciers would melt by 2035 was wrong by a factor of ten. The glaciologists (experts) spotted the error and notified the IPCC but no effort was made to correct it: how can one have any confidence in the 'assessment reports' that emit every five years or so from the IPCC – huge documents that are treated as tenets of the 'new religion'. As a point of comparison this is how the tenets of cancer research arose, where the so-called independent bodies, became the Orthodox Church and 'religion' of cancer treatment. If one questioned those basic tenets one became a heretic and not quite burned at the stake – but at least hounded until silenced. Global warming may or may not be *man- made*, but it seems the earth has in the past gone through geological and climatic cycles of warming and cooling even ice ages and magnetic reversals and yet the public are not informed on these cycles. To do so, might bring to the deceived public's awareness that cycles govern this universe including earth.

The case for climate action must be made from the ground upward and not the other way round. Similarly the case of cancer must be looked at from the ground upwards, which I tried to achieve with my Petition, asking for a panel of **independent multidisciplinary scientists** to look at my research paper and the accompanying '*Second Millennium Working Report into Cancer,*' now for the main incorporated here in Part 2. One comes to understand that new approaches and ideas would only rock the boat of vested interests and myths can only be maintained by excluding sceptics from the argument by levelling the label of "conspiracy theorist" at them to avoid looking at the evidence. To maintain a myth, this necessarily includes blocking any media coverage the sceptic might attain, which might wake up the sleeping populous. There should be more openness and willingness to discuss new approaches and research like my own, but I am afraid this is the sane route and sanity and objectivity is not something you will find, as it depends on reasoned argument and careful observation. In the longer term more open ways of reviewing science should be explored and independence of committees and panels must be assured.

There must come a point, when government and scientists realise that cancer has not been cured, but is in fact increasing and therefore the debate and science is not closed. Cancer is a killer disease, it is also an emotionally devastating one and we must expect and demand that taxpayer's money and charitable donations are not being used to support a myth that with just a little more money a cure is round the corner. In struggling with a bludgeoning deficit the government should look at the whole case of cancer, because the myth, is one that requires huge costs by the NHS to maintain. Iraq's WMD turned out to be a myth and goodness knows how much the war has cost this country, as quite incredibly no-one sees fit to publish the accounts, even though one suspects it must have hugely contributed towards the massive deficit, in which case I propose 'The Angel of Death' be sent the bill and not the British taxpayer. *Man- made* global warming may be a myth, where the earth's cycles may be of more importance in climatic change, the jury is still out and cancer may be another Greek mythical tragedy.

Who stands to benefit from these myths other than vested interests? In the case of global warming there is now the fast emerging carbon trading business and the climate catastrophe business, wind turbines, energy efficient cars, not to mention the jobs, lure of money, fame, grants academic acknowledgement and so on. I am all for taking care of the planet, giving other generations or indeed

156

a person's future lives a chance, but one should realise that ultimately the planet will not survive when the Sun runs out of fuel; and it seems from the *Theatre Earth* research that there are also in addition to geological cycles – conflict cycles which may be related and eventually two kings of different racial origins square up in a nuclear battle – thus ended the last conflict cycle. Even now countries like China are buying up farms in other countries and are about to lift their one child policy. Food and water resources are already targeted and earlier this year, *The Observer* reported that the total area being bought up by rich nations was more than double the size of the UK. A recent forecast rise in food prices prompted crisis talks at the United Nations and increased speculation in the commodity and land markets. It seems highly likely if not entirely probable that a war over resources will occur, repeating the demise of the last conflict cycle on earth. Further conflict may also arise over resources in the Antarctic.

The defence industries made huge profits in every war and Vietnam was quite a money-spinner as I expect Iraq and Afghanistan are. Lives are cheap however in any war even in cancer. Soon global warming like cancer will become a large industry and no one will be allowed to question whether it was all just a case of the 'Emperor with no clothes.' Yes the climate is changing, but that has occurred cyclically many times on this planet, when mans' input was not possible.

I am in favour of looking after the environment and countries like China and India need to look at the consequences. Recently (*June 2010*) I was dismayed by the judgement in the case against Union Carbide, the US based company that built and operated a pesticide plant in the central Indian city of Bhopal. In 1984 around 8,000 people died within hours of 40 tons of deadly methyl isocyanate gas being accidentally pumped into the air. Directors including Chief Executive of Union Carbide - Warren Anderson, were not prosecuted but lesser officials were, but even so only got two years. Rachna Dhingra who voiced the on-going health problems of those who survived and their dismay at the ruling said: 'This is what comes after 25,000 deaths'. This is an open invitation to multinational corporations to come and pollute and then leave without (responsibility). Campaigners say successive Indian governments have declined to act more firmly against the US Company because they do not want to frighten off the Americans or potential overseas investors. In 2001, Union carbide was taken over by the mighty American Dow Chemical

Company. Belated efforts to extradite Warren Anderson, the chief executive of Union Carbide, and other US officials, failed.

Global pollution has focused on carbon dioxide, because it has the possibility of profit, whereas the focus has been taken off, equally damaging sources of pollution. *The Guardian* [9] recently carried an article - *In China's 'cancer villages, residents pay the price for a dirty revolution.'* The breakneck economic growth in China has been at a price. Nationwide, cancer rates have surged since the 1990s to become the nation's biggest killer. In 2007 the disease was responsible for one in five deaths, up 80% since the start of economic reforms 30 years earlier. Whilst the government insists it is cleaning up pollution far faster than other nations at a similar dirty state of development, many toxic industries have simply been located to impoverished, poorly regulated, rural areas. These people do not have access to expensive lawyers in order to fight for their right to a clean environment and life.

Chinese farmers are almost four times more likely to die of liver cancer and twice as likely to die of stomach cancer, compared with the global average, according to a study commissioned by the World Bank. Reports of 'cancer villages' – clusters of the disease near dirty factories, are now becoming more frequent. The majority of these villages are on the richer eastern seaboard, the first area in China to accept 'outsourced' dirty industries from overseas. Toxic chemicals from these 'dirty industries' are finding their way into streams and rivers and from there, into the water table and into the food chain. A doctor at the village clinic - Zhan Jianyou, said he has noticed an increase in cases of cancer among the 3,000 residents. 'The pollution has definitely had an impact. I have been here 43 years. In the past cancer was not obvious, but in recent years it has become a very evident problem'. Zhang said that when residents tried to protest, the authorities blocked them because the chemical factories contributed to the local economy. Growth at all costs and one has to consider whether this planet's resources will run out, at the rate they are being utilised. The planet-hopping aliens may indeed be unknown amongst us – perhaps as the retained genetics of the Nephilim!

As I said there is no point protesting when you are up against policy and as unpalatable as it is, that policy places little value on the life of the poor as in the case of Bophal. In a recent study of 'cancer villages' Lee Liu, of the University of Central Misouri, said the problem was exacerbated by the

158

government's tendency to focus on urban development at the cost of rural areas: a once beautiful planet being destroyed by greed and the lust for products along with depletion of the world's resources. Do I really want an electrical gadget made by some exhausted worker in a factory in China? Do I really want to expose whole communities, which recycle electronic waste, to toxic cadmium, mercury and brominated flame-retardants? There again do I want to stay on this planet any longer? I suspect that this cycle of greed has occurred before on the track of time and resulted in a nuclear war between "two kings" who were of different racial origins; the evidence for which was given in '*Theatre Earth*'.

You might ask whether it has all been worth it on a personal level. If one believes in only one life, then obviously no, but as I believe in reincarnation then yes it has been most definitely worth it. When I am old, I should like someone to ask me: "When were you happy on earth?" I would say: "when I was in Arcadia and I found the Holy Grail". It was more than happiness it was a truly momentous and joyous moment. To celebrate I sought the river Alpheus in the Peloponnese – the alpha and beginning, before it forked into two streams - paths. Driving through the pretty mountainous village of Andritsana, no one seemed to know where the beginning was, but finally I found it and in celebratory baptism of re-birth, I dived naked into the Alpheus river at its source and *the beginning*: as I swam in the clear sparkling water, for a moment I thought I saw a goatherd watching me with his flock and then he was gone. Pan the god of nature and peddler of panic had been defeated. I had crossed the abyss.

'Et in Arcadia ego...'

He took my arms and folded them in grace
Gently over his pyramid the heart
Spring waxing moon's protective embrace
Love at peace and not thorny with his part
No King, Lord or octopus did I see
Through surf of indigo rippled silver
Wisdom serene no square sarcophagi
Golden body arching as sun's healer
Gently withdrawing as a crane in flight
Eyes still and through me rhythm of lyre
Arms hold in millennia memory tight
White light spirals woven to their pyre
No distance pain loneliness of battle
Fade our pyramid or patient yearning
Freedom's flight dolphin as dove with apple
Moon's love waning broken shell returning
New moon waxing the serpent is learning

R. Henry
(In memory of my fellow traveller)

16 How the Mind Works

The ultimate threat to a person's survival is pain, physical and emotional and death. Whether we know it or not, each day we carry out activities which are vital to our survival. It would seem that a basic motivation in life is to survive.

A warning of non-survival and death is emotional pain. There is an active thrust away from pain and death towards survival and life. I knew a man who when he experienced that terrible emotional pain, got up out of an armchair where he had been sitting for two years, to pick up a phone and cry for help. Emotional pain was something I could relate to. I had always known that it was the central clue in my search for an answer.

Pain is always a loss and emotional pain is a warning of impending loss. The loss can be physical for example an arm or leg, or it can relate to relationships, possessions, people, jobs etc. Loss is perceived as a loss of survival potential. One confuses physical pain and the loss of survival of the body or objects with emotional pain. So there is such a thing as "mental pain".

A man then survives to attain activity and happiness and when his hope of these diminishes, so does his survival potential. Survival is not sharp i.e. life and death, but graded. At the lowest end of the survival scale, would be death and at the other end of the scale, would be immortality and ultimate happiness and pleasure.

The maximum amount of pain exists, just before death, which I experienced in my Near Death Experience. Pain in one great sweeping shock brings about an immediate death. A shock means that a person can be broken down on the emotional scale so steeply, sharply and suddenly, that they can be killed. All losses I had ever experienced caved in on me, which resulted in the Near Death Experience. The ultimate pleasure is perceived as immortality and when I left the body in the NDE experience, the feeling of tremendous peace and joy was the recognition that I was an immortal being as a spirit. The spirit does not die it is immortal.

We are powered by the pain of death towards life i.e. the further away from pain one is, the greater the survival potential. The ultimate survival potential might be described as being one where you would be entirely successful, you would know, be serene, trust and be in perfect health physically and mentally: a state where you would be at cause and not effect in one's life. The cycle of survival is conception, growth, attainment, decay, death, conception, growth, attainment, death, etc., over and over again, which means we have lived continuously in so called past lives. There is also an activity learning cycle within a person's life of action, attempt, success and a conclusion to that action i.e. success or failure. There is also an emotional cycle, with happiness round to failure.

It would appear that death and failure are synonymous, with the chance to return and learn again. Failure is perceived by the organism as a loss i.e. loss of success, felt more acutely by men. A number of male patients in the clinic were company directors terrified of failure. Women I noted in many ways are more prone to loss through relationships, where that relationship holds survival value. It is well known that marriages that are built upon mutual respect and care of another's well- being are likely to increase longevity.

If a person fails often, his survival potential is seen to decrease and the nearer they approach death. Orthodox psychoanalysis concentrates a great deal on self and therefore neglects the much broader aspect of a healthy individual. Some redress for this is now available through group work, where people are encouraged to help and support one another. The survival of mankind is dependent on cohesion and commitment to survival of the family (a small group) and the larger group of one's community and country and then to the whole of mankind, including the animal and plant kingdoms.

If the mind solves the majority of the problems presented, the organism achieves a high level of survival. If the organism's mind fails to resolve the majority of the problems the organism fails. The mind is one of the best computers ever to be built, why would it not resolve problems? After all it has a trillion years of bioengineering behind it. In order to answer this question, let us look at the mind in two parts: the rational and thinking mind and the irrational primitive mind.

The rational mind *may* exist in the pre-frontal lobe and cerebral cortex area of the brain. This is not to say that at some future date the mind may be more accurately described in terms of energy fields. However for our purpose here, let us describe it as a computer, which is concerned with the input, filing and the output of data. It is also responsible for analysing data. The rational mind is the best computer ever invented and does not make mistakes: the rational mind records data from the environment using the senses or perceptions, such as taste, smell, auditory, visual, tactile etc. In fact there are around fifty or more perceptions, which we can record, some of the more unusual ones are, bodily sensations i.e. pressure, balance, co-ordination rhythm, kinaesthesia (weight and muscle motions) and importantly emotion.

The data in the environment is recorded in the rational mind as a complete overall record and picture or hologram if you like. If you remain stationary i.e. if you are the static or the cameraman, then life is recorded as a moving picture just as a movie reel is recorded. For the purpose of this chapter, your life is recorded from the moment of conception as a series of pictures of motion. You might refer to such pictures as your memory. When one recalls these memories, generally the pictures are remembered in terms of the perceptions of taste, smell, visual, auditory and emotion: it was a lovely sunny day and I walked through the bluebell wood, which smelt of spring and I felt happy etc. However the pictures themselves or the memories contain far more information than you are immediately aware of; they do in fact contain *all* perceptions at the time of recording and there may be as many as 51 perceptions.

Your life span is recorded in minute detail as a series of motion pictures of your experiences, which are then stored or filed if you like in memory banks. Computers in fact work like this. The experiences also include conclusions of the experience. Let us take a car crash on a particular bend in the road. You survive the crash, but thereafter when you approach that bend you do so with more care, because in your mind is a picture of that bend and resultant conclusion that it is a dangerous bend. In this way we learn from experience. People who can recall their past experiences or memories easily have a good recall or good memory. Your memory ability is your ability to recall the correct picture from your motion picture filing system. Unfortunately the education system is obsessed with the accumulation and recall of these pictures as facts. Generally children who have upset in their lives, experience poor recall for reasons I will come to discuss.

Your experiences or memories are recorded twenty-four hours a day, asleep or awake. They are also recorded during periods of anaesthesia such as during operations. I was able to access complete tracks of conversations held, whilst undergoing the operation for cancer; an interesting point for surgeons and nurses to observe. Interestingly I also was able to approach the recorded memory of radiation. The extra-ordinary experience in recall was felt and perceived as a complete static, where at some energy level; I was completely 'pinned' in space. This recall of the experience of radiation only emerged when I encountered the physical 'pinning' to the cot as a baby. One was a physical pinning; the other was definitely a pinning in terms of a field of energy. Perhaps I could liken it to a rabbit pinned to the spot by the headlights of a car. The memories of being "pinned" or "trapped" evidently were stored under the same headings or type of experience.

The experiences or memories are filed in the mind in consecutive chronological order giving the time and date of recording, extraordinary as it may seem one can date past lives. Those experiences thus accurately dated record every detail. They are in fact a motion picture of your existence in three dimensions with over fifty perceptions also recorded. A person is aware and fully conscious of the content of the rational mind i.e. all the pictures in the rational mind are known to you, if you can remember or recall them.

The following is an example of the way the rational mind works. Perhaps one day you saw a cat, you recall (very fast) pictures from your past memories that resemble that animal, which you then recognise as a cat. Children are taught to read, by presenting them with a picture of a cat, with the word or phonetics below. They come to associate the word with the picture, which they then remember. You might also from past memory recall what breed of cat it is e.g. Persian or tabby etc. The rational mind is the perfect computer, and never gives a wrong command.

I have already remarked that an organism can and does fail to resolve some problems when posed: as the mind fails to avoid pain and discover pleasure, so the mind fails for itself, the family, the community and ultimately for mankind. Murder is an irrational solution and arises when an individual or group has failed to find a rational solution to their problem. A mind working well using the rational mind correctly computes and solves problems and puts solutions into action. This is a winning mind.

The survival of the organism is assured. However the mind on occasions does not function rationally and sometimes it computes wrong or irrational answers and in such cases the mind and hence the organism is thrown into confusion and doubt. We all know that despite better judgement we sometimes do make the most ludicrous decisions, or act in the most ludicrous way. This is due to the irrational mind.

When the mind loses control it is unable to direct the organism away from pain and ultimately death. The mind that computes badly or tries to solve problems with irrational answers begins to survive only for itself and as such is doomed. Death is a means of removing obsolete organisms. It is questionable whether man will become extinct at some point, through his inability to compute rationally and solve his problems. We know from evolution that those organisms, which cannot overcome their environment or compute correct solutions towards survival, become extinct and are removed from life and interaction with others. This is Mother Nature's way of removing dangerous organisms. I do not include man's effect on survival of species as a natural mechanism and in fact man may be writing his own swan song, by doing so as biodiversity is a critical component of ecosystems.

The irrational mind then is the cause of the computer not functioning properly. Unlike the rational mind, which is the sane and pro-survival mind, the irrational mind is primitive and computes survival in terms of primitive programming, to take the analogy of a computer. It is as though you have an old floppy disc from the eighties to deal with and have to switch programmes.

Importantly the individual, who cannot recall those memories with ease, does not immediately know the contents of the irrational mind. It is a primitive area that Gurdjieff referred to as the 'Reptilian Mind'. It is a legacy of our own evolution from more primitive organisms. In those more primitive types it has a high survival advantage, in that it is a reactionary mind, requiring the organism not to think about danger or non-survival, but merely to speedily react to that danger. Whilst this mind had some value in primitive forms, it has become non-survival for man. We know from evolution that any organism, which cannot react to danger, is doomed.

The contents of the irrational mind are filed in the same way as the rational mind, with all perceptions, dates and conclusions. The individual has no control over this mind if he or she is not aware of its contents or memories. The mind reacts outside of the person's influence and may be considered to be entirely reactionary. The main difference between experiences filed in the rational mind compared to this primitive mind, is that the experiences are all

165

threats, perceived or real against the survival of the individual. This mind contains **pictures of loss** such as death, injury, bereavement, loss of jobs, divorce etc. The pictures are essentially those times when you experienced a loss or some physically or emotionally painful experience.

As the unfortunate song played at my wedding in Las Vegas went: 'memories too painful to remember, we simply choose to forget'. As Pam the recovering alcoholic remarked, when asked on truth day to recount the worst thing she had done whilst under the influence she humorously stated: "well you come in here to forget all that". In fact the saying goes, that you can tell an alcoholic by looking at their family. The alcoholic or drug abuser often has no memory of their actions, which they vent on others to experience, because the entire recording of those events is retained in the primitive mind. The alcoholic or drug abuser by definition is trying to forget by taking drugs in the first place.

Thus, the primitive mind contains a permanent record of all the bad events in your life. *The spirit retains memories and importantly conclusions, from consecutive lifetimes.* The 'camera' in the primitive mind, only 'switches on' if you like, or records, in moments of unconsciousness or painful moments derived from injury or emotional loss including shock. At this point the rational mind is not working and the entirety of any such event is recorded faithfully by the primitive mind. Severe traumatic states such as a severe illness, sudden news of a death or a shock also cause the rational mind to 'cut out' and the primitive mind to 'cut in'. Later in this book, I will discuss the rates of vibration, which I believe trigger such 'switches'. The mechanism might be considered protective, similar to an overload safety cut out switch, but in terms of evolution, as a scientist, I prefer to take the view that evolutionary development and vibration rates are linked through the musical scale of the spinal column, which I more fully covered in volume 3 of the *'Theatre Earth'* series.

The irrational or primitive mind is more rugged and durable than the rational mind, which is at a higher stage of evolutionary development. The irrational mind is the source of all irrationality and departure from logical and rational behaviour. It may be unnecessary to list such irrational actions, but the majority if not all crimes are due to this mind. The educational system at least in Britain, whilst acknowledging the 'Reptilian Mind', certainly has given it free reign in our schools, because it is not understood or known how to deal with it. Children from upset backgrounds then are allowed to destroy others education, whilst they behave purely in accordance with the irrational mind. Schools at one time never tolerated this mind and its behaviour, no matter what background you came from and you were taught to control this mind.

The irrational mind is also the source of many illnesses or common ailments and as I will explain later, the psychology of cancer lies in this mind, which can and does affect the course of the disease.

Gaps occur in the rational mind memory banks: pictures are missing in the consecutive moments of time. These gaps are the periods of unconsciousness or shock or injury, which I will from now on refer to as traumas. These traumas contain painful emotion and physical pain differing from the pictures in the rational mind, which do not contain these traumas.

As in Janov's system, there are levels of trauma, with the first level being the more serious. Level 1 traumas are the source of mental and physical abnormalities. These traumas have a great deal of charge or power locked up in them, which when released gives great relief. Level 1 traumas sometimes create turmoil in a person undergoing recall, often evoking in replay the very strong emotions felt at the time the trauma was received. However as the trauma is recalled again and again in therapy the charge dissipates, until the person can view the incident without emotional upset and can place the trauma in a rational context. Many therapists in counselling simply stir up the emotions of incidents without fully erasing them and this certainly worsens the person's condition. The emotions of fear and terror in patients undergoing the Gerson Therapy derive from the re-stimulation of these level 1 traumas, but since the patient has no access to the events of the trauma itself, unless regression is undergone, then only the emotions will be felt in present time. The patient of course as I myself experienced, has no idea where the feelings of terror and fear come from. Usually these traumas involve past life deaths but also moments of great loss in this life.

Let us take an example of the functioning of the irrational mind. Suppose you have been bitten badly by a dog, when you were a baby. This is sufficiently traumatic to be recorded as a Level 1 trauma in the primitive mind; in that physical pain and loss occurred with unconsciousness. As you grow up, what little if any conscious memory you have of the incident submerges and since the incident itself almost entirely has been filed in the primitive memory files, then you would have no conscious memory of the incident. However, you tell people you don't like dogs, you are nervous around them and for no reason that you can rationally explain, they create anxiety and even fear or terror. The primitive mind is in effect steering you clear of what was a non- survival incident *in the past*, which is remembered in order to protect you from any similar encounter *in the present*.

Irrational actions occur when a person unknowingly *acts out his past in present time* and cannot discern the difference. Was it then? Or is it now? The frightening thing is this – 99% of the population do this and may be considered neurotic. Fortunately only a small percentage acts out their past violent memories as psychotics.

The primitive mind has a very low computing ability. In the example above of the dog bite, it would compute something like this:

DOG = PHYSICAL AND EMOTIONAL PAIN=NON SURVIVAL= ALL DOGS

In other words everything is equal to everything else or in computing terms A=A=A.
The outcome of such a computation is that dogs are non-survival, since everything in the picture or recording of the trauma equals everything else. So let's say in the incident an aeroplane passes at the time of the bite, then the primitive mind records this:

DOG= PHYSICAL AND EMOTIONAL PAIN = ALL DOGS=AEROPLANE = NON SURVIVAL

So now aeroplanes give you a sense of impending doom, you are afraid of dogs and flying makes you nervous. The strength of the emotions at the time the trauma was received, will dictate the level of emotion when re-experiencing the trauma.

In computing terms we can describe the computation of the irrational or primitive mind as one that operates on:
A = A =A =A

Whereas the rational mind can discern differences or A does not equal A etc. If the rational mind considered the incident it would be able to discern between aeroplanes and dogs.

One can immediately see how ludicrous this primitive mind is, in so far as everything in the recording becomes a threat against survival and thus makes such computing irrational. In an attempt to procure your survival this mind seeks to warn you and remove you from the perceived anti survival incidents in the past, which did threaten survival. This mind is incapable of identifying the actual cause of the non-survival element. This mind does not reason, for which reason it is primitive and of a lower evolutionary level.

This method of survival has value in lower forms. A fish for example might react fast and swim away from shaded water. It has learnt that shade equals danger and often the banks of rivers are places predators including man lurk. Shade then is registered as non-survival.

Unfortunately in man's development came speech where the traumas are accompanied by language as another perception in the recording. Words spoken over unconscious people, or those in shock or under anaesthetic can later act as commands directing behaviour and even health, without the person knowing anything about it. "She can't help it" was in my case recorded in the primitive mind as a sympathy trauma during the asthma attack. Later when threatened with loss, asthma keyed in justified by the thought "I can't help it".

Sympathy traumas are linked to continuing illness, because they have some survival value. You were sick, you got sympathy for it, which is close enough to love or empathy to be perceived as having some survival value. You are again threatened with a loss, such as a cold relationship and you pull in the sympathy trauma and become ill, which attracts sympathy with some affection within that. It is better not to talk over people who are very ill, in shock or under anaesthetic, or severely injured.

If at a later date in what is a current situation, a similar experience arises to a past trauma, if it approximates enough to the content of the Level 1 trauma, then the trauma itself will come forward and be re-stimulated enough to create anxiety and negative emotions. Let us take a dysfunctional family, where a child climbs a tree, which is a natural childhood game and he falls and whilst unconscious, his father says to his mother: "See I told you he was useless and no good". The child will have that command phrase recorded in his primitive mind, along with tree climbing. If the child accumulates similar phrases in his life, recorded in moments of loss, or emotional upset, then his desire to be adventurous will decline and he will come to think of himself as "useless and no good". This may in later life be a phrase in his head, which he applies to any situation where he feels he failed. He may even marry a wife that constantly nags him and tells him he is no good. Of course there is behavioural re-enforcement and the later one discovers the traumas, the more difficult it is to retrain what might be termed ingrained 'habits' or 'personality traits.'

Level 1 traumas then are mental image pictures, recording a time of physical pain and unconsciousness. The irrational mind stores up all these bad experiences or traumas and then throws them back at you in moments of danger and upset and so dictates your actions irrationally and along lines that you would not consciously have chosen, if you were not upset. I would suggest that with serious illness including cancer on the increase and millions of people reporting mental health issues inclusive of stress then it is time to confront the mechanism of this mind. You *never* speak to or attempt to have a rational discussion with anyone who shows anger, rage, or grief or apathy because the rational mind is turned off and they are dramatizing or acting out pictures of loss in their irrational mind.

There is another type of trauma, which I will call a Level 2 trauma. The real pain in this type of experience is emotional and the real mental pain of it is caused by incidents 'resting' on an earlier Level 1 trauma, where there was actual physical pain and unconsciousness. A Level 2 trauma *re-stimulates* an earlier Level 1 trauma, which contains similar data, but real physical pain. Let us say a marriage is failing. It is emotionally painful and there is a fear of being left or abandoned. In my case, this Level 2 trauma was compounded by the death of my father (Level 2 trauma) and also rested upon a Level 1 trauma of being tortured in hospital as a child and tied down to a cot in physical pain with chronic eczema and then left like that for 6 months until my skin re grew – effectively abandoned. All of that time would have mainly been recorded in the primitive mind to which I had no rational access. To have expressed anger at my ex-husband's behaviour, would have challenged the conclusion I had made as an eighteen month old baby, watching my parents leave after their weekly Sunday visit: "don't cry or be a trouble, or they will never take you home and love you". Goodness knows how many other children like myself, treated for chronic eczema in the 50s are still walking around unknowingly with the same trauma dictating and even ruining their lives. It's tragic. Years later when I heard about the Romanian orphans tied to their cots, I was overwhelmed with a sense of grief for them, understanding fully what hell they went through. Many of them never recovered from psychological problems.

A Level 2 trauma then is a mental image picture of a moment of severe and shocking loss or threat of loss, which contains unpleasant emotions such as anger, fear, grief, apathy or terror. It differs from a Level 1 trauma only in that it does not contain *physical* pain and unconsciousness. A Level 2 trauma is a mental image recording of a time of severe mental distress. The loss of a loved one feels painful because of its association with the very real original Level 1 trauma upon which it rests and the presence of real physical pain. A man once described the breakdown of his marriage to me as: "like having my right arm cut off". The Level 1 trauma was virtually unveiling itself and one suspects it involved a right arm injury in this life or a past life.

One woman, who had cancer in this life, had always stated a phrase whenever she was very upset: "I just want to put my face to the wall and die". She had no idea why she said it, but whenever she felt moments of loss, she would automatically repeat this phrase. She had in her last life been a concentration camp victim of the Holocaust and had died when she placed her face to the wall and had just given up. One considers very carefully what actions one gives others to receive, because the law of karma is more harsh and just than you will find in a court on earth. One has to be *very* careful with karma. The problem with actions, which cause another pain and loss is that there are ramifications in terms of energy and one may spend thousands of years looking for just one individual to reverse the karma one has caused, let alone the ramifications of actions during that time.

There is also a Level 3 trauma, which is an emotionally painful experience, which does not contain unconsciousness neither does it contain physical pain. A Level 3 trauma may re-stimulate a Level 2 trauma for example the sight of a coffin may re-stimulate a Level 2 trauma of the death of a loved one, which in turn may then re-stimulate a Level 1 trauma with actual physical pain and unconsciousness in a death. It's rather like a set of dominos falling in a line. The reason one aims to bring to the cognitive rational mind all past lives and level one traumas (normally deaths), is that they no longer have any command value over your actions and thinking in present time.

A person ought to be able to look at all past experiences in his life including traumas and do so without difficulty or upset. People, who are counselled for upsetting circumstances in their lives, are often asked to go over and over, Level 2 traumas, which then unknown to them and the counsellor in many cases is merely stirring up a Level 1 trauma. It is actually quite harmful to do this, without locating the Level 1 trauma. Once you have stirred up a Level 1 trauma, it will take around three days to recede during which time a person is actively affected and directed by it. By attending counselling sessions once a week and continually 'poking' a Level 1 trauma, means that for most of the week you will not be fully conscious or in control of your actions. Children who live in upset families will often 'miss' the first three days of the school week (after a weekend with their parents) because they have been re-stimulated upon the subject of loss and what is worse, that upset and irrational thinking is then spread through the rest of the class. Unfortunately too the education system at least in the UK, puts up with this where half the school week is lost through children being re-stimulated and being allowed to act out their primitive mind freely in class – tantrums, shouting, rudeness, surliness etc.

As a point of caution, one should never in serious illness approach Level 1 traumas and even Level 2 traumas. A person, who is very ill as in cancer, must focus on *gains* and not losses. Only when a person is on the road to recovery can one cautiously approach Level 2 incidents and only when a person is stable, can Level 1 be approached. The problem with the Gerson Therapy is that it does stir up Level 1 traumas particularly in the first 3-6 months and these have to be dealt with.

The more a person avoids confronting their past experiences, especially bad ones in their life, then the less well that person will be. A person who is totally unable to look at any aspect of their life may live in a Walter Mitty world of no confront. Sanity is the ability to look at all aspects of your life good and bad. Psychoanalysis recognises this in aspects of drug use recovery programmes.

Since a person's experience in his irrational primitive mind dictates what a person must avoid in order to survive, then the more a person avoids those mental image pictures and memories, the less willing the individual will be to experience life. This individual has to avoid looking at or experiencing so many situations and aspects of life in order not to re-experience the pain of the past, that there may be little left in life to experience.

The person who is continually let down by others in life, continually experiences loss and these losses are recorded as Level 3 traumas, which will constantly re-stimulate Level 2 and 1 trauma. A person like this may eventually end up incapable of adjusting to his environment or people around him. He may become reclusive, shutting himself away so that he may never experience pain again. On the other hand a person may through active *choice* seek isolation, which is different. Humans however are social animals and require contact and certainly research shows mortality is linked to warm and loving social contact, through relationships and friends.

Illness is on the increase and one cannot discount that loss in our daily lives contributes to that far more than we recognise. In a society where 'dog eats dog' has become the normal rather than the rarity loss is inevitable. Each day it seems one is picking up some pieces of loss caused by another's lack of ethics or plain nasty behaviour. My philosophy has always been 'if you would not like it done to you, then don't do it to another.'

If one suggests that there is a psychosomatic component acting in illness and cancer, people immediately become agitated and shout: "How dare you suggest that I brought this on myself!" Despite the objections there is a respectable body of scientific literature implicating emotional and psychological factors in the onset of cancer and some other diseases.

Psychosomatic illnesses are those which have a mental origin but where the symptoms of the illness manifest themselves physically. Many factors are now implicated in cancer such as smoking and lifestyle, but the psychosomatic component has been neglected, for not altogether ethical reasons as will be seen later. Environmental toxic factors such as smoking, chemicals etc. are also perceived as loss – to a body.

One cannot be responsible for traumas that are hidden in the primitive or irrational mind and thus the meaning of psychosomatic has been misinterpreted. Psycho refers to the mind, whilst somatic refers to the body. Psychosomatic illness is an autogenetic disease in that it originates from within the body and mind itself: whereas an exogenetic disease would originate from factors coming from the outside of the body e.g. bacteria, virus, environmental factors etc. Cancer is a disease which develops when there is threat to survival and other disruptive environmental factors are present: thus cancer is a combination and summation of anti- survival factors both autogenetic and exogenetic.

Some people even doctors have great difficulty accepting the power of the mind over the body even though the placebo effect has long been known. It is easy to demonstrate such power in hypnosis experiments. A suggestion such as: "your heart rate will rise when I snap my fingers" can indeed produce elevated heart rates. Positive suggestion can inhibit blood flow to an area and more importantly, the endocrine system, the system of glands producing hormones e.g. the male hormone testosterone and the female hormone oestrogen can be affected by positive suggestion.

In a person with an unbalanced hormone system there are normally Level 1 traumas in re-stimulation. Once the Level 1 trauma has been contacted and seen in a rational light by the rational mind, then it no longer has the power to direct the individual including disruption of the endocrine system. Level 1 trauma is the basis of psychosomatic illness. Instead of spending millions on fertility techniques it would be easier to first erase any level 1 traumas that are affecting the endocrine system.

Gerson Patients often report a "woolly" or "not here" feeling which is due to the constant re-stimulation of the primitive mind, which records moments of unconsciousness and physical pain. Their rational mind is not fully in command. Further patients often report a pain and disturbance in the lower part of the back of the head. The hypothalamus is the area of the mind controlling the body and is often referred to as the life function regulator or master control area. It seems that the healing reactions of the Gerson Therapy 'switch' through this area, translating traumas or mental image pictures through the hypothalamus into body reactions, which include hormonal release or inhibition.

The hypothalamus is the diencephalon brain; this is the part of the brain between the cerebrum and the mesencephalon. The main structures of the diencephalon are the thalamus, the hypothalamus and the pituitary. On a crude level the thalamus plays an important part in receiving information from the body and associating this information with feelings of pleasantness or unpleasantness for example pain, temperature and touch: it also plays a part in the arousal or alerting mechanisms. The hypothalamus on the other hand although small and weighing little more than seven grams, is vital and critically links the mind and body, via nervous and endocrine systems. It also links to the cerebral cortex i.e. the psyche or what psychologists call the 'I' of existence. It is the place where the 'I' controls the body. Critically however it is the route by which emotions can express themselves in changed bodily functions.

The hypothalamus therefore along with the pituitary is the most likely area involved in the manifestation of a psychosomatic illness, linking mind to body. Some of the neurones in the hypothalamus function as endocrine glands. Their axons secrete chemicals, called releasing hormones into the blood, which circulates to the anterior pituitary gland, releasing hormones from there such as growth hormone and other hormones that control hormone secretion by the sex glands.

A hormone called somatostatin is secreted by the hypothalamus, which has been shown to switch off the production of somatotrophin (growth hormone) by the pituitary gland. It would appear logical that in cases where an animal's survival is threatened, then growth is 'shut down' in favour of reducing energy demands on the body. Our ancestors were much smaller than us and whilst one might argue that intermix and evolution has increased height, it can also be argued that our ancestors may have suffered continual threat from the environment and would operate mainly from the primitive or irrational mind. As an aside it might also be interesting to note that man resorts to violence, when under threat of survival and certainly violence is a reaction dictated by the irrational and primitive mind.

The hypothalamus also plays a part in maintaining the waking state. It keeps the individual alert. If this area is the region most affected by the primitive mind, then sleeplessness and the constant chewing over of perceived survival worries or stress related issues would in terms of survival make sense. Under perceived threat the animal must remain alert and not fall asleep. The antidote to insomnia such as reading a book requires a rational mind and therefore 'switches off' the primitive mind replaying its old Level 1, 2 and 3 traumas, with emotions of fear, terror or grief etc.

Hypothalamic disorders, produce the same mental effects as those reported during Gerson "flare ups" or the healing reactions: a feeling as I described it in my own experience of "wading through mud" or a "cotton wool feeling in my head" and loss of perceptions: as Charlotte Gerson told me: "as you proceed on the therapy, you will become more yourself". This might be more technically described as not being subject to the constant re-stimulation of the primitive mind and more in control as the rational mind 'switches on'.

The hypothalamus also functions as a crucial area regulating appetite and the amount of food uptake. People often mistake morbidly obese people as being greedy. However if the primitive mind is 'switched on' due to perceived threat of survival, then food consumption may be linked to an irrational computation such as:

FOOD = COMFORT = LOVE = SURVIVAL

Perhaps a failed relationship or some loss has caused the individual to be re-stimulated on the Level 2 and 3 traumas, which then re-stimulate a Level 1 trauma. It may be that the individual suffered physical pain and injury or unconsciousness and food became a way back to health or provided comfort. If that were the case then the Level 1 trauma and its conclusions would act to direct the individual in present time: the so-called 'comfort eater'. In the reverse case of anorexia, then not eating would irrationally become in the mind of the individual a survival action. Glamorous celebrity size zero women in magazines may represent high survival to a young girl, who perceives her own survival threatened in some way e.g. by parental divorce.

It is quite probable that the hypothalamus is involved with monitoring and coping with stressful situations. In severe physical pain or in intense emotional states then the cerebral cortex especially the limbic lobe is thought to send impulses to the hypothalamus. In turn the hypothalamus stimulates via releasing factors the pituitary gland, which secretes hormones and releasing factors, which further stimulate other endocrine glands. Thus the hypothalamus links the nervous system to the endocrine system and is subject to stress (loss). When survival is threatened, then the hypothalamus through its releasing factors can take over the commands of the anterior pituitary gland and hence from there, the thyroid gland, the adrenal cortex and sex glands (ovaries and testes).

Through hormones, the chemical messengers in the body, the brain can influence via the nervous system, all the cells in our bodies. This is a two way process and information on the body is fed back to the brain, by what is called biofeedback loops, again involving the nervous and hormonal systems. In this way the state of the body can and does influence mental processes and mental processes can and do influence the body. Environmental toxins then can easily not only lower survival of body cells, but can induce mental depression by this route.

People like to talk of "stress" but it is really a perceived survival threat, which then re-stimulates the Level 1, 2 and 3 traumas, with their emotional content, which then manifest in present time. A person feels overwhelmed or threatened in their job and they become increasingly nervous, they suffer the physical symptoms of nausea, perhaps diarrhoea or heart burn; blood pressure may rise or they may experience headaches. Such physical responses are created from the interactions of nervous, circulatory and hormonal systems in response to the perceived threat of non-survival. People take time off work and remove themselves from the threatening non-survival situation and feel better, but have not dealt in most cases with the source of the stress and the Level 1 and 2 traumas.

Post-traumatic stress is really a Level 2 trauma (a shocking incident) or a Level 1 trauma (unconsciousness and injury), which remains in re-stimulation and requires erasure by full recognition of its content inclusive of emotion. Let us take a person who has returned from war and experienced the flashing of guns and the noise of war, or they suffered an injury, or saw a friend die. Anything in present time that approximates the content of the original trauma will re-stimulate the entire content of that trauma and the person will experience a "flash back." In other cases the person becomes 'stuck' in the trauma itself as it constantly replays in their mind.

Sympathy traumas can be very tricky. Take the example where a child is very ill and under those conditions the child was severely physically and mentally distressed and where survival is threatened. The whole of the incident now is recorded by the primitive mind and the child is only semi-conscious. However whilst the child appears to be unconscious, in fact everything including muscle tension, body position, smell and sound etc., are being recorded by the primitive mind, including conversations.

The parents, worried and fatigued argue over the child. One parent threatens to leave. The primitive mind also records conclusions, thus if one parent wins the argument the primitive mind will conclude who won and the personality of the

177

winner: thereafter the personality of the winner may in fact be used and acted out rather as if they had claimed another's identity for themselves. The primitive mind makes conclusions for future survival. Later in life the child now an adult may encounter a similar threat e.g. their spouse may threaten to leave. Unknown to the adult (since the childhood experience was recorded in the primitive mind) the Level 1 trauma (pain and unconsciousness and the illness) will be re-stimulated. The adult will unconsciously 'act out' the past trauma by becoming ill. Suppose his father won the argument in the childhood experience then the adult will start to take on the personality of the father. Suppose the father was aggressive and shouted - then this personality will be adopted. The person in present time 'plays acts' or mimics the winning personality of the past incident. He can't remain himself as the child, as this was non-survival and thus he assumes the role of the winning personality in the incident. In fact this is the way that the worst traits of parents are perpetuated through their children, apart from the role models they provide. If violence was part of the Level 1 trauma then violence will be 'play acted' in present time. If sexual abuse was part of the trauma, then this too will be 'play acted' if in later life a similar situation arises. This is, apart from and in addition to past life experiences, which can also form a significant part of actions in the current life.

Furthering the example of the child that is ill, then suppose he had severe food poisoning with accompanying abdominal pain and where one of his parents has threatened to leave. This is a Level 1 trauma. If later as an adult he becomes re-stimulated perhaps by his spouse threatening to leave, then he will try to assume the winning personality from the Level 1 trauma. If a person is prevented from acting out the experience or prevented from assuming the role of the winning personality e.g. his wife may tell him if he doesn't stop shouting at her she really will leave him, then under such threat he will have no alternative but to 'play act' himself in the incident, which means he will experience the abdominal pains and he may even become genuinely sick. He now has no option left when threatened with the loss of his relationship, which of course will be perceived by him as life threatening. The Level 1 trauma with its life threatening illness is the real source of his emotions, but this is not recognised by him, since it is stored in the primitive irrational mind. He will now experience tension of muscles in his abdomen, which were the Level 1 trauma physical perceptions of the food poisoning. The illness will again manifest as a psychosomatic pain. He may blame this on his wife, but in fact the pain has its origins in the Level 1 trauma as a child. With abdominal muscle tension, he may experience other effects due to that as blood flow will be restricted and over a period of time he may develop a chronic disease – even cancer.

The crucial point to be made is that a person will not allow himself or herself to suffer from the illness content of the past trauma, unless that illness becomes a means by which the individual can survive, however illogical that is to a rational mind it appears to make sense to a primitive mind. Let us say the incident contained some sympathy from the parents, who normally showed little love or perhaps attention. Sympathy has some survival value and thus at any point in future, when the person feels unloved or abandoned, they will pull in illness based upon a Level 1 trauma, to gain sympathy based on the conclusions of the Level 1 trauma filed in the primitive mind which computes on $A = A = A$ or:

ILLNESS = SYMPATHY = SURVIVAL

This mind moronically computes that all things are equal and equal survival. His mother may have given him chicken soup when he was ill and thereafter if he feels unloved, abandoned or threatened by abandonment, or becomes ill, he will eat chicken soup. Chicken soup is equal to survival or:

ILLNESS = SYMPATHY = CHICKEN SOUP = SURVIVAL

This is the way the primitive mind computes and obviously one immediately observes its moronic illogical nature compared to a more highly evolved being like us that can compute logically, where illness does not equal survival.

Again the critical point here is that the chronic psychosomatic illness, which a patient displays, will be based upon a past trauma containing sympathy. The child might conclude that the person, who stayed with the child under threat of loss, is the personality with high survival value. Children can become 'clingy', when they perceive threatened loss or abandonment.

The worst trauma you could have is one, which contains physical illness or injury with threat of loss and a sympathy element, accompanied by words spoken. At the time that a trauma is recorded, 51 perceptions are also recorded and it is conceivable that the biochemistry of the body at the time is also recorded. Later in this book, I will explain that cancer is an embryological biochemistry and return to that biochemistry, or to put it another way cancer is the biochemical manifestation of a type of embryological growth - regeneration.

17 Emotional Scales

There is a scale, which plots the ascending spiral of life from death, to half vitality and consciousness, to vitality. *The behaviour that a person exhibits will depend upon his position on this scale*, which is remarkably accurate. In the *Theatre Earth* series I showed that the spinal column and nerves are arranged as a musical scale. It appears that during evolution as certain levels of command centres evolved, those centres or positions on the spinal cord and column were subject to different vibratory influences at the time they evolved. Cephalisation or the formation of a head is a fairly recent event in terms of evolutionary history and the spinal cord in vertebrates (animals with backbones) has a slow evolution from lower invertebrate types (animals without backbones), where command centres developed mainly along the main spinal nerve axis.

I have remarked that in my own experience, the depth of fear and terror I experienced could never be expressed in words and only by music, or in my case Elgar's concerto in E minor Opus 85 with Jacqueline Du Pre on cello.

A person who has suffered too many losses, too much pain, tends to become fixed at some lower level of the spiral or emotional range and with only slight fluctuations, becomes stuck there. His behaviour and speech will reflect his position on this scale. A person who is winning life's game generally shows a high ethic level, is hardly ever ill, exhibiting a good attitude to children and is open to communication of different ideas inclusive of belief systems. These people are logical and have a high level of reality. Since they show a good interest in others and because they are keen to help their fellow man they make good friends. They don't lie and are truthful.

As a person begins to experience losses in life, they begin to descend the spiral or scale. Consciousness decreases along with reality, as the rational mind 'switches' to the primitive mind, where they act out past incidents and are easily re-stimulated. Further down the scale the person becomes unethical, has a poor attitude to children, hates helping others and views life from the position of self. This person cannot tolerate new ideas or communicate freely with others. They are argumentative and hostile and this turns to apathy, the further they descend. At low levels paedophilia and abuse of children sets in as does lying and harm of others through that. These people are actually a liability both as friends, managers or part of a relationship.

As the individual descends the emotional scale, he first begins to lose his confidence in trying to reach out and control his environment, as he begins to confuse yesterday's losses with today's losses. He goes from an ability to listen to other viewpoints and allow others the freedom of those viewpoints, to conservatism or some willingness to listen, provided that his world is not challenged or threatened. Dropping further on the scale, he will arrive at boredom, where he does not actively seek others views, or communicate his own. Further down he rejects other viewpoints and becomes hostile and aggressive, denying another's viewpoint entirely. Here you have 'my way or no way.' This person is virtually psychotic where they compute ' I must be right or I die.' If you tried to point out how wrong this person was he would probably feel totally threatened and may even become violent.

A person can be at an emotional level of boredom, open hostility, anger, covert hostility, grief or apathy. At all of these levels the primitive mind is operating on a scale reflected by the level itself and the inherent behaviour. Actions will be irrational to the degree, with which the primitive mind is re-stimulated. The behaviour, views and emotional tone of individuals are connected. By recognising at what emotional level an individual is operating, one can *predict* behaviour and views held. It is a very precise psychological assessment. Unfortunately people are often selected to run companies, or even countries, without regard to their position on this scale, which is often quite low down and therefore subject to irrational behaviour, unethical behaviour and sexual promiscuity along with a limited tolerance of others viewpoints. It seems amazing to me that neurotics and even psychotics are allowed to run countries.

A person may fluctuate briefly up and down the scale, if they are still subject to re-stimulation of traumas. This is acute and of short duration unless their environment poses a constant threat, which will cause a person to become chronically stuck in any one of the negative emotional states such as grief, anger, apathy, hostility etc.

Where a dominant member of a family or a workplace displays a chronic low emotional state, such as anger or hostility, then the whole family or workforce no matter where they are on the scale will eventually succumb to the lowest state of the dominant family or workplace member. A hostile and angry parent, who criticises constantly, will pass this on to be mimicked by the children. The children then will arrange themselves in a hierarchy of suppression according to age, with each child exhibiting hostile behaviour towards the child below and so on.

When a parent's emotional low tone comes to dominate a family, you will also see illness and where family members are failing and not succeeding. At low emotional tones, the primitive mind 'switches on' through re-stimulation and this mind contains mental image pictures of illnesses, injuries etc., which will come forward to be 'play acted out'. Whole families can look awfully unlucky until you find the smiling 'Mona Lisa' who has created the highly re-stimulative environment within the family through their own case and chronic low tone: but nobody would have ever suspected them, as people around this person go up in smoke in an upset state. The smiling 'Mona Lisa' can easily convince people the upset has nothing to do with them.

People can be quite artful at hiding their true chronic low tone. You meet someone, they seem nice and high toned, but then you say something controversial or make what I call a purposeful comment in order to 'test their psychological button' and watch the reaction. Antagonism or hostility may suddenly reveal itself and you realise this person is actually quite low down on the scale. Someone lies artfully and you know that you are dealing with a person very low down on the scale and yet his colleagues think he is a nice guy, but he secretly plots and no one would ever suspect this person is actually quite dangerous and at least harmful.

In the case of illness or cancer then, one must check one's environment for any low toned individuals who have a negative and re-stimulatory effect. Constant invalidation and suppression, critical and hostile comments are all stock in trade of the 'Anti-Social Personality' and no one will regain their health by remaining in the vicinity of these people. One has two options if such a person is found – you either handle them or you remove yourself from any further contact. One cannot expect to regain one's health, whilst a low toned person constantly stirs up loss through re-stimulation.

PART 2

THE CANCER FILES

THE AUTHOR'S RESEARCH

"An eagle's old age is worth a sparrow's youth"
(Greek saying)

"Not even the gods fight necessity"
(Simonides, 8, 20)

THE CANCER SYNDICATE

To understand how orthodox treatment of cancer works, you have to understand how tumours grow. Normal healthy cells, divide in a controlled way, where their growth is checked by a mechanism or complex set of interactions between cells. Cancer cells however do not grow in a controlled way, where intercellular communication does not occur and the growth-inhibiting mechanisms no longer work. As a result the cells reproduce endlessly and a tumour forms. Metastasis or spread of cancer occurs when a tumour reaches a certain size and cells break off and are dispersed in the blood stream or lymph system to other organs, or tissues, where they may form new tumours.

Orthodox doctors often apply the term survival time, rather than cure, because the disease can reoccur, as long as 20 years after a cure. However doctors deem you to be cured if you are cancer free for 5 years. I think that eventually cancer will be seen as a managed condition and cure is relative to whether you maintain a healthy lifestyle and how you deal with the psychological component of cancer - loss.

Survival figures (statistics) can be misleading since a patient can die of cancer after 6 years but will still be counted as a cure in government generated statistics. Governments are very good at manipulating statistics, especially around times of Cancer Day or large fund raising events, or in the run up to elections, or if any criticism appears in the press over orthodox cancer mortality rates. The proverbial expert is then wheeled out to support the orthodox view and assure the masses that one day, scientists will solve this enigma, with just another billion in funding and so on.

Oncologists rush people into surgery for small cancers as it is deemed most successful, but if the cancer has spread or metastasised, and is no longer localised it will be treated by chemotherapy or may be deemed inoperable. Even so many so-called inoperable or terminal patients have survived using the alternative methods. So being told by orthodoxy that there is nothing more to be done does not mean there is no alternative. However the problem alternative therapists have is that the patients they normally see are those who have been left to die by orthodox doctors and are at a late stage in their disease. The cases then are hard to reverse but even so 10% of these cases do make it.

Survival times are lower for metastasised cases, and so surgery is not the answer or a definitive solution. Once the cancer has spread, the option is chemotherapy, which doctors will use to try and kill all the cancer cells in the body, which have spread. Chemotherapy is not specific and will attack healthy cells too. The rationale is that the cancer cells are weaker and more prone to chemotherapy attack. Orthodox medicine sees the cancer as *the cause* of the disease. The tumour or growth to orthodoxy must be aggressively attacked and removed. No other underlying cause as such is sought because in orthodox medicine the cancer or *tumour itself* is seen as *the cause* of the disease. In alternative medicine the tumour is *not* seen as the cause, only *the symptom* and therefore the underlying causation, is sought.

As far back as 1970 Sir John Bruce, Regius Professor of clinical Surgery at Edinburgh University and past president of the Royal College of Surgeons, said of cancer treatment: 'The future lies elsewhere than in the operating room'. Alternative therapists and doctors claim that surgery merely releases some of the cancer cells into the bloodstream or lymph system, thus increasing the likelihood of spread. Surgery then is better when directed at small tumours.

Radiation is also often recommended following surgery. Radiologists now try to narrow down the ray so that it focuses on the smallest area of cancer cells, claiming to leave healthy cells less affected. The theory is that cancer cells will be affected more than healthy cells and die off when radiated. Often patients are not told, as I was not, of the possible side effects of radiation. Conditions such as lymphedema arising from breast cancer treatment can be devastating and there is no guarantee that radiation itself will not - say in 20 years cause cancer from genetic mutation of the radiated cells. There is a 10% chance of lymphedema occurring with radiation alone and up to 30% when radiation is carried out with surgery. Personally since I suffered side effects I now totally regret having had radiation and admonish my stupidity at ever agreeing to it. However, the point is that you are bamboozled into treatment in a state of shock and in that state, a patient does not ask questions, ask for statistics, survival times, side effects etc. In my case I was not told of the side effects and therefore did not give informed consent. I was also given wrong data on survival rates.

So how stupid was I when agreeing to radiation? Well let me quote an extract from Morris Bealle's book entitled *The Drug Story* (11) written in the 1940's.

'Because the price of radium increased 1,000%, when some enterprising medical business men started a fad in using it on cancer victims, too much money is tied up in radium now for those who own it to give up cancer futility without a struggle'.

Whilst it is claimed today that radiation increases survival times several high profile doctors in the past have refuted that claim. Doctor W. Powers Director of Divisional Radiotherapy at Washington University School of Medicine in the 80's stated: 'Although pre-operative and post-operative radiation have been used extensively for decades, it is still not possible to prove equivocal benefit from this combined treatment'.

Doctor P. Rubin, Chief Divisional Radiotherapist with the University of Rochester Medical Department backed this view when he said: 'The clinical evidence and statistical data in numerous reviews are cited to illustrate that no increase in survival has been achieved by the addition of radiation'.

When asked to comment one scientist from the NCI (National Cancer Institute) in the States explained:

'Look, when you've got 10,000 radiologists and millions of dollars' worth of radiation equipment you give radiation treatment. Even if study after study shows a lot of it does more harm than good, what else are they going to do? Like surgeons: they've been trained to cut so they cut'.

Whilst I was updating this data I noted an article in the press (*The Daily Mail 14.09.2010*), which claimed: 'Radiotherapy saves millions but can inflict cruel damage.' The article also claimed that radiotherapy is an "effective cancer treatment," which contradicts past research quoted from the University of Rochester, which shows no increase in survival times. The article however stated: 'Experts say it increases survival rates by about 50% - it can damage healthy tissue around the tumour site'. There was no quote or research reference indicating where they took the value of 50% from and whether that figure is accurate, as it clearly contradicts Dr P. Rubin's claim. This is the sort of un-referenced reporting that people then base life decisions on.

The press article went on to say that the most vulnerable to radiation damage are the 12,000 patients a year who have pelvic irradiation for bowel, cervical and womb cancer, and those who are treated for head and neck cancers. Dr Jason Lester, an oncologist at Velindre Cancer Centre, Cardiff stated: 'We think that about 50% of patients who undergo pelvic irradiation will suffer some radiotherapy damage'. If we consider the 'damage' then it covers 'a change in bowel habits, but others may have distressing symptoms such as bowel ulcers, rectal bleeding, pelvic pain and a lack of bladder control. Some will need a blood transfusion, or even end up with a colostomy bag'. Personally I don't see the point of surviving cancer, if one ends up with a whole raft of problems and even a colostomy bag. In the case of bowel cancers, which are often caused by diet, then the alternative dietary therapies have had very good success, with no side effects or damage.

It is yet to be seen whether proton beam therapy, an advanced form of radiotherapy that claims to target cancers with minimal damage to healthy tissue, will improve matters. However access to proton beam therapy may only apply to 'high-priority patients,' that generally means children and it is doubtful whether older sufferers will be included in that group.

Doctors now have to send their patients for treatment for radiation damage, such as HBO therapy or hyperbaric oxygen therapy. The NHS then spends millions of pounds in treating patients for damage *created* by orthodox cancer treatment in a never-ending spiral of costs. Dr Phil Bryson, director of the Diving Diseases Research Centre in Plymouth says the principle behind HBO therapy is simple: 'We know the protein which controls cell growth and healing depends on oxygen. HBO delivers a huge amount in a short time, and research shows it stimulates this protein to work more efficiently. This is particularly relevant when you consider that radiotherapy damage is characterised by the death of the blood capillaries, which feed oxygen to the damaged area.' I will cover research later, which shows that oxygen is essential to *prevent* (and treat) the biochemistry of cancer and it seems ridiculous to actually through radiation create damage to the blood capillaries, which carry blood and therefore oxygen: a procedure then likely to *assist* cancer metabolism. You may remember in my own story of how during an intense healing reaction of the radiotherapy area, it turned purple indicating increased blood flow, almost certainly indicating as Dr Gar Hildebrand stated that radiation had caused capillary damage and in my case muscle and bone damage.

The Daily Mail article, which covered the case of one patient given radiotherapy for prostate cancer in 1993, who then 15 years later began to suffer symptoms of radiation damage, went on to describe how: 'He went from being a fit, highly-motivated businessman to someone in constant fear of incontinence'. The poor man was wetting himself and had to wear incontinence pads. He also suffered painful cystitis and bowel problems and passed blood in his urine: as the article stated: 'All these symptoms are text book radiotherapy damage'. Yet no one told the patient exactly why these symptoms had appeared. The patient stated: 'I thought I was simply living with the effects of having had cancer'. The article then went on to say: 'While the damaging side-effects of radiotherapy have been recognised for decades, until recently patients weren't told of the risk. Partly this is because of concern that patients may refuse treatment if they knew the risk of damage. This attitude has left generations of radiotherapy patients struggling to get a diagnosis – let alone treatment – for their problems'. Is it not deeply unethical that patients are not told of possible side effects, in order to push them uninformed into treatments that can cause huge damage, just because it is government policy?

I had symptoms of radiation damage straight away, but you will remember that on the Gerson Therapy I suffered enormous healing reactions of damage due to the radiotherapy. I was not told of either the risks or informed of the cause of the damage. I was alerted by the Gerson doctor whom I rang in Mexico, but did not find out definitely until I saw a newspaper article on a group of patients who had been damaged at the Royal Marsden Hospital by over- radiation – I belonged to that group. The solicitors Russell Jones and Walker explained that the orthodoxy i.e. the Royal Marsden would win any legal case because a court would accept the legal argument that the situation of cancer is so desperate that I would have taken the radiotherapy even if I had been warned. The fact that I did the Gerson Therapy and refused chemotherapy presumably had no bearing on their legal argument. Here we have the syndicate at work – the monopoly on cancer treatment and the arrogant assumption that you had *no choice* - because there were no alternatives. I just walked away to save my sanity.

It was not until years later also, when I had to have extensive dental work that I was told by my orthodontist that radiation often causes teeth to crumble.

Chemotherapy entails the use of drugs and hormones to treat cancer. In 1947 the late Doctor Sidney Farber of the Children's Cancer Research Foundation in Boston, treated 16 children suffering from leukaemia with an agent called aminopterim and achieved temporary remissions with 10 of them. On that the era of chemotherapy really started to take off.

The reason there are successes in treating cancers of the rapidly dividing lymph and blood cells, the leukaemia's, the lymphomas and Hodgkin's disease (a type of lymph cancer) is that these forms of cancer often occurring in children, show rapidly dividing cells and chemotherapy aims at destroying all newly formed cells. Whilst healthy cells can divide again, cancer cells die and do not divide further: however the majority of cancer drugs basically work by poisoning (all) cells. Initially chemotherapeutic agents were used singly, but since cancer cells develop resistance to drugs, then today several drugs are used in combinations – 'cocktails' in drug treatment plans called protocols. What is not generally pointed out to patients is that chemotherapy and radiation are actually carcinogenic, responsible for *causing* cancer even some five to ten years after the therapy has been completed.

I was appalled when I discovered that research had shown in one study that the incidence of secondary cancers in sites treated by radiotherapy was as high as 17% after twenty years. In one Swiss study where patients had been treated with chemotherapy there was a 68% reoccurrence of cancer in those patients who had been given chemotherapy compared with only 40% incidence in the control group or those who had received no chemotherapy after periods ranging from three and half years to five and half years. In addition 63% of the treated group had died while only 39% of the control group had died. An increased incidence of acute myelocytic leukaemia (AML) was seen in patients receiving adjunct chemotherapy for breast and ovarian cancer. The leukaemia appeared connected to the use of the cancer drug – melphalanalome and chlorambucil. It is hard to say also, how much do the pain, disfigurement, toxicity and depressing nature of orthodox treatment affect survival times, where people sometimes loose the will to live under the onslaught.

Chemotherapy was hailed in press stories throughout the sixties and seventies as the great new hope in cancer treatment, with little mention of the now well-documented serious side effects that these powerful drugs have. In 1973 Dr Dean Burk, head of the Cytochemistry section of the National Cancer Institute or NCI in the USA, sent an open letter to the then NCI director Frank

Rauscher, charging that virtually all the conventional anti- cancer drugs had been found to actually *cause* cancer in the NCI's *own* studies. Whilst the general news editors at Associated Press and *Time* Magazine enthusiastically accepted this story, science and medical editors killed it - an action, which is part of the *Cancer Blackout*, where any contradictory news on cancer, which threatens orthodox methods, is simply erased from public view.

It is true that incredible suppression of innovative ideas that threaten the orthodoxy of the time has always occurred in the history of science. William Harvey the new thinker in town in 1657 had terrible trouble explaining blood circulation, which the orthodoxy mainly under the views of Galen thought flowed due to the ebb and flow of tides. This caused a wit of the time to remark: "I would rather ere with Galen than be right with Harvey" - Galen's theory was the prevailing orthodox view.

Poor old Galileo about a hundred years earlier fell foul of the Catholic Church, when he brought in his new idea of rotation of the planets and challenged the geocentric orthodox view that the Earth was the centre of the Universe. So you see there is nothing as troublesome in science as a new idea and those who dare to put forward new views are still viewed as heretics to be subjected to 'witch hunts.'

Most research that does exist on alternative cancer therapies was carried out between 1920s, 30s and early 40s. The connection between diet and cancer was an era of vigorous scientific inquiry, accounting for an estimated one-third of all research. In both laboratory experiments and epidemiological surveys, scientists learned that excessive fat and calories as well as the relative amounts of protein and vitamins exerted major influences on the origin and course of cancer. These encouraging findings however were covered up and never applied because, in the words of Dean Burke PhD., founder of the American National Cancer Institute: 'After World War II, along came chemotherapy,' which represented a more profitable and fashionable area of investigation. Not until the mid-1970s was research on diet and cancer again acceptable, but again big pharmacy was to dominate the allocation of research grants.

Economics and politics intertwine in shaping conventional medicine's approach to cancer. By the 80s and into the 90s the concern of big business was to wring vast profits from everything that could have a value put on it –

even human life. It was found that *treating* disease was enormously profitable, whereas *preventing* disease was not. The most frightening notion to the big pharmaceutical companies was the prospect of a cure. The established cancer charities at least in the U.K. now saw their assets as more important than their mission. Highly organised and sophisticated they virtually dictated and controlled the way cancer care and research was conducted. The umbrella of various co-ordinating committees meant that 'solidarity and uniformity,' was to ensure a consolidated response. The cancer establishment found that 'singing from the same hymn sheet' was necessary to avoid the rogue maverick scientist.

Rogue mavericks made countless efforts, to show that the impression these organisations created - that cancer would soon be cured, but more money was required, was in fact false. Their voices however would soon be silenced by a monolithic power, which maintained the loyalties of members, by offering large salaries and secure pension pots: nobody would want to stick their neck out. A doctor had to decide whether to take the safe route or have his livelihood threatened, if he questioned the edifice on which this monolithic power was built. When Professor Kenneth Calman, head of clinical oncology at Glasgow University raised concerns over orthodox treatment saying that: 'some forms of cancer treatment, notably radiotherapy and chemotherapy, may actually induce cancer,' he was silenced. But if comments like this cause embarrassment to the orthodox cancer establishment, there is a further revelation, which may make them positively squirm; and that is the extraordinary and deliberately suppressed discovery that many patients would live longer if they refused to submit to harmful treatment and underwent no treatment at all. This does not mean you would recover if you did nothing at all, it means you would simply live longer. To recover one has to take a pro-active approach and undertake an actual alternative programme. The cure time of five years is purposefully set, because that is about the time you would live anyway without orthodox treatment.

Suppression in the field of cancer did not notch up a ratchet until after World War II, which coincided with the rise of the powerful petrochemical industry. The first enlightening investigation on cancer ever done in the U.S was a series of articles written in 1978 and 1979 by reporter Robert Houston in close collaboration with the famous radio commentator Gary Null. Unsurprisingly given the cancer blackout, the articles were rejected by every important newspaper office in the States, only finding acceptance in the relatively obscure publication of *Our Town*, New York's municipal paper and thus not dependent on advertising. Another unlikely medium for this medical news was *Penthouse* magazine whose five and half million voyeurs made this magazine equally independent from any advertising pressure. But then what has advertising ever done for mankind?

To quote a piece from the Houston-Null analysis:

'As a multibillion dollar experiment in how to solve a disease organised cancer research has released its major finding, it has disproved itself. The climax of its failure was the 'War on Cancer.' Began as a PR cause by the Nixon Administration in 1971, the 'War' was acknowledged lost in late May 1978. News of the defeat appeared on the front page of the New York Times; with a banner headline "Cancer Research now Shifting Away from War Policy". With Dr Arthur Upton, Director of the National Cancer Institute, as herald of disaster... The rout was in the flow charts. A river of gold had been pumped into a mammoth establishment whose lush survival depends on the state of no cure. Absurd? Or is it?'

Houston and Null in fact came up with a disturbing speculation. To quote from their analysis:

'A solution to cancer would mean the termination of research programmes, the obsolescence of skills, the end of dreams of personal glory, triumph over cancer would dry up contributions to self-perpetuating charities and cut off funding from Congress, it would mutually threaten the present clinical establishment by rendering obsolete the expensive surgical, radiological and chemotherapeutic treatments in which so much money, training and equipment is invested. Such fear, however unconscious, may result in resistance and hostility to alternative approaches in proportions, as they are therapeutically promising. The new therapy must be disbelieved, denied, discouraged and disallowed at all costs, regardless of actual testing results and preferably without any testing at all. As we shall see, this pattern has in actuality occurred repeatedly and almost consistently'.

Houston and Null went on to say:

'The American Cancer Society or ACS as the medieval church of the current Dark Age of Cancer, has managed to black list the most innovative and promising lines of cancer research, the FDA (Federal Drug Administration) has added muscle to the witch hunt, harassing and persecuting proponents of alternative therapies and road blocking all reasonable attempts at fair testing...The truth eventually must be confronted that the real enemy is not cancer – a natural phenomenon – but the cancer establishment itself, which consistently moves to destroy whatever is hopeful against the disease, and to enlarge its predatory position as a parasite on human suffering'.

The journalists' cynicism was hard to avoid:

'The ACS and the NCI, as a showcase project of the 'War on Cancer', co-sponsored a massive X-ray screening program for breast cancer- on 260,000 women – the notorious mammography follies. With kind smiles and Pollyanna counsel, women were encouraged to affirm their virtue on the altar of technology by exposing themselves to periodic radiation known to increase the risk of the disease...Emphasis was placed on radiating women over 50 – the very group that would be most vulnerable to induction of cancer by radiation...The American Cancer Society seminars are essentially the spring fashion shows of cancer research, letting health and science reporters know where the big money is going though in actuality the expense has yielded almost complete failure...There is always a 'breakthrough' or two announced, and this right round contribution time, which neatly and coincidentally dovetails with the science writers' conference. This annual spectacle exemplifies how some health reporters become engaged in not so much journalism as advertising, thereby boosting the profits of the medical establishment. From the conference, the public receives a barrage of 'progress on cancer' articles, through which its cancer consciousness is raided and its resistance softened by paraded false hopes. Then the fund raising is put into high gear, and cheques by the millions are raked in for the avowed purpose of furthering research to the imminent triumph that lies 'just over the horizon' – where it has remained stuck ever since the ACS began in 1913 as an 'emergency temporary organization'. The alternatives have been covered up by those science writers of the national news media who ride shotgun for the medical establishment's solid-gold cancer train'.

Well that was in 1978/9. However, when I attempted to submit my Ancient Right of Petition to the British Parliament in 1997, all I had asked for in redress was for a panel of multi-disciplined scientists from across the broad spectrum of science disciplines and who were *independent* to read my research paper and the accompanying report and answer 'Yes' or 'No' to the question 'Do you think that this research may represent a solution to the mechanism of cancer?' If the answer was 'Yes,' I asked that a *fair test* be conducted in *fair* clinical trials overseen and maintained *without bias*. However, since only Sheila my co-author and I knew how the mind worked in cancer, I doubt whether unless people were trained in the programme, whether it could be repeated. Further where does one find any independent experts? - By definition they all work for orthodoxy or they would not receive their honorary title of 'expert'. To quote the famous physicist Niels Bohr: 'An expert is a man who has made all the mistakes, which can be made, in a very narrow field'.

Having spent many years working in the British Foreign Office, the thriller writer John Le Carré knew well the mechanics of big business. In his book *'The Constant Gardener'* made into a Hollywood movie, he gave some account of how it *actually* works. Le Carré stated: 'Big Pharma is engaged in the deliberate seduction of the medical profession, country by country, worldwide. It is spending a fortune on influencing, hiring and purchasing academic judgment to a point where, in a few years' time, if Big Pharma continues unchecked on its present happy path, unbought medical opinion will be hard to find'. In actual fact this precise prediction has already come about.

So I could do little more than offer my own story, which was covered in small part by the journalist Liz Hunt in *The Independent* newspaper in *October 1989*. Even so, the article was followed by the obligatory disproof by orthodoxy. The BBC World Service picked up on the story, only to drop it, when I understand Miss Hunt had given some negative comments.

We are victims of the media's regular announcements that the ultimate breakthrough, the one single, sure, safe cure for all types of cancer, is on the verge of being found. These misleading stories probably start in cancer research public relations departments, since the coverage encourages the public to go on raising money. At about the time Liz Hunt was finally persuaded to run my story, a Press Association report published in *The Independent* [10] raised false hopes of a cure. Near the end of the article it was noted that the most spectacular case the article claimed was a cure had survived 18 months. The minimum survival time, required to claim a cure is accepted as five years. Any holistic approach claiming such results after so short a time would be laughed at. In fact my own research paper showed

195

patients with longer survival times – even 5 years - and those patients were classed as terminal! The story stated: 'A new cancer treatment which homes in on cancer cells has saved *two* terminal cancer patients. The treatment, which consists of one injection, has led to a full remission of brain tumours, which had failed to respond to chemotherapy and neurosurgery. The treatment was pioneered in Britain by the Imperial Cancer Research Fund' (*author's emphasis*).

In my own published research paper, despite that some patients had actually survived for more than 5 years, we noted the research was not statistically significant, because some patients were still on-going with the therapy at 18 months and there was not enough patients in the study to prove statistical efficacy – points which did not worry the ICRF in their rush to report their research based on a couple of patients only. In fact our 'cures' were better than those of the reported study from the ICRF, but no newspaper would have dreamt of making a fanfare of our results, even though all patients were classed as terminal!

Well I guess Thomas Jefferson in 1812 was on target when he said: "I was bold in pursuit of knowledge, never fearing to follow truth and reason to whatever results they led." My research was too bold and not politically correct and certainly challenged a multi-billion industry and thus despite a couple of doctors referring to the research paper as "brilliant", it sits collecting dust in the British Library Archives [3].

When a person is diagnosed with cancer, what they are not told is there is a significant body of research and qualified opinion in some cases that represents an alternative to orthodox treatment. Orthodoxy would have us believe that these methods to quote one of the letters in *The Times* in response to Michael Gearin- Tosh's account are the product of greedy 'charlatans', when in fact many alternative practitioners were and are compassionate, qualified medics or scientists – or like myself biochemists. In actual fact the research over a number of years virtually bankrupted me. The 'quackery' accusation is the main accusation that has been aimed since the 1940's and is now a recognised propaganda line. When a person is labelled as such, it has the same effect as labelling a person a "conspiracy theorist", it removes them from public debate, where the tables are turned and you are questioned: this deflects the accuser away from having to confront the evidence. The 'Angle of Death' (Tony Blair) in the Chilcot inquiry in 2009 effectively evaded evidence by labelling his detractors as "conspiracy theorists". I have even had this label thrown at me in a court of law, in order to evade evidence in court.

Houston and Null listed an impressive number of therapics that were not approved by the official medical bodies, which therefore defined such methods at least in the U.S. as quack methods. They claimed:

'Files on unorthodox therapies are kept by various medical agencies as lists of taboo areas to guide funding and funding policies. The central index of heretics is maintained by the American Cancer Society or ACS, the Vatican of the cancer establishment'.

The reporters went on to say:

'ACS Incorporated appears to conceive its mission to be that of axing discoveries that seem too good to be true. As a protection agency for the status quo, the Society issues a widely circulated blacklist, entitled 'Unproven methods of Cancer Treatment,' defaming approaches that have deemed to deviate from the standard cut-burn-poison school of healing.

It seems odd that an organization supposedly devoted to encouraging research by definition the study of the unproven, should use 'unproven' as a pejorative and promote the cardinal error in science of confusing 'unproven' with 'disproven'.'

Exactly, they won't test these therapies and when they do, they set out to *purposefully* make them fail, by various means – the *doomed trial*, which I will return to in the case of the Bristol Cancer Help Centre in the UK - a case that occurred in 1990.

There are many facets to this scene, which hold back new ideas especially in the alternative field. Young doctors start learning their profession only when they leave medical school and their real contact with patients' starts. Junior doctors begin their real pharmacological education, when drug manufacturers flood them with glossy brochures. High-pressure salesmen from the Chemical Syndicate often visit General Practitioners but doctors do not write the brochures, which are written by copywriters and art directors for advertising agencies or by 'In House' teams of the pharmaceutical company. The advertising men and women don't understand the product but they produce convincing copy and certainly no serious side effects will be listed.

Even the so-called 'safe' painkiller paracetamol and aspirin can hospitalise you and recently it has been questioned whether codeine should be removed altogether. The cancer drugs are not only in most cases carcinogenic but many can have serious side effects. Drug companies test their drugs in animals in order to gain a licence, which deems the drug safe for clinical trials. However the animal method of testing is not assured. Apart from the horrendous experiments on innocent animals, dangerous drugs like thalidomide can slip through the safety net. Hans Ruesch in his anti-vivisection book '*Slaughter of the Innocent*' [12] gave animal testing as the causation of the thalidomide tragedy. The animal model does not equate in many cases with the human model.

Ruesch's exposé of the Chemical Syndicate covering the interlocking nature of the big industries from steel to oil to aviation to armament was radical in its time. Ruesch claimed that the Medical Power enables the Chemical Syndicate to palm off on the world's population, conditioned through brainwashing, a never-ending line of 'New' medications that replace those whose uselessness and danger can no longer be concealed. As any advertising executive knows the word 'new' removes the necessity to look at the old efficacy figures. Ruesch in his second book entitled '*The Naked Empress*' [13] stated:

'In every country, the ruling Medical Power is one of the Syndicate's most reliable collaborators, the more efficient for being unrecognised by the ignorant, misled majority. The Medical Power has today the role that belonged to the Church in the Middle- Ages'.

Through its immense wealth and ruthless tactics the Chemical Syndicate influences not only domestic policies but also foreign governments. It is well known that Food Aid financed by taxpayers is used as a method of imposing chemicals, be they drugs or vaccines, agrochemicals or genetically modified food on Third World Nations.

Kurt Bluchel author of '*The White Magicians*' [14] published in Germany in 1974 defined the Chemical Syndicate as: 'A business Association, a very strict form of Cartel with its own legal structure and administration' and further as a 'criminal organisation masked as a legitimate business enterprise'. Bluchel noted that the essential ground structures of both types of Syndicate are identical and that the statutes of our Medical organization can correctly be defined by this term. He went on to say that what marks the Syndicate in a commercial sense is *the monopolization of all products and services of a particular type*. Whoever needs products or services of this type, can get them only from the Syndicate. From this derives the immense power of the Syndicate, whose monopolistic nature enables it to blackmail markets and society. The lion's share of the Syndicate's revenues goes to a very small group of directors, who dictate how all the internal and external Syndicate affairs are to be handled. On the other hand, the Syndicate ensures for each one of its ordinary members a very good income and pension – well above the national average and even into the stratosphere. A small board of directors makes the big money; the ones who never rock the Syndicate's boat.

The banking system also operates like this, where we have seen the obscene salaries and pension pots these men walk off with; along with bonuses to keep the next generation of board managers in line. The greed and disregard for the consequences to the greater part of humanity is certainly not recognised, as the boss of Goldman Sachs illustrated in *The Sunday Times* newspaper [15]. Goldman Sachs, the bank that is set to pay a record £12 billion in salaries and bonuses in 2009 told the newspaper that banks serve a 'social purpose' and do 'God's work'. As with the banking profession, the medical hierarchy and the Chemical Syndicate there is an illusionary view of monolithic and monopolistic power, justified by claiming it oils the capitalist system and pays for jobs and salaries that keep the rest of us alive.

Doctors may be misguided, or even uneducated in alternative methods, but they are not the real issue. It is the Chemical Syndicate, the small number of Chief executives that effectively blackmail governments and even ordinary members of the medical profession. Bluchel pointed out that the Syndicate has all the features of a *secret society* and considers itself outside the law of the land, or rather above the law of the land. I did go on to research the history of the secret groups in 4 volumes of *The Theatre Earth* books.

Doctors can no longer confront their profession. I once asked an oncologist to look at my research. He told me that if he looked at my research, he might have to question what he was doing and he was not prepared to do that. I was fairly jaw hung at the time because what he was really saying was that if I had discovered the mechanism of cancer, he did not want to know about it, because it would threaten his world and his job. "We certainly can't solve problems by using the same kind of thinking we used to create them" as Einstein once remarked.

Dr Vernon Coleman in his book entitled '*The Medicine Men*' [16] in 1975 wrote: 'As it stands, the drug industry seems to be ruining the medical profession. Doctors are pushed around and bullied and bribed by the Drug industry. They have undoubtedly lost control of their own profession and must consequently be held responsible for all the disasters and errors which bad prescribing produces. It is not fair simply to blame the drug industry (whose sole purpose is to make a profit) for not having strong ethics. The responsibility must be laid fairly and squarely on the medical profession'.

Doctors have studied hard and completed long hours as junior doctors, before they rise up the ladder. They are very well paid so they are not going to risk all that and their pensions by rocking any boats that would bring them into conflict with the medical hierarchy or government. History is scattered with the ruined lives of 'whistle-blowers' and scientists are particularly vulnerable. Even as I update this, one doctor is being sued for libel by an American Drug Company for reporting adverse reactions of a drug *at a scientific meeting*! In the UK several doctors and lawyers are calling for an inquest into the death of Dr David Kelley the British scientist and weapons expert, who they claim could not have committed suicide over the Iraq Dossier, by cutting his ulna artery. Dr Kelley effectively blew the whistle on Tony Blair's government over the Iraq dossier which claimed Saddam Hussein had Weapons of Mass Destruction with a launch and strike capability of '45 minutes,' a claim now known to be false.

Then there is the case of Dr Wakefield in the UK, whose only crime it seems was to put patients first when he published a *Lancet* article expressing reasonable fears about the triple MMR vaccine and autism. The General Medical Council (GMC) in what many viewed as the Establishment's spite struck off Dr Wakefield.

What is evident from these cases as with the early pioneers of alternative medicine is that no scientist can afford a conscience, or propose new ideas, which threaten the orthodoxy and vested interests or government policies. Whistle blowing in the public interest if it conflicts with vested interests is subject to a degree of revenge that few scientists are willing to confront.

Science is no longer the pursuit of truth; it is merely the whore of capitalism. For my part for 23 years I stood on the front battle line and I can assure you the battle has been formidable.

A GCSE science course book, printed in 2009 in the UK, discussed the case of Dr Andrew Wakefield, stating that Wakefield's research had been 'completely discredited'. It had certainly been attacked at the time the book was printed, but it was not until the start of 2010 that the ruling Medical body the General Medical Council ruled against Dr Wakefield and discredited his research. This poses the question as to the impartiality of his hearing, when the outcome it appears had already been printed in children's' science course books in 2009! The journalist who reported this stated: 'This 'completely discredited' tastes to me like establishment bullying of a scientist who said something unwelcome' [17].

What is noticeable is the speed with which orthodoxy move to imprint their views on the young – the next generation of compliant witless sheep. Even though the global warming debate is not over and still open, virtually all science courses even the very early Key Stage 3 courses present *man- made* global warming as a statement of fact, with regards to man- made carbon dioxide emissions. Ah yes brainwashing starts early – catch them before they can think independently, or form a scientific argument based upon research and two opposing views, which is the history of science *innovation.*

The case of Dr Barry Durrant-Peatfield mirrors that of Dr Wakefield. In 2001 Dr Durrant-Peatfield had his license to practice medicine suspended for 18 months by The General Medical Council (GMC) in the UK. The doctor claimed: "If I'd had the Pope there to defend me, it would have gone the same way. This is purely their excuse to get me off the register to practice thyroid and adrenal medicine". Dr Durrant-Peatfield was in fact practising alternative thyroid care and the GMC took a predictable stance in support of orthodox policy. He came to the attention of the GMC not through any complaint; far from it he had hundreds of satisfied patients who supported him. It was claimed that the GMC was really opposed to his success and the fact he worked with the *natural* prescription thyroid drug - Armour thyroid and his treatments were sometimes considered unconventional by the National Health Service's highly restrictive approach to thyroid treatment. It was claimed that the GMC was not seeking to act in the public's best interests through handling complaints or other information, which casts doubt on a doctor's fitness to practise, since there were no complaints. It was suggested by Dr Durrant-Peatfield's supporters that he was no "threat to the public" as the GMC claimed, but instead the GMC had conducted a witch-hunt to weed out unconventional doctors.

Such proceedings sound like a process that is far too familiar, even in the United States where vilification of alternative practitioners, and in some cases, efforts to remove alternative or unconventional doctors from medical practice is part of policy. Between anti-alternative medicine site *Quackwatch*, which labelled America's most popular alternative medicine experts – such as Andrew Weil, M.D. Deepak Chopra, M.D and Bernie Siegal, M.D. as 'quacks' – to the effort to take away the license of a New York holistic physician Serafina Corsello, M.D, conventional medicine has been on the offensive, since the rapid rise in interest of alternative therapies mainly dating from the 80's.

Dr Robert Sinaiko in the year 2,000 was one of the more recent in a long line of California medical doctors to be persecuted by the California Medical Board (CMB) for using effective therapies not sanctioned by organized medicine. Shula Edelkind of the Progress in Medicine Foundation (PMF) met Sinaiko when he was a medical advisor for the Feingold Association, which developed a dietary regimen similar to the Gerson Therapy that allows toxic food additives to be removed from the diet and purged from the body. Use of the Feingold program has helped thousands of adults and children recover from behavioural problems without the use of addictive psychotropic drugs such as Ritalin. There lies the problem for the pharmaceutical industry. Despite that Sinaiko is a board-certified internist and allergist/immunologist who has been in practise for 29 years without one reported incident of harming a patient; he underwent a court hearing, based on one father's complaint who was seeking custody of his son and therefore sought to use Sinaiko as the means to that end against his former wife. Unfortunately even in my own case this is depressingly familiar where I was dragged through Wardship proceedings with my ex-husband. Sinaiko was effectively put out of business as Edelkind said: 'The CMB disciplinary process shows that evidence does not matter, expert testimony does not matter and logic, reason and truth do not matter'. Certainly in courts of law in the UK I have experienced the same – you can kiss goodbye to evidence where there is a policy and bias and you might just as well be in a court of Alice in Wonderland.

Edelkind claimed the California Medical Board has been at the forefront of impeding medical progress in the U.S. since it was used to discredit the use of Laetrile in the treatment of cancer throughout the 1950s and 1960s The CMB was so concerned about advances in medicine that were allowing doctors to successfully treat cancers and other degenerative diseases holistically and inexpensively that it lobbied and passed "anti-quackery" laws in 1964. These laws have been used to professionally assassinate and criminally prosecute physicians who choose to heal their patients without the approval of the state board and the FDA.

As far back as 1961 Dr Walter Modell of Cornell University's Medical College, whom *Time* magazine described as one of America's foremost drug experts wrote in the journal – *'Clinical Pharmacology and Therapeutics,'* 'when will they realize that there are too many drugs'. He went on to add, 'At the moment the most helpful contribution is the new drug to counteract the untoward effects of other new drugs'.

J. Ehrenreich in his book *'The Cultural Crisis of Modern Medicine '*[18] commented that the claim of efficacy of drugs is also dubious. A National Academy of Sciences panel, studying the effectiveness of prescription drugs in the USA in the mid-sixties, found that 50% of these drugs were either ineffective, or ineffective in the form normally prescribed or at best 'possibly effective'. Today one would never gain grant funding to test this and certainly no one would publish the results as drug companies have taken to issuing libel writs. Science is no longer free to carry out research, which looks at either efficacy or safety. To find a newspaper or media outlet that is willing to question the very foundation on which the health services lie and methods used would be unthinkable: and certainly a public brought up on a diet of drugs for the treatment of illness and brainwashed via the science curriculum, would squeal if that were to happen and so the dog chases its own tail.

We will always need some drugs, such as penicillin, which have been proven to work and have saved many lives: and surgeons are brilliant craftsmen and their skills will always be required. However it is the overload of drugs and the dependency on those, which is in question. J. Williams in his book *'Nutrition Against Disease'* [19] stated:

'The basic fault of drugs is that they have no known connection with the disease process itself...drugs are wholly unlike nature's weapons... They tend

203

to mask the difficulty, not eliminate it. They contaminate the internal environment with the side effects, create dependence on the part of the patient, and often complicate the physician's job by erasing valuable clues as to the real source of the trouble'.

Many support groups who could assist people, are guided by orthodox medicine. In the case of arthritis and rheumatism the line of approach in treatment is the use of Non- Steroidal Anti-inflammatory Drugs or NSAIDS. Despite the cost to the Health Service and often-elaborate claims Charles Medawar in his book '*The Wrong Kind of Medicine*' [20] claimed that none of them are superior to aspirin: as the authors of the *Health Action International Drugs Pack* pointed out: 'The development of products of this type accounts for a substantial part of the total investment of the pharmaceutical industry and the number of compounds available has multiplied within the last two decades, though without a proportional advance in the quality of treatment they can offer'. Further, 'an obvious reason for concentrating on the development of NSAIDS is the large number of people who will use these products. In Northern Europe some 5% of all adults are at any given moment undergoing treatment for one or another of the rheumatic disorders, which comprise the main indication for NSAIDS'.

The sales of NSAIDS in some 40 countries in a twelve-month period in 1983-1984 accounted for more than $2,500,000,000 at manufacturers' prices, excluding sales of various brands of aspirin and other painkillers. These figures give some idea of the kind of money we are talking about and when you compare rheumatism and arthritis to the business of cancer and chronic heart disease then profits escalate. One begins to see why a solution to the problem of chronic degenerative disease and especially cancer is always just around the corner – the blunt truth is that it has been more profitable to look for a cure than to find one.

Iatrogenic illness or illness created from drug side effects is indeed responsible for hundreds of thousands of people hospitalised each year. The reason this battle never reaches the ears or eyes of public is because of that interlocking web of interests. Journals, newspapers, magazines, commercial TV and radio stations, beholden to advertisers or subservient to government do not wish to upset their own applecart. Houston and Null defined the problem very clearly in the 1970's:

'The American Cancer Society lends its support to prominent science writer Jane Brody of the New York Times. In 1977 she co-authored an article entitled '*You Can Fight Cancer and Win*' with Arthur Holleb M.D and Vice President of the American Cancer Society. In the same year the society awarded Brody its Merit award for 'excellence in communications' for her gushingly pro-chemotherapy article entitled '*The Drug War on Cancer.*' As President of the American Society of Journalists and Authors, Science writer Pat Mc Grady Jr., wrote a celebrated article on the success with Vitamin A and enzyme therapy for cancer at the Janker Clinic Bohn in Germany. The piece, which many felt is one of the classics of American journalism, finally appeared in *Esquire* after 5 years of rejection by many other magazines.

As for Pat's father Patrick Mc Grady Sr., he had resigned from the ACS for reasons of principle and summed it up: 'Nobody in the science and medical departments at ACS is capable of doing real science. They are wonderful pros who know how to raise money. They don't know how to prevent cancer or cure patients'.

The true history of innovation in scientific thought, never came out of the academic institutions, the main advances came from men or women working in garden sheds, or performing their own private experiments like NikolaTesla who very nearly brought down a high rise apartment block in New York with one of his experiments. Einstein never formally qualified and was a shipping clerk.

Even in 1981 Dr Robert Nefferberg and Robert Taylor in their book entitled '*The Cancer Conspiracy*' stated:

'The directed research practises and other activities of the National Cancer Institute (NCI) and of the American Cancer Society (ACS) have been scandalously counter-productive in the conquest of cancer, in spite of the billions of dollars expended. The cancer establishment is closed to new approaches and ideas, thus creating a self-perpetuating system with no clear objectives remotely in sight'.

As we remember though in a Syndicate a small number of people at the top receive big salaries and maintain the status quo. It is hardly surprising that the Cancer charities make slow headway when the majority of funds go towards staff salaries, plush buildings and pensions etc.: further celebrities eager to be seen as philanthropists or just to be seen, will attend fund raising events and appear in commercials. Care is taken to promote in advertising only those who themselves or a relative have overcome cancer by orthodox means. Success stories and tear stories bring in funding.

Try as I might to raise funds for the research study I carried out, applying to no less than 30 cancer research funding bodies for a slice of the solid gold gravy train that is available and setting up a charity – Karnak, a pub quiz brought in £400 and that was it – research on a shoe string you might say. This did not account for my own considerable outlay. 'Charlatans' are we? By 1993 I had enough, I shelved the hope of an alternative cancer research centre and fed up with legal battles took off for Greece to set up a healing centre in the Greek tradition. No one can quite believe me when I say that I was walking in Holborn in London, near to the law courts in 1989, when a barrister turned and said to me "Just remember that from now on Big Brother is watching you". I thought he was joking but he was not. I replied: "So is God" – which left him temporarily mute.

Professor Ian Kennedy and Dr David Greaves wrote a forward to a small booklet by *The Natural Medicines Society* entitled '*The Health Crisis*' authored by Chris Thompson and Denis Mc Eoin [21]. Professor Kennedy who headed the Centre of Medical Law and Ethics at King's College London had this to say: 'Over the past 30 years a succession of commentators has put forward various critiques of modern medicine. The common theme has been that the system of western medicine is in crises'. The authors in their introduction stated: 'Indeed the World Health Organisation, in examining the relative merits of professional and lay health care, found that modern medicine appears to have contributed little to the overall decline in mortality. Not only this, the World Health Organisation also concluded that, beyond a certain basic provision of health-care services, there appeared to be a *negative correlation* between medical services and health'. Note my emphasis – 'a negative correlation'.

There is now a body of research to support this view. In America for example, the health of the average person has, if anything deteriorated over the last thirty years or so, yet the amount spent on health care rose from 3.5% of gross National Product in 1950 to over 10% in 1980. Basic health care is now an open argument in the States, but they should consider carefully which way they want to go in terms of the type of provision – expensive orthodox or

206

cheaper alternative. Agreed there is probably a basic repertoire of drugs that are considered essential such as penicillin, but do we really need thousands, some of which are incredibly expensive and may provide no better outcome than complementary therapy. The fact is that capitalism will continue to dictate policy on treatment and that includes cancer.

Clearly to say that modern medicine may be a factor working *against* health is a serious charge and yet there is now evidence in support of that view. Serious illness and particularly cancer is on the increase and ultimately we are going to have to accept that health versus disease in many cases is a life-style choice. In a consumer driven society you will always have a high incidence of disease and mental illness, because the majority experience constant loss when confronted with the great divide of the 'have's' and 'have not's'. Loss is a killer - as I will cover in the section on the mind in illness.

Brian Inglis in his book entitled *'Diseases of Civilisation'* [22] noted that it was assumed that the demand for health services would rise sharply as soon as the free National Health Service (in the UK) came into being, because so many people who had lived with their lumbago or rotten teeth would now be able to be treated. But surely as soon as the backlog had been worked through, the Welfare State's benefits – free maternity services, free advice on prevention linked with free immunisation procedures would mean that fewer people would fall ill? By the mid 1950's when initial demands on the National Health Service were expected to decline, living standards were rising more rapidly than ever before, which in itself, might have been expected to lead to considerable improvement in the Nation's health. In fact the opposite was true and real spending in the NHS rose year by year to its current astronomical level of 121 billion pounds.

In the case of Britain, as the Empire collapsed in the 40's and 50's a large influx of Commonwealth immigrants occurred and this has not been factored into Inglis's account. Following further massive influxes of European Union immigrants the NHS has struggled to cope with demand: and where in a recent newspaper article it was reported that Britain had dropped to 14th in the World in its standard of health care, just above countries that were always considered to have poor health facilities. That fact was not widely reported. There is no data to show whether the NHS would have been cost effective, if there had been low-level immigration. A radical re-think is now required on the goals of the NHS as clearly the premise on which it was set up has changed.

The NHS must consider its options of whether to go on buying expensive drugs or provide other cheaper services. Drugs however for common day illness are now ingrained into overall expectations of what health care consists of – medication. A person goes to the doctor and expects a 'quick fix' and leaves with a prescription. Melvyn Werback in his book entitled '*Third Line Medicine*' [23] had this to say: 'The assumption has been that the body can be regarded as a machine whose protection from disease and its effects depends primarily on internal intervention, an approach which has led to indifference to the external influences and personal behaviour which are the predominant determination of health'.

Recently through various TV programmes and health initiatives, people are more aware of the effect of diet and lifestyle upon health, but very contradictory views often emerge from media such as informing people that diet has little if any effect on cancer, which is not true. Cancer if one includes the mechanism of the mind is a unique personal disease to each individual. There are in each case unique mind traumas, triggers, allied environmental causative factors that come together and which have to be addressed as *a whole*. This holistic approach to cancer however is expensive in terms of *time* and therefore is not cost effective compared to orthodox treatment and use of high technology and drugs, where patients are processed for speed. It takes time to sit down with a cancer patient and deal with all the causative factors, but particularly the mechanism of the mind. Counselling is beyond the economic reach of many and because counsellors do not understand the mechanism of the mind, they are often not effective in dealing with cancer or chronic degenerative disease.

In the 80s The London Food Commission a pressure group catalogued many examples of excessive official secrecy. In their list of the 'Secret Seven' they gave seven areas in which the government in the UK had conspired to keep data secret.

'1. The results of the Government/Health Education Council/Industry Working party on Nutrition NACNE, were kept secret for two and half years because its message for dietary improvements were opposed by powerful industry interests.

2. The preliminary result of a 1983 DHSS survey of Schoolchildren's diets, commissioned after the standards for school meals were abolished showed that many children ate a poor diet.

3. The Official Secrets Act, regardless of whether members have signed, covers much of the data examined by government committees on food. The government claims this is necessary to protect commercially sensitive data from competitors.

4. For over 20 years all evidence relating to pesticide safety was an official secret. After a public outcry the Advisory Committee on Pesticides published its first report in 1986 but still kept basic data on pesticide toxicity a secret.

5. The DHSS repeatedly refused to reveal the amount allocated for food in its welfare benefit payments.

6. With the exception of the 1979 report on colour additives, the Ministry of Agriculture, Fisheries and Food (MAFF) did not published estimates of quantities of additive consumed: yet such data was used by the government to interpret safety studies and to give clearance to additives. Requests for this data received the reply: "As for consumption figures, we do not have them".

7. MAFF misleads even the scientific 'experts' who supervise its work. Its own evidence suggests that at least 30% of food has detectable pesticide residues. However the chairman of MAFF's scientific sub-committee said on radio that only 1% of foods sampled had detectable residues'.

In the 80's none of these "secrets" would have been damaging to national security. When finally in the year 2,000 the Freedom of Information laws were introduced in the UK, information became easier to gain, but certain safety issues are still not placed in the public domain. Food was a subject where massive publicity and transparency was needed, not maximum security: and still is now with the GM debate.

Jonathan Aitken then M.P told the House of Commons in 1985: "The lack of information and secrecy causes the consumer to have little confidence in government decision-making on food. It is a myth that these protected secrets are damaging to national security – you mean we might all panic? The USA and many other countries operate freedom of information legislation. Why don't we follow suit?"

Britain was always one step behind when it came to 'freedom to know' and it was not until TV chef Jamie Oliver took up the cause of British children's school meals some 20 years later that the issue was opened up. I mention this background since at this time in the late 80s, I was trying to get my cancer research looked at, which obviously was a hopeless quest.

In a retrograde step going back to this era, I note an article in *The Guardian* newspaper (16.11.2010) 'Inquiry urged over industry role in shaping health policy'. To quote:

'Diane Abbott, the shadow public health minister, is calling for the health select committee to launch an inquiry into government moves to put Mc Donald's, PepsiCo and food manufacturers such as Unilever and Kellogg's at the heart of writing policy on obesity, diet-related disease and alcohol misuse in the UK.

Abbott said she was "shocked" by revelations that the health secretary, Andrew Lansley, has set up five networks dominated by the food, alcohol and retail industries to write "responsibility deals" between business and government to tackle the crises of public health.

Professor Philip James, who was the lead adviser to the government on the setting up of the Food Standards Agency, and until recently chair of the International Obesity Task Force, said he was 'scandalised' by the government inviting industry to help draft public health policy. 'It is a major setback for the health of the nation. The sabotaging of public health by the food industry is universally recognised'.

This is what has happened in the case of cancer where the pharmaceutical industry has taken over as the 'experts,' where business interests are placed above public health and valid research.

To further quote from the article:

'Capewell, of Liverpool University, was on the public health commission Lansley set up before the election to make recommendations to the

Conservatives on diet-related diseases and alcohol abuse, but said that he now believes the commission was set up to suit business interests.

Capewll is gagged by a confidentiality undertaking from describing the detailed discussion of the commission. However, he said he felt the process had been "carefully stage stage-managed" – the health representatives were always in a minority, and those individuals were put under intense pressure to support the party line when it came to the wording of the report. Specifically, he says, describing foods high in fat, salt or sugar as junk food was brusquely ruled out'.

Presumably then in line with vested interests profits, we can also expect a rise in the incidence of heart disease and cancer in lower socio-economic groups where austerity cuts will mean a diet of cheap food, with no expensive fruit and vegetables – and junk food promoted by the manufacturers.

I met up with the American Jeremy Rifkin in 1988 who was a long-standing critic of the biotechnology industry then emerging. He was in London to spell out the potential risks associated with the new generation of GM food or biological products. One of his major battles had been the four-year battle in California to prevent the release of a genetically engineered microbe called 'Frostban', which was designed to protect strawberries from frost damage. Rifkin argued the threat to biodiversity and thought that by knocking out a naturally occurring microbe by the Frostban microbe, that this ultimately might threaten rainfall. He lost the battle however and the courts finally granted the company – Advanced Genetics Incorporated, permission to proceed with trials. Rifkin argued at the time: "The scale of risk is enormous". He warned of the more frightening prospect that the US patent Office was extending patenting laws to include all higher forms of animals: "altered or mutated by genetic engineering or other techniques". Rifkin said to me at the time: "It's a step nearer to a brave new world". He fumed: "How can you own a species that's been around thousands of years just because you tinkered with it – a horse is a horse – right? The guy at the Patent Office said: no that's not quite right. A horse is just a temporary situation – it only represents a certain amount of information, and that can now be changed". Meaning as we all suspected that everything was up for grabs - all for commercial exploitation and profit – unbridled greed definitely emerged in the 80s. It is difficult to imagine now the sense of astonishment, urgency and total outrage we all felt in 'The Movement' as it was called back in the 80s. My own feelings as a scientist were one of outrage that instead of remaining custodians of this planet, scientists were seeking to profit from the creation of "Frankenstein" products changing genetic codes that had successfully evolved and adapted over billions of years. One could not help comparing such products to the cautionary tale by Mary Shelley – Frankenstein or 'The Modern Prometheus'. In the novel the scientist Victor Frankenstein learns how to create life, in the form of man-monster, which eventually kills off everything Frankenstein holds dear to him.

Even as I updated this, I noted an article in *The Times* (*July 12th 2010*) – *'Antarctic 'disaster' as China moves in for the krill'*: 'Conservationists are warning of a potential disaster in Antarctica as China seeks to exploit the world's last untapped ocean'. Penguins and seals depend on the krill, which is a basic component of the Antarctic food web and therefore fundamental to the survival of that food web. You find yourself thinking 'God what now!' The exploitation on this planet is itself a food chain and web, with the few powerful predators at the top and the man in the street is merely the krill. Eventually when man has exploited all resources to the point of extermination, he will turn on his own species - as the last conflict cycle ended with a nuclear war.

You might say that in the 80s the change to rabid commercialism and the greed was starting to rapidly surface and there were a few people, who started to wake up and fight, but the majority slumbered on. In Britain the GM story was yet to unfold and the worry then was the secret trials of the hormone Bovine Somatotrophin or BST – bovine growth hormone (BGH), which promote the increase of the milk yield by as much as 40%. Because of my concerns on the mechanism of cancer, I took up the issue. In the UK secret trials of the hormone had been carried out by the old Ministry of Agriculture, Fisheries and Food (MAFF) on behalf of a number of drug companies. Rifkin had managed to stop this in the United States. In fact the hormone in milk was already being sold in British outlets and entering the food chain, but 'guinea pigs' were not allowed to know where it was sold. All my enquiries on safety studies were simply ignored and I was given curt responses merely stating the hormone was safe to the public even in milk given to babies. Now we have cloned animals and their products such as milk entering the food chain.

Geoffrey Cannon in his book *'The Politics of Food'* (1988) had this to say:

'Any public health problem must necessarily be a political issue, and in good times, a political opportunity. Anybody concerned with public health in Britain today is however, faced with what may prove to be an intractable problem, which is there is no evident vested interest in good health. In the cold gloom of short-term economics, which is a good as we generally get nowadays, a healthy citizen is a wretched proposition'.

The problem was always what is called the 'revolving door', where a majority of the scientists who advise government on official food policy are linked in some way with the manufacturers of highly processed foods. These links may take the form of research grants, consultancies or membership of food-industry funded organisations. In the 80s I worked out that 250 Members of Parliament also had links with the food industry, which took the form of consultancies, present or past employment within the food industry, or simply a constituency interest.

The Annual Report of giant pharmaceutical Smith Kline Beecham (SKB) in 1999 illustrated the principle of the revolving door and the interlocking nature of directorships, where a number of board members were linked through directorships to other companies, banks and organisations. Sir Peter Walters the Non-executive Chairman of SKB was also Deputy Chairman of HSBC Holdings plc. and Chairman of the Institute of Economic Affairs and Director of Saatchi and Saatchi plc. Sir Christopher Hogg also a non-executive Director was also a non-executive Chairman of Reuters Group PLC and Allied Domecq PLC and Chairman of the Ford Foundation. Donald F McHenry as a non-executive Director also held non-executive Directorships at Coca-Cola, Bank Boston and AT&T Co. He previously served as Ambassador and U.S. Permanent Representative to the United Nations. Sir Ian Prosser another non-executive Director was also Chairman and Chief Executive of Bass plc. and non-executive Deputy Chairman of BP Amoco plc. The list continues but in terms of connections to powerful organisations Peter Sutherland the Non-Executive Co-Chairman of SMKB in 1999, it is interesting to note that he was also on the Council on Foreign Relations, Chairman of the Overseas Development Council with further connections to GATT and World Trade Organisations and the Bilderberg group which has often been dubbed 'the Secret Government of the World'. In effect the Board of SKB as with the Board of any blue chip multinational contains powerfully connected people with interlocking interests and directorships.

The mission statement from SKB – to improve the quality of human life, illustrates the conflict of interest when board members hold senior positions with corporations that do not have mankind's best interests to heart, including directorships of alcohol, tobacco and chemical-pollutant conglomerates and even in companies like Rio Tinto who once had an appalling human rights record, continually exposing its workers to toxic fumes, lead, arsenic and radioactive materials, leading to serious illnesses including cancer.

The Food and Drink Federation (FDF) was set up in the UK to protect the industry in Whitehall, Westminster and Brussels and it became the 'talking head' of the industry, with which the government negotiated. The outward mission of the FDF was to protect fresh food for the public, but it was found to be an association working on behalf of the big manufacturers. When I looked into the FDF I found 30 leading scientists serving on this committee, eight of whom also served on government advisory committees – those links were never acknowledged in government reports. Thus the ludicrous position arose in 1986, when The Scientific Technical Committee a think-tank for the British Food-Manufacturing Committee, helped the FDF to set up a campaign to *defend* chemical food and additives and also championed the legislation for food irradiation. The media then set about convincing the public that chemicalised food was not harmful and the position is still retained today. The label "conspiracy theorist" arose at about this time in the 80s, to hide evidence and cover up effectively the big whopping lie. By labelling someone as a "conspiracy theorist" you effectively removed from them any credibility and justice they might seek in provision of evidence. It is a label used by vested interests to protect their lies and a method of social control.

Barbara and John Ehrenreich in their book '*Medicine and Social Control*' [24]; and Irving Kennet Zola in his book '*Medicine as an Institution of Social Control*' [25]; and Thomas Szasy in '*The Theology of Medicine; the political philosophical foundations of Medical Ethics*' [26] all argued that modern medicine was a way of producing conformity. It might seem reasonable in a democratic society to allow a small minority of 'awkward' individuals to indulge their unconventional convictions by choosing to opt out of orthodox cancer treatment, but the hostility I encountered from doctors when I did so, was proof at the time of a more powerful kind of state, more akin to Communism or Fascism.

In 1974, Kurt Bluchel the author of 'Weisse Muger'- *The White Magicians*' [14] was forced to remove his book from the market. He exposed the

214

pharmaceutical racket in Germany's Federal Republic and proved it to be the foremost culprit for the rise of chronic diseases, malformations and cancers. As Bluchel pointed out, the tenet of multi-national corporations is more or less: 'look buddy we are the main taxpayers and principle employers in the land. We keep the state on its feet. It is we, mainly who keep you boys. So it's only fair that we should have a say in how things are run. If you make any kind of trouble for us, we simply shut down our factories and move to some underdeveloped country, which will receive us with open arms. Anyway, yours and the people's welfare are close to our heart, as we work for the benefit of mankind'. The Indian Government in the enquiry into the Bhopal disaster, in 2010, refrained from prosecution of Directors including the Chief Executive of Union Carbide - Warren Anderson, because they were worried western companies would not set up businesses in India: basically then the tenet of economic blackmail from the 70s still holds and today bankers use much the same argument.

The orthodox view of illness rests upon two assumptions that firstly all illness can be classified into specific named diseases and secondly that each disease should have a specific cause and preferably can then be treated with a specific drug. Labels are often hung around children's necks with this or that illness and which might be considered as a behavioural problem, but more often is a result of life-style choices of the family. Poverty however provides few life-style choices. We have been educated in applying labels for each disease and the expectation is that the pharmaceutical industry can provide a cure in the form of a tailor-made drug or vaccine for each label. The Gerson Therapy is non-specific in so far as it can cure a number of apparently non-related illnesses and diseases, which implies that the root cause of many illnesses lies in a common causation at the biochemical and metabolic level.

As I updated this, I noticed an article in *The Guardian* (*1ˢᵗ Oct. 2010*), which reported drug companies were accused of attempting to turn the loss of sexual desire that some women experience into a medical condition that can be treated by pills. Although drugs, from antidepressants to variants of Viagra have been found ineffective, the companies were charged in an article in the British Medical Journal with inappropriately trying to create a market for pills to treat a condition that is as much psychological as biological, and which may need the intervention of a relationship counsellor as much as a doctor. Indeed and even a regressive counsellor.

If illness and cancer is to be regarded as an enemy, then the appropriate course of action must be to destroy that enemy, even if some harm is done to one's own forces at the same time – collateral damage. In such a context as this, it would be inconceivable that illness should instead be viewed as a helpful, though often severe, a reminder that perhaps there is something at fault with one's lifestyle, attitudes and environment. It is precisely because this latter possibility has largely been ignored that so little attention has been paid in the past to the whole concept of health promotion. There is no question that basic health care is the sign of a civilised society, but one should be careful on how much responsibility is withdrawn from the individual and given to the State. I feel that the angry letters in the London *Times* in response to Michael Gearin - Tosh's story, may stem from the attitude that the Welfare State said it would look after us from cradle to grave and there really is no need to think for yourself in between or take responsibility: we are assured that we are looked after by "experts" and it is not for you to question them. Governments then appear to be in a tug of war with themselves: on the one hand they ask the citizen to take responsibility and then fight him if he does!

However, the main problem is paying for alternatives, when the National Health Service does not in many cases provide the spectrum of therapies that are available in the private sector of alternative health care. The problem could be overcome by issuing people with a 'credit' for any one illness, to spend according to their own choice and where hospitals or clinics offer those choices.

There is in some respects more awareness now of prevention than when I developed cancer in 1986, but the drug mentality is still with us. Instead of seeking to find out why a patient is ill they are classified according to textbook medical descriptions of their disease – cancer types etc. Doctors no longer have the training or attitude in most cases to deal with patients in human terms. To be fair to them they are allocated so little contact time with the patient, which at least in the UK is 10 minutes and about to be reduced to 6 minutes that a personal approach is impossible. The personal approach requires time and personal qualities, whereas in 10 minutes the government expects the GP to identify the illness and write a drug prescription. The distance the doctor takes from his patient also allows him to process them without becoming emotionally involved. Until we accept the individual as a whole, rather than just the symptoms, which present themselves at the physical level, we can never understand illness. The first question that a cancer patient often asks themselves is "Why me?" They may be absolved from answering that question honestly by orthodox medicine, but it is a question that the alternative therapist will require *you* to find the answer to.

The tumour is really a symptom that all is not well in your world: getting rid of it will not rectify the underlying cause. If one honestly reviews one's life one can see that there were many warning signs, before a tumour manifested but they were not acknowledged or acted upon. You really do have to be brutally honest with yourself, when diagnosed with cancer or a chronic degenerative disease.

In holistic medicine, the view is of the whole life of the person as important in the onset of any disease. One cannot take any one isolated factor in this approach - one considers all factors, which have brought the person to illness. Importantly this includes psychology or at least mental attitudes and experiences. Sometimes a cancer patient has said to me: "Oh yes, I can see now where I was doing fine and then this happened"... and so on. The slippery slope as I call it. In my own case I suspected very early on what had happened and set about ruthlessly eliminating those factors and persons, which I knew to be contributively linked. Unless you make those vital decisions, and take control over your life, it would be difficult to survive a serious illness like cancer, where as if to give you a major clue the cells are out of control and not communicating with each other. So if you pass total control of your illness to someone else, that is denying *your own ability to take control and communicate with yourself.* You might be considered one of the awkward squad, but becoming involved in your treatment or therapy, be it orthodox or alternative is vital. For those who decide to take orthodox treatment Professor Jane Plant wrote a good book entitled '*Your Life in Your Hands* [27].

Professor Hardin Jones, Professor of Medical Physics and Physiology at Berkely California made a study lasting 25 years of the life span of treated and untreated cancer patients and came up with the astonishing conclusion that untreated patients don't die sooner than patients receiving conventional treatment and even indicated they live longer. Dr Jones reported his findings to the American Cancer Society's Science Writers Seminar in 1969 in which he confirmed what he had written as far back as 1955, in his classic paper on the subject published in *Transactions of the New York Academy of Sciences*. Surprisingly Dr Jones found that survival in breast cancer was 4 times longer *without* conventional treatment. He controversially stated: 'People who refuse

217

treatment lived for an average of twelve and a half years. Those who accepted surgery and other kinds of treatment lived an average of only 3 years'. Since drug improvements have allegedly been made since this time, a worthy study would have been to check these results in a modern setting and matching groups very carefully according to what therapies they *actually* undertook. For instance those people in the group, who turned down orthodox treatment or were not offered it, might have undertaken other therapies. Equally the orthodox group may have undergone additional therapies in conjunction with orthodox treatment. This would have been a valuable study, but I am sure as the authors Houston and Null pointed out, no funding for such a study would occur and if it did, there are considerable ways it could be manipulated by the unscrupulous.

Whilst governments particularly in the U.K. in the light of difficult financial times are considering cuts in all services, they have stated that they intend to ring-fence health care services; but it must be asked whether the type of Health Service we have here in Britain is constitutionally incapable of dealing with the volume of illness. We hear that services are often over run with binge drinkers and drug addiction problems, which is a warning sign of a sick society. This would have been unheard of in the 50's. The shift in emphasis in the last 20 years has been towards health promotion, rather than disease management. However that promotion is still tied to vested interests. A recent study heralded in headlines in 2008 claimed that organic food had no beneficial advantage over chemicalised food. Anyone with an ounce of common sense would realise that food without chemicals has to be more beneficial. This study merely reflected the strong arm of the petro-chemical industry attempting to protect their share price by having us believe that their chemicals – or genetic modifications are not harmful. Indeed the results of imbibing genetically modified food, may not in the laboratory of human evolution be known for centuries, but I think it is remarkably foolish to think that one can tinker randomly with the human genome or with the genome of plants and animals that are a part of ecosystems and the food chain.

The journalist George Monbiot at the Watlington, Oxfordshire rally protest against genetically modified food in 1999, painted a familiar picture to cancer when he stated: "We might look to the government to do things about the terrifying spread of these threats to human kind, but it has proved again and again that when faced with a choice between what the electorate wants and what big business wants, it will side with big business. We might appeal to

218

international treaties protecting the environment, but those pursuing coercive trade at any cost have overruled them. If we do not take responsibility for what is happening to the environment no one else will. It is time we stopped wondering what are THEY going to do about it, and start thinking what are WE going to do about it".

Sadly this is a point, that I realised over the years meant there would be few comrades on the front battle lines and certainly no help. The few scientists and doctors, who do make a stand, get worn down when faced with continual bankruptcy, prosecution and all the other methods used to gag and professionally ruin them. One of the best methods used is to attack your employment and make damn sure you don't have any vital finances to continue.

Currently the American company Monsanto is hoping to market, with the Maharashtra Hybrid Seed Company, a genetically modified aubergine in India, where aubergines are a major crop and staple diet, especially for the poor. If permission is given the aubergine will become the first GM foodstuff to be grown in India. As India seems to defer to the US as evidenced by the Bophal disaster, it seems likely Monsanto will win. The aubergine genome will contain a gene from the soil bacteria Bacillus thruingiensis, which is toxic to boring insects, but not it is claimed harmful to humans. Environmental Campaigners question the evidence, and argue that commercial interests have overly influenced the regulatory process. They claim that 2,000-odd varieties of aubergine cultivated in India would be threatened by the genetically modified variety.

Monsanto provoked uproar by taking a patent over nap hal wheat particularly suited to chapattis, but saying it had no plans to exploit the patent. VS Achuthanandan, claimed GM foods would lead to the 'colonisation of the food sector' and 'we should not be a part of a system that will destroy traditional seeds and crops and allow multinational corporations to infringe on the agriculture sector.' In Britain whilst fighting off GM crops for years, the first GM potato will be planted. It has been made very clear the public do not want GM foods and yet time and time again that view has been ignored.

Government 'experts' have assured the Indian government that the genetically modified variety poses no threat and now comes the unbelievable bit: "Our experts examined the science behind Bt Brinjal" (the genetically modified variety of aubergine) 'and concluded that it is absolutely safe. *The only thing that hasn't been done is human testing*' (author's emphasis). One could not make it up! The fact is any fungicidal gene (and we don't know the consequences of bacterial genes) would lead to a decrease in immunity: thus whilst genetically modified food may not kill humans directly, who is to say that the *indirect* action would be to induce cancer or other diseases through lowered immunity?

In 1989 I campaigned outside Sloane Square tube station in London, warning about the first genetically modified strawberry – Frostban. People looked at me as though I was mad and could not see the urgency, with which I urged them to sign a petition banning GM food. I and Jeremy Rifkin spoke of biodiversity before it had become a buzzword and warned that ecosystems may collapse. It even crossed my mind then that one could theoretically kill people by inserting a gene, which would be a form of population control. One hates to be always right and say "I told you so" – but the emergence of Monsanto's 'terminator gene' which meant crops only lasted one year and any farmer would have to buy (from Monsanto) new seed every year, was one such occasion when a shiver went down my spine. Could that technology be applied to humans? A bit far-fetched you might think, but then hasn't cancer become a form of population control? I am reminded of the economic background to the biblical Egyptian famine, I recounted in the first volume of *Theatre Earth*, where the citizens cried out "give us seed to sow". Jacob had locked up the seed in a case of government speculation; and I note the Jacob's of this world are still repeating such evil actions in 2010 – Traders are now gambling on food as a commodity, causing people in some poorer countries to riot crying out for food. Incidentally the Freemasons used this method i.e. of pouring grain into the rivers, such that Parisians had no bread to eat, precipitating an orchestrated revolution.

Even as I write this paragraph I note an article in *The Independent* (*12.07.2010*) – '*Population explosion scrutinised as scientists urge politicians to act*'. 'Britain's premier scientific organisation has launched a two-year study into global population levels. A growing body of scientists believe the time has come for politicians to confront the problems posed by the future increase in human numbers. The Royal Society has established a working group of leading experts to draw up a comprehensive set of recommendations on human population that could set the agenda for tackling the environmental stress caused by billions of extra people on the planet'.

Roger Martin of the OPT (Optimum Population Trust) said: 'Overpopulation is a much used and abused work, but we believe the index helps to anchor it firmly in the realm of sustainability: of people living within the limits of the place they inhabit'. Nobody explained that to a banker.

Much of the coming increase in human numbers will be in the poorest developing countries, notably in sub-Saharan Africa, where the population is set to rise by about 50 per cent over the coming decades. Some of the poorest nations in Africa could see their population's triple. Although I will briefly discuss AIDS in relation to cancer later, there are some people who believe AIDS was part of a population control programme. Some may find that accusation ridiculous, but when you have been on this scene for over 20 years, some find it perfectly plausible. Certainly little has been done in the last half century to raise the self-reliance of these countries as they drift from one famine and crisis to the next – self-reliance means empowerment and therefore loss of control by multi-nationals.

The further problem is that since the 70s multinational companies (and governments) have discovered PR. Before the 70s it was a case of 'mind your own business.' In the past there was very little information given to public, but since the explosion of the Internet, PR has become a necessary tool for big business. The ruse soon became that big business was 'listening" to the concerns of the consumer and government was "listening' to its citizens. In the 90s Monsanto had become deeply distrusted and was already under attack from pressure groups. Robert Shapiro, the CEO of Monsanto suddenly stated: "We forgot to listen...our confidence in biotechnology has been widely seen as arrogance and condescension". One can see the PR brief at the back of such statement – cynicism and hypocrisy I'm afraid comes with the territory. It was a surprise to me that Patrick Holden, of the Soil Association fell for it and he should have known better: "I emerged from the meeting with a very clear impression that they are prepared to re-think their position fundamentally out of an awareness that Europe has said no to genetic engineering and perhaps a fear that the North American public might follow suit".

Monsanto however, were playing the waiting game and soothing their critics and attaining more favourable press, with the emphasis on their reasonable and listening concern to arguments over safety. The implication from press articles in 1999 was that Monsanto was considering abandoning genetic engineering and using its detailed knowledge of plant DNA to help traditional

221

and organic plant breeders develop better hybrids. This revelation emerged from 'stakeholder dialogue' between Monsanto and four consumer and environmental associations. Charles Secrett of Friends of the Earth fell for it and said: 'they were wanting to learn...You could see closed minds beginning to open'. Which must account for the fact that in 2010 Indian environmental groups are fighting the battle of aubergines and Friends of the Earth are fighting over the planting of genetically modified potatoes in England, but this time the crops are not being torn up – as I said protestors finally get worn down and move on and the multinationals know this. The last point is significant in that as with other big issues e.g. European Union and cloning and animal vivisection, protesters are not only worn down, but since the government of Tony Blair, activists are now more suppressed than ever. The decline of civil liberties under the Blair government in the UK was a disgrace to democracy.

One can't help but be cynical about Monsanto's alleged interest in helping organic farming. In the US, they are destroying organic farming through genetic contamination and the promotion of genetically engineered maize and cotton, which has already been showing resistance to Bt spray, an organic pesticide. Furthermore Monsanto's genuine desire to be perceived in the British media as a 'caring and sharing corporation' does not sit well with the other under-reported activities such as the rapid acquisition of water companies in Mexico and India. So whilst Monsanto cares so much about organic farmers in Britain, presumably gagging people like Prince Charles, they are making a guaranteed profit from the water crisis in the southern hemisphere. There is no doubt that Monsanto see themselves, as the rightful inheritor of the world's entire food chain: just as the Biotech companies see themselves as the rightful inheritors of the human genome. Further it seems that as the rich nations like China seek to buy up farms in other countries, the position of resources and food and water, is perhaps going to produce future violence and perhaps wars over resources – Antarctica being another critical issue.

Another Machiavellian PR strategy is 'divide and rule' which has the effect of dividing the diverse alliance of NGO's and campaigning groups that come together to challenge any GM technology. By offering concessions to individual groups, their particular fears be they consumer choice, or organic farming practises or 'the Third World' can be allayed, and the alliance will come apart.

Ultimately however, once any organisation, government or company becomes powerful enough the pretence of the Trojan horse is discarded and the true intention is revealed. I am reminded of how once in power; Hitler showed little interest in the details of policy – not for him files or cabinet meetings, let alone parliamentary style debate. The resemblance to Tony Blair Prime Minister in the UK for a decade was uncannily familiar as were the loss in civil liberties and persecution of dissidents.

The British government of Tony Blair had already agreed with companies like Monsanto that gene technology was to be pursued. In the year 2,000 a secret cabinet report followed the PR line of Monsanto; that the technology could win the war against hunger in the Third World. Much the same argument for the use of drugs to win the war against cancer had been used before – big technology to solve man-made problems. Such claims in 2010 were not proven to be the case and in fact some genetically modified crops had worsened production, by interfering with ecosystems and causing more pests to multiply, with consequently *more* pesticide use needed.

Tony Blair, quick to respond as the chameleon to mounting anger by pressure groups and public concern, admitted in Japan at the 2000 G8 Summit, just a few weeks after the secret report that there was: 'potential for harm, both in terms of human safety and in the diversity of our environment, from GM foods and crops.' Together with Bill Clinton, Blair called for a debate based on 'facts not prejudice'. The point is that none of those who support GM crops or the ministers themselves will volunteer in clinical trials to eat the stuff for 10 years to find out scientifically whether any harm is caused in humans. Nothing immoral however is seen in pushing on to some of the poorest citizens in the world a technology, which has a huge safety question mark hanging over it and where no long-term safety trials in humans have ever been conducted. The cavalier attitude by scientists is 'let's suck it and see.' I seem to remember when they first exploded the Atomic bomb they had no idea of whether it would set light to the biosphere!

Hypocrisy isn't new however. Doctors when they get cancer, often turn to the alternatives in a somewhat hypocritical stance. Dr Wakefield who was involved in the MMR vaccine controversy in the UK, was forced to resign by the GMC (General Medical Council); but Tony Blair when asked whether his young son had received the supposedly "safe" vaccine, declined to answer. Perhaps privately, the Blair's looked up the MMR research and references. If so, they will have discovered that MMR is actually a direct assault upon the child's delicate immune system.

Michael Gearin-Tosh noted a survey conducted by Dr Ulrich Abel of Heidelberg published in the professional *Journal of Biomedicine and Pharmacotherapy* in 1992: 'It should arouse concern that, according to opinion polls, many oncologists would decline to accept cytotoxic therapy in their own case'. Ten years later, Dr Julian Kenyon MD MB ChB, who uses alternative approaches to cancer wrote to Michael Gearin-Tosh: 'I am somewhat bemused by the number of doctors who consult me, many of them with cancer, and so far as they are concerned they apply the arguments you have applied to your own illness in *Living Proof.* The doctors seem to reserve the approach espoused by conventional oncologists for their patients only. This is a curious state of affairs'. There is a saying that goes – 'if you want to find the best restaurant then watch where the locals eat.'

Just as people who can afford it eat organic food then those cancer patients, who can afford it, invariably use alternative methods alone or in combination with orthodox medicine. However the majority of cancer patients cannot afford adjunct therapy or counselling and orthodox treatment is their *only* option.

Reusch pointed out that the poorest undeveloped countries had become the lushest land of conquest for the Drug Cartel. As a case in point in Chile a medical commission nominated by President Salvador Allende in 1972 himself a doctor, had come to the conclusion that there were not more than a couple of dozen drugs with therapeutic value and the international pharmacopoeia should be reduced accordingly. But most of the minority of Chilean doctors who wanted to translate these findings into a practical programme were murdered within one week after the take- over by the junta, which with CIA support (later acknowledged by Washington) toppled the Allende regime on September 11th 1973. The date at least is a reminder. The result was the institution of a far more ruthless dictatorship, but one that was wide open to American trade and the products of the petrochemical industry. There was no conclusive evidence that the American CIA had a hand in the murder of those Chilean doctors who opposed the flood of American drugs. On the other hand, nobody explained why in a political revolution so many medical doctors were murdered.

A similar case occurred in Italy. In 1975 in Italian medical commission was set up and a list of several thousand drugs was issued that the commission wanted removed from the catalogue of the National Health Insurance because they had been proven useless or dangerous. The Italian press then published the list. A higher body the so- called Superior Institute of Health, overruled the medical commission's demand and decided the products should remain, favouring industry at detriment to the public health and purse.

In an article by Anthony Lewis entitled: *'The Price of Secrets'*, that appeared in the *New York Times* and *The International Herald Tribune* on *August 22nd 1980* he stated:

'The arrogance of Kissinger's words, when seen in print, was no doubt embarrassing to him. But what he said at a meeting of the 40 Committee was more than a personal matter. It reflected what was and had been for years a prevailing attitude in the CIA and the White House, an almost casual willingness to intervene secretly in other countries with arms, money and murderous plots'. As we all recognise the dollar marches before the army in any war. It seems the disastrous wars in Iraq and Afghanistan have followed the same mentality.

The case of Chile was far from unique. When in 1978 the Socialist government of Sri Lanka, following the recommendations of a medical commission, was about to reduce the number of imported drugs, the American Ambassador threatened to stop U.S. Food Aid. So much is spent by Third World countries on western drugs, that there is little left for prevention.

I can still remember the anger I felt in the 80s, at reading an article in *Mother Jones* an American magazine, which someone in the States had sent. A November 1979 article entitled *'The Corporate Crime of the Century'* covered the practise of the Chemical Syndicate in dumping on uninformed populations in underdeveloped countries chemical products that had often been banned in the country of origin. Health warnings were omitted that products are obliged to carry in western countries. Dr Milton Silverman, a lecturer in pharmacology at the University of California Medical Centre in San Francisco compared how certain important prescription drugs were advertised to doctors in the U.S and in Latin America. Whereas drugs in the U.S were quoted with adverse reactions, in poorer countries the reactions were not publicised. Pope John Paul II went as far as he could when he stated: "This Continent suffers from

225

interior and foreign assistance subordinated to certain conditions." The story continues today with AIDS drugs and recently it has been posed that the billions of unwanted swine flu medications should be distributed in third world countries. Does this mean that such countries will be forced to buy unwanted swine flu vaccine, in exchange for food aid? Presumably the safety concerns over the vaccine will not be detailed. Finland suspended the vaccination programme following reports of narcolepsy in people who had received the jab. Narcolepsy is a condition where people suddenly fall asleep. There had been 27 reports by 2010 of suspected narcolepsy in people across Europe who had previously been vaccinated with Pandemrix, the H1N1 swine flu vaccine made by GlaxoSmithKline. *The Daily Telegraph (27.08.2010)* reported that the European drugs regulators were to investigate the safety of the vaccine, but there is no report to say whether the vaccine had already been distributed to third world countries.

In this respect it might be interesting here to give you the story of Morris Bealle in the 1930s. He was former city editor of the old *Washington Times* and *Herald,* and later ran a county newspaper in Maryland. The local power company brought a quarter page advertisements every week, an account that was important to Bealle for the survival of his newspaper. Bealle ran a story on behalf of some of his readers, who received poor service from the Power Company. The paper was out on the stands for a couple of hours, when Bealle received a mafia-type phone call from the advertising company, which handled the power company's account. Needless to say they threatened to cancel the advertising contract if any more articles appeared. For good measure they also threatened to remove accounts for the gas and telephone company.

Bealle was one of those old-time principled men that are so hard to find now. He decided to sell the paper and get out of the business. He went on to write a brilliant exposé entitled *'The Super Drug Story'*. He couldn't get it into print and had to found his own publishing house in order to do so. Bookstores would not stock it and newspapers would not review it. So they made sure it never reached the bestseller list. You might say well that was back in the 30s but I had exactly those problems with the *'Theatre Earth'* series and had to publish the lot myself as I will have to do with this book. In the late 90s I had paid a fair amount of money to take out a quarter front- page advertising my cancer research in the local newspaper *The Brighton Argus*, part of the Newsquest media group whose parent company is the US giant Gannett Co.

Inc. The advertisement appeared in the morning edition but was pulled before the afternoon edition, where a department store got free advertising on my money! I wasn't refunded and letters of complaint were ignored. The Syndicate don't believe that laws apply to them.

Bealle was a brave man in tackling the Rockefellers, when he gave the true history of the cancer quack. According to Bealle thirty years ago the Standard Oil Company became impressed with the methods of the pig-packing houses, which used, processed and sold every part of the pig but its squeal. To quote Bealle:

'Their sales research department went way back to the 1860's when "Old Bill" Rockefeller, the itinerant pappy of John D (the first) and a patent-medicine showman used to palm off bottled raw petroleum on the yokels as a cure for cancer. Old Bill called his bottled petroleum Nujol (meaning new oil) and sold it to those who had cancer and those whom he could make fear they would develop it. This sounded good to Standard's researchists. The druggist paid about 21 cents for a 6-ounce bottle of Nujol, which cost Standard Oil around a fifth of a cent. Instead of calling it a cure for cancer they called it a cure for constipation. Soon after Nujol was put on the market it was discovered by physicians to be harmful. It robbed the body of fat-soluble vitamins and caused serious deficiency diseases apart from oil being highly toxic. Standard Oil checked the loss in sales by adding Carotene to Nujol claiming this overcame the injuries'.

To quote Bealle: 'For some years before his death Senator Copeland of New York used to set up a radio microphone in his Senate Office building quarters in Washington, furnished by the American taxpayers and plug this greasy product for $75,000 a year'. And here we have yet another method of the Syndicate, the so-called 'revolving door', where people in power use that position to gain directorships, promote products and generally gain a lucrative income from such associations and connections. There is no shame, integrity or responsibility.

By the 1930s in Bealle's time Nujol was made by Stanco Incorporated, listed at the time as one of the many subsidiaries of the Standard Oil Company. Again to quote Bealle: ' The breath-taking profits from Nujol made it inevitable that America's largest and most ruthless industrial combine – the Rockefeller empire, would emerge'.

It wasn't until 1939 however, that the Drug Trust formed and the upward curve in their profits began to assume the present gigantic proportions, which in 1948 made 10 billion a year. How the American Drug Trust was formed by an alliance with its opposite number in Germany is almost a story in itself. When Hitler began to plan his one thousand year Reich, the powers that were in Germany didn't know that American politicians were going to solve their acute employment crisis by forcing the U.S into the Second World War, which would save Rockefeller's oil.

Germany's huge chemical cartel the IG Farben Industrie enjoyed a monopoly on all chemical products manufactured in Germany. German IG made an alliance with American Standard Oil in order to control important patents. So when in 1939 it became apparent that Germany would soon be unpopular in the United States, Standard Oil helped Hitler's Reich cover its American holdings in the drug and chemical field. The American IG was formed. Standard Oil took 15% of the stock in the New German-American Chemical Trust. Among the directors of this cover-up company were Walter Teagle (President of Standard Oil), Paul Warburg (a Roosevelt-Rockefeller stooge) and Edsel Ford.

I.G Farben's ethics were clearly portrayed, when they used slave labour from Auschwitz – where approximately 300,000 concentration camp workers passed through I.G. Farben's facilities at Auschwitz and at least 25,000 of them were worked to death. Twelve of I.G Farben's top executives were sentenced to terms of imprisonment for slavery and mistreatment offences at the Nuremberg war crime trials.

Shortly after the Pearl Harbour attack, which has been greatly questioned as yet another atrocity that would persuade Americans to go to war, the American IG Farben decided to camouflage its German parentage and sympathies with the help of Standard Oil. It changed its name to the General Aniline and Film Corporation after purchasing an undisclosed number of shares in various large American companies, including Schering & Co., Monsanto Chemical, Dow Chemical, Standard Oil of New Jersey, of Indiana of California and the du Pont Company. It took over the privately owned Hoffman-La Roche Company.

After the war when the Americans reached the industrial city of Frankfort they were amazed to find intact all the buildings and the huge plant of the German

IG Farben Chemical Trust. Everything else had been targeted and demolished by bombers. Once this enormous monopoly Drug Trust had been formed along with others it became impossible to carry out any true and meaningful cancer research, which threatened the Drug Cartel. The tentacles from the Chemical Syndicate and Drug Cartel reached through just about every sector of government. The Drug companies as they still do allocated generous donations to Universities for research funding just to ensure that everyone was 'singing from the same hymn sheet.' The next generation of science managers, had been well and truly brainwashed not to 'think outside the box', to become politically correct and stay 'on message' (adhere to policy). As I have stated any new thought, especially if it threatens share prices, rarely comes from such places and is more likely to occur on kitchen tables or in garden sheds.

Even in the 1930s Bealle warned that the Rockefeller interests had developed into the most far reaching industrial empire, where the Rockefellers owned the largest drug manufacturing combine in the world and where their other interests would be used to bring pressure to increase the sale of drugs. The wealth of such companies meant they had the power to threaten governments and manipulate them. It is against this highly suppressive background that the alternative cancer therapies were pitted. Many of the alternative cancer therapies emerged prior to the Second World War and had the Drug Cartel not taken over, no doubt research and funding would have been channelled down this promising route. The alternative therapists and doctors who developed alternative therapies, were usually if their methods were successful continually harassed, threatened and some were imprisoned and threatened with removal of their licence to practise medicine. Many alternative cancer therapists in America in fear of lawsuits had to practise across the border in Mexico.

Hoechst and Bayer, the largest and third largest companies in world pharmaceutical sales respectively, are descended from I.G. Farben. The Rockefellers gave billions of dollars- worth of gifts and research grants to colleges and public agencies within the United States who taught Rockefeller drug lore. In 1927 they formed the International Education Board, which similarly 'donated' millions of dollars to foreign universities and politicos; this allowed the Rockefeller Empire to expand. Morris Bealle the US investigative reporter stated: 'The keystone of this mammoth industrial empire is the Chase National Bank with 27 branches in New York City and 21 in foreign countries (now renamed the Chase Manhattan Bank with over 200 branches in the US and abroad). Not the least of its holdings are in the drug business'.

The American Medical Association (AMA) and the Federal Drug Administration (FDA) acting alongside the multinationals have been instrumental in the United States in attacking and silencing any small operation that looked promising. How did America go down this route, after the grand words of the Founding Fathers and many great Presidents? As Bealle pointed out Rockefeller interests financed Roosevelt's original forays into politics and Rockefeller naturally called in the debt, when Roosevelt came to power directing major policies that were in the interests of the multinationals. This of course still goes on today in lobbying and through the 'revolving door.' In Britain honours are still shamefully doled out for such activities.

As the great man himself Thomas Jefferson said: "If people let government decide what foods they eat and what medicines they take, their bodies will soon be in as sorry a state, as are the souls of those who live under tyranny." He also warned: "If once the people become inattentive to the public affairs, you and I, and Congress and Assemblies, Judges and Governors, shall all become wolves". The problem now is that it is virtually a full time job following the wolves.

Keith Lasko in 1980 in his book entitled: '*The Great Billion Dollar Medical Swindle*' put it this way when he spoke of the American Medical Association.

'Superficially, the American Medical Association seems to represent the medical profession. Historically hardly more than a trade union, and presently a barely functioning lobbyist organization, it stands in patients eyes for what it truly is: a bulwark against socialized medicine'.

Bealle claimed the AMA had actually damaged the doctors' image. The fight against Medicare in the 50's and 60's Bealle said stripped them of all pretence and revealed them as not caring a damn about patients' welfare and where instead they were dedicated to the preservation of doctors' excessively high incomes. Even today as President Obama wrestles with the problems of American deficit, social welfare and Medicare, he has been accused of giving in to the far right and their capitalist masters. Unfortunately people fail to understand just who runs countries and it certainly isn't the one on television, giving political broadcasts.

The past U.S President Woodrow Wilson was ordered by the Chemical Syndicate to enter World War I. Ferdinand Lund a history professor in his book '*The Rich and the Super Rich: A study in the power of money today*' (*1968*) claimed: 'As to the role in the 1914-1918 war, of the industrial tycoons, American and foreign, far from saving the world they were the chief operative factors in producing World War I, as a wealth of research conclusively shows. Again it was the American business leaders who pushed the United States into that war'.

Even in 1930 James Gerrard former ambassador to Germany had listed 64 names that ruled the United States. In the banking crisis today we still recognise some of those historical names including J.P Morgan. Professor Lundberg even claimed that Woodrow Wilson's Administration was little more than an adjunct of J.P. Morgan and Company. The position has not changed and corporate power and the banking system is still the dominant force in our society and yet naively Americans expected Obama to take on this monster of the banking system and admonish him for allowing Wall Street to write their own self- regulation rules. One can expect nothing and definitely not conscience or responsibility from the spiritually bankrupt.

Against this background then, what cancer patients are told is based upon a convenient and lucrative way to treat cancer. The inconvenient truth is that cancer is no longer a medical problem but a socio-political one.

Nobel Prize winner (double Laureate) Dr Linus Pauling PhD went on record as saying: 'Everyone should know that most cancer research is largely a fraud, and that the major cancer research organisations are derelict in their duties to the people who support them.' Samuel S. Epstein, M.D., in his book '*The Politics of Cancer*' (*1982, updated 1998*) stated: 'We are dealing not with a scientific problem. We are dealing with a political issue'.

In 1964, the World Health Organization estimated that 60 to 80 per cent of human cancers are caused by factors in the environment (including diet and lifestyle) and hence the disease should have been largely preventable. Since then scientists have listed a catalogue of products and social practises that contribute to cancer: such as chemical and food additives, denatured fibreless diets, excessive fats, drugs, medical and dental X-rays, occupational chemicals, air pollution and chlorinated/fluoridated water. However virtually all these causes represent profitable vested interests and in a competitive capitalist market, getting rid of such causes and thus preventing cancer, is probably impossible unless consumers are able to drive the market.

Chemotherapy drugs are markedly immunosuppressive which means that they reduce the native resistance of the body to a variety of diseases, including ironically the ability of the body to fight cancer cells. Recently in 2009 a patient was killed in the U.K after the wrong dose of chemotherapy was administered. Had that occurred in the alternative field could you imagine what a field day the press would have had with stories about quacks and charlatans. Why do people accept that in allegedly getting well, their hair must fall out or any one of the following will occur – vomiting, nausea, bone marrow damage, bleeding, increased infections, liver and kidney damage, numbness, impotence, sterility, scarring of the lungs, shortness of breath, weakness, fall in blood pressure, diarrhoea, sores in the mouth, rashes, fever, sensitivity to sunlight, allergic reactions, phlebitis, disorientation, lethargy, bladder irritation, heart damage, skin ulcerations, loss of balance, mental confusion and even death. These are just some of the reported side effects of orthodox radiation and chemotherapy. Is this really a body getting well, or is this a body under onslaught, where it is hoped that the cancer dies before you do?

I am reminded of Michael Gearin-Tosh's account where he was told not to take chemotherapy otherwise he was "a gonner"; this comment more than anything upset *The Times* readers, some of whom had already gone down that route. Well things *may* have improved since then with less appalling side effects, but I remember being at the Health Show in Olympia in London in the mid 90's, when an elderly couple came up to my stand. They told me how the husband had inoperable bladder cancer and were told that there was nothing more they could do for him in orthodox medicine. His wife said that they had heard about the Gerson Therapy but for various reasons mainly financial they could not do the whole therapy. The wife however, had made a quart jug of carrot and apple juice every day for her husband and that was 10 years ago!

Perhaps twenty years ago, I was fortunate not to be confronted by the mass of information on the Internet. Thousands of links come up on "alternative cancer treatment" and an anxious patient, in panic, will be overwhelmed by the sheer quantity of information. The patient then has to make serious life decisions and without a science background is incapable of sorting the wheat from the chaff and it is no wonder that patients, then return to their oncologist, as the 'safest' bet. As Phillip Day author of *'Cancer: Why We're Still Dying to Know The Truth'* (*1999*) stated: 'many people just gulp, enter the cancer tunnel and hope they come out the other end'.

Only by sweeping the board clean and undergoing a complete review would unearth some of the very harsh facts, I have revealed here. Dodgy research as I term it, is rife not only in cancer research but in other areas, where such research continues to be used as the basis of government policies today. The way it *actually* works is that a policy is decided and then facts that support the policy are chosen, whilst those that contradict it are ignored. The verdict is still open as to whether this applies to the science of global warming.

Fluoridation of drinking water (a known cancer link) is a prime example. *Prevailing Wind* a small magazine in the U.S published a sensational-but-suppressed story about how the U.S. government twisted and suppressed the truth about fluoride's adverse health effects because hydrogen fluoride was part and parcel of the top-secret atomic bomb project between 1944 and 1945.

Alternative circles have been aware for five decades of the dangers to health in fluoridation of water. The government, stonewalling on fluoride and its attendant dangers, helped to create the mythology about fluoride being good for children's teeth. There is actually no "science" to support this toxic water treatment program, but the mainstream media has neglected this topic. Joel Griffiths and Chris Bryson, the investigative journalists once commissioned by *The Christian Science Monitor* to probe the atomic project's relation to fluoride highlighted these five facts:

1. A-bomb project scientists, who had been secretly ordered to provide "evidence useful in litigation" against defence contractors for fluoride injury to citizens, generated much of the original proof that fluoride is safe for humans in low doses. The first lawsuits against the U.S. A-bomb program were not over radiation, but over fluoride, the documents show.
2. Human studies were required. Bomb program researchers played a leading role in the design and implementation of the most extensive U.S. study of the health effects of fluoridating public drinking water –

233

conducted in Newburgh, New York from 1945 to 1956. Then, in a classified operation code-named "Program F" they secretly gathered and analysed blood and tissue samples from Newburgh citizens, with the co-operation of the State Health Department personnel.

3. The original secret version – obtained by these reporters – of a 1948 study published by Program F scientists in the *Journal of the American Dental Association* shows that evidence of adverse health effects from fluoride was censored by the U.S. Atomic Energy Commission – considered one of the most powerful of Cold War agencies – for reasons of national security.

4. The bomb program's fluoride safety studies were conducted at the University of Rochester, site of one of the most notorious human radiation experiments of the Cold War, in which unsuspecting hospital patients were injected with toxic doses of radioactive plutonium. The fluoride studies were conducted with this same ethical mind-set, in which "national security" was paramount.

5. The U.S. government's conflict of interest – and its motive to prove fluoride "safe" – has not, until now, been made clear to the general public in the furious debate over water fluoridation since the 1950's, nor to civilian researchers and health professionals or journalists.

An article in the *March 2000* issue of *Acres USA*, the nation's leading eco-farm journal, featured an interview with Dr Albert Burgstahler, an emeritus professor of biochemistry at Kansas University and the editor of *Fluoride*, the journal of the International Society for Fluoride Research. Professor Burgstahler in the article, independently confirmed how the cities of Newburgh and Kingston, N.Y., were part of the fluoridation control experiments starting in 1945 and how the results were suppressed so that the agenda could not be stopped on scientific grounds. He said:

'At the time, the argument was that the tooth decay rates were comparable in the two cities – actually that wasn't quite true- but in the event, they collected data for 10 years following the fluoridation of Newburgh. Proponents claimed there was a 50 to 60 per cent lower tooth decay rate in the children they examined. The same was argued for Grand Rapids, Mich.; Brantford, Ontario; and Evanston, Ill. And so forth. But following that 1955-1960 period, tooth decay rates in Kingston were also going down, and in the mid-1990s tooth decay rates in the non-fluoridated control city of Kingston were actually a little lower than in fluoridated Newburgh, but the dental fluorosis rates in Newburgh were twice as high.

On the medical side, the Newburgh blood samples were sent to the University of Rochester where atomic bomb research was going on. Scientists there were concerned because they had seen some toxic effects in the uranium workers handling uranium hexafluoride for the isotope separation. They were looking to see what kinds of biochemical parameters would be found in that general blood sampling. That was all suppressed. We don't really know what they did find, but some things did leak out: cervical bone abnormalities in the boys in Newburgh were twice what they were in Kingston. The onset of puberty was advanced by some five months for girls in Newburgh, so there were some suspicious things that they should have looked into more closely'.

In the *Prevailing Wind* article, Griffiths and Bryson told how the atomic project had serious liability problems staring them in the face and how they had to cover up the fluoride poisoning at all costs. The secrecy of the atomic project caused the cover-up and it served to propel the fluoridation mythology.

The research of Dr Phyllis Mullenix has shown that fluoride causes hyperactivity and lackadaisical effects on animal subjects, particularly the young and had depressive effects in older animals. The research has vast implications as America struggles (as with Britain), with uncontrolled hyperactivity in children, while the mental sluggishness of millions of average Americans and indeed Britons, is evident. Also at least in the UK girls are reaching puberty earlier.

In the interview, Burgstahler offered an anecdote from his own experience that tied into the findings by Dr Mullenix:

'What we lack is a comparison of children with a low fluoride intake versus those with a high fluoride intake. I can give you one anecdotal story that's very relevant. A woman called some years ago about her 16-year old son who was experiencing real problems in school. He couldn't concentrate; he was always jumping around, and was generally unmanageable. I met with her and her child and suggested she try distilled water for a few weeks and see what happened. She called back and said that it was "amazing" as he had become a normal child'.

In very familiar action Professor Burgstahler describes what happened to Dr Mullenix and her research when she took responsibility:

'As a result of that research, she became very concerned and prepared a paper for publication, but she was told that in order to publish she should clear her findings with the Public Health Service. She went to Washington, D.C., to give a presentation, where they were rather shocked and wanted to know what her publishing plans were. She knew at this point they were trying to suppress publication, but she went ahead and published anyway in *Neurotoxicology and Teratology Journal* in 1995.

As soon as that happened, the lid blew off. She was then informed that her services were no longer required. The Forsyth Institute admitted bluntly that if she were to continue there, their funding, which was practically the entire source of support for their research institute, would be cut off by the Public Health Service in retaliation'.

This is no surprise to me as I have experienced loss of employment due to my research and books. Certainly one way they can get rid of the 'nail that sticks up' is to make sure you don't find work anywhere else.

Griffiths and Bryson showed Dr Mullenix the documentation that the researchers uncovered about the "top secret" version of the research that was published in the August 1948 *Journal of the American Dental Association:*

'The secret version reports that most of the men had no teeth left. The published version reports only that the men had fewer cavities.

The secret version says the men had to wear rubber boots because the fluoride fumes disintegrated the nails in their shoes. The published version does not mention this.

The secret version says the fluoride may have acted similarly on the men's teeth, contributing to their tooth-less-ness. The published version omits this statement.

The published version concluded: 'the men were unusually healthy, judged from both a medical and dental point of view.

...After comparing the secret and published versions of the censored study, toxicologist Phyllis Mullenix commented, "This makes me ashamed to be a scientist". Of other cold War-era fluoride safety studies she asked, 'were they all done like this?'

Radiation treatment of cancer in my view fits into the same category. How can you 'treat' cancer, with radiation, which is known to CAUSE cancer even years later? The legal argument is that cancer is a desperate situation and you had no choice anyway, so you would have taken it, even if you had been warned of the side effects. Don't even try to legally argue - that well no you would not have taken radiation and in fact would have done and did do, the Gerson Therapy. The legal argument remains that no matter how much they harm and maim you even to death, you would have agreed to it whether or not those consequences had been explained to you, because there is *no choice* in cancer treatment and orthodoxy is the *only* option and accepted correct opinion: welcome to Alice's Tea Party folks!

To underline the madness Andrew Lansely, the current government Health Secretary in Britain (2010) besides astoundingly handing over Public Health to big business, has introduced a new mantra: "no decision about me, without me" but the minute you accept orthodox treatment, decisions without you have already been made – it's called policy!

The Daily Telegraph (08.11.2010) reported a trial at the University of Cardiff led by Professor Malcolm Mason, which showed deaths from high-risk prostate cancer, can be cut by giving men radiation treatment as well as hormonal therapy. The combined treatment led to 43 per cent fewer deaths after seven years. Men then must weigh up this trial with the fact that radiotherapy is not a "soft option" for prostate cancer. It has long-term effects that may not be seen for three or four years, including a risk of impotence. Given the mechanism of the mind and loss, which operates through the hypothalamus altering hormonal and neural responses, then it is unknown what effect regressive therapy would have in bringing these responses to normal thus removing the hormone that drives the cancer. The drugs used to treat prostate cancer aim to prevent testosterone feeding the cancer and yet it may be possible to use regressive counselling to achieve the same result. However no money is available to test my theory. So, as I realised when I developed cancer, you are on your own and your survival not only from the disease itself, but also from the side effects of orthodox treatment, really depends on how much you know, the decisions you take and what you do.

In Britain it was reported in *The Times* (*12.07.2010*) that 'GPs may control £80bn in shake-up of NHS funding'. 'Millions of pounds in NHS funding could be diverted to private consultancy companies and health mangers as GPs are offered more control of local health services. Plans for a reorganisation of the NHS (National Health Service) that would give much of the multi-billion NHS budget to family doctors were due to be published by the British Government.' Under plans set out in a government White Paper, up to 500 GP networks will control about £80 billion of public money: this coming at a time when the public finances are in disastrous array. One simply could not make it up!

Several private companies are thought to be keen to work with GPs under the proposals – you bet they are! The predators already circling one might note. As Katherine Murphy, director of the Patients Association, said: 'GPs are generalists, trained to diagnose illness and treat patients to the best of their ability. They are not so used to being financial managers or commissioners responsible for a huge amount of public money'.

Who stands to benefit most from this public money – the 'Big Pharma' companies. So whilst people lose their homes and jobs as the age of austerity hits the man in the street, the Big Pharma companies stand to make a tidy sum and it's all left to GPs or those private companies.

The observant Polly Toynbee pointed out in *The Guardian (02.11.2010)* 'Forget patients. Lansley is the servant of big Pharma', a point evidenced by Lansley's transfer of Public Health to big business. Toynbee went on to say:

'In taking away the power of the National Institute of Health and Clinical Excellence (Nice) to select only cost effective treatments, Andrew Lansley appears to be offering a health service without limits just when the NHS is to cut back as never before.... The Nice saga is just one telling example of Lansley folly. This time he seems to have been bowled over by a toxic combination of Daily Mail anecdotes of dying patients desperate for a few more months of life and intense lobbying by a pharmaceutical industry that has campaigned long and hard against the one body that kept NHS drug costs under a modicum of control.... Lansley is bringing in something instead called value-based pricing, where the pharmaceutical industry and government officials negotiate over the price of drugs'.

Professor Alan Maynard fears the lid will be off both the prices charged and the number of ineffective drugs prescribed. As Toynbee pointed out: 'Nice was the first coherent check on runaway drug costs, but value-based pricing will re-open it all, to the industry's delight'. In fact Nice (National Institute of Clinical Excellence) was one of Labour's achievements.

Representatives from drug companies play a big role – only 7% of doctors don't see them. But the main source of doctors' knowledge is the medical press, which consists of half a dozen profitable publications plus a few unprofitable ones – many more publications than are usual for one industry. They are overwhelmingly funded by drug company advertisements. Most of these publications are sent free to all GPs. As Toynbee commented:

'A glance at the history of how well drug companies manipulate, bribe and bamboozle busy doctors into prescribing their most expensive products instead of cheaper and equally effective ones tells why the pharmaceutical industry is throwing its hats in the air at Lansley's infinite gullibility. Big Pharma has run a ferocious campaign against Nice because it has become the trusted international standard by which other countries agree to buy drugs in their health services...'

President Obama in the US is confronting a similar dilemma. Tea Partiers protest that Obama's health plan means "death panels" to decide who lives and who dies at what price: but again as Toynbee pointed out: '...every private health insurance plan was always rationed too, according to price of policy. Without rationing treatments, any system would go bust'.

The importance placed on advertising by the drug companies is apparent from the careful readership profiles they assemble. All research breaks doctors down by age, sex, number of people in the practice, year of graduation, and number of scripts written a day. Advertisers of course favour publications that reach doctors who write scripts readily, which under Lansley's scheme they will be forced under their medical ethics to do. They are also the ones who get invited to the dinners and symposia. Increasingly symposia occur in exotic fully paid up destinations.

An important promotional tool is the medical magazine supplement. Sometimes drug companies would like to make claims about their product but cannot find references to support them from the literature. In this case they may sponsor a supplement, which will carry research of such a minor nature it would not normally make it into the main part of a reputable journal. Editors, whilst saying everything that appears in the supplement is true, admit a lower standard of scientific importance applies. At stake is an enormous industry and you can bet that at least in Britain if GPs are the source of money, they will be heavily targeted.

Doctors are the point of intersection between the drug companies' products and the patient. In Japan, drug companies have developed a unique relationship with doctors. Japan spends more on drugs than any country in the world: in 2,000 it was $228 per person each year, compared with $169 in western Germany, the second most prolific pill popper. Japanese doctors not only prescribe drugs; they also dispense them. The doctors' buy their drugs from wholesalers who typically sell them at a discount on the official prices set by the government: doctors are reimbursed by the government for the drugs they prescribe – but at the official price. The system encourages doctors to use lots of expensive drugs and pocket the difference between the discount price and the official price. As a result, the average Japanese general practitioner earns £327,000 a year, most of which is made by selling drugs, compared with the average $213,000 a year earned by the average US doctor.

AIDS

I don't want to spend too much time on the topic of AIDS, which deserves a book in itself. I will just limit this section to my connections and research notes in the 80s. AIDS or acquired immune deficiency syndrome in humans is known as HIV (previously LAV or HTLV 111)

The last progressive state of AIDS is cancer and that underlines the fact that cancer progresses, where the immune system has failed. AIDS therefore like cancer is a progressive degenerative disease. HIV in healthy people with robust immune systems does not give rise to the full-blown disease. Likewise cancer cells in healthy tissue with high immunity would not be allowed to grow. The AIDS virus flourishes in degenerative systems.

The AIDS type, which occurs in monkeys, is Simian AIDS. In the 80s the National Vivisection Society, who at the time resided at 51 Harley Street in London, contacted me, when they forwarded a booklet entitled '*Biohazard*'. They claimed:

'All over the USA during the 1960s and the 1970s vivisectors have deliberately transmitted Simian AIDS from animal to animal and species to species, laboratory to laboratory, watching it develop in secrecy and speed of action. No attempt at all was made to contain the viruses, for at this stage the human consequences of such work were unknown'.

In short the group claimed that the virus was spread through cancer research experiments in monkeys and gave considerable evidence to back this claim. I spoke to T. Rattigan who wrote '*An Apple a Day – The Threat from orthodox Medicine*' for the group Nemesis, who at the time were in Lincoln UK. He felt that the two main sources of the AIDS "holocaust" were the New England Primate Research Centre and The Davis Primate Research Centre in California. Both he informed me were involved in extensive monkey vivisection and had been using viruses, although he could give no further details, but felt it was possible that a member of staff had taken the virus into the outside world.

Having worked for fifteen years in research, I can see how scientists did not at least in that time period take great safety precautions and Rattigan's claim

241

seemed a possibility. I was working on suicide brain research in the late 70s and had to collect brains from the deceased, whenever I was contacted by a hospital, which for some reason usually occurred during the rush hour. My professor was too 'tight' to allow money for taxis and thus I had to take a canister on the tube across London. In order to get a seat, I found yellow and black 'nuclear warning' tape around the flask came in handy. As I remarked to a colleague, today I would probably get six bullets in the head!

In fact the U.S. Physicians' Committee for Responsible Medicine had warned of the risk in injecting HIV into animals, because of the risk of mutations across species barriers, which could then infect humans. The mutations cannot be controlled; neither can the new viruses be prevented from escaping. They can be virulent within the human body and can mutate again. A human leukaemia virus has been proven to have been accidentally created from ape virus in cancer research experiments and a particularly nasty form of herpes virus.

AIDS became prevalent in Africa and it seems that those with broken immune systems are then more susceptible. Max Gerson reported his conversation with Dr Albert Schweitzer who had worked in Central Africa. Gerson in his book stated in 1954:

'Many natives, especially those who are living in large communities, do not live now the same way as formerly – they used to live almost exclusively on fruits and vegetables, bananas, cassava, ignam, taro, sweet potatoes and other fruits. They now live on condensed milk, canned butter, meat and fish preserves and bread'.

The enormous deluges of drugs, which have been forced onto the poorer countries including Africa since the late 50s, probably also, contribute to broken immune systems. Hans Reusch in his book '*Slaughter of the Innocent*' (*1978*) gave a fuller account. There are also currently a number of books that claim the AIDS virus was deliberately used to infect people, but space does not permit any lengthy analysis of the veracity of that position.

Given how AIDS in all probability arose from irresponsible research, then I would at least warn from a historical point of view of the unknown territory and potential for devastating harm, once you start genetically modifying species or placing cloned animals in the food chain.

242

The book *Full Disclosure: The Truth about the AIDS Epidemic* by Dr. Gary Glum (*1994*) is a good account and Patrick Rattigan still operates NEMESIS with useful information on AIDS.

ALTERNATIVE THERAPIES FOR CANCER AND CHRONIC DISEASE

It should have occurred to any reasonably minded person that conventional approaches have not brought us further to a resolution of cancer. To keep pursuing these conventional approaches may no longer provide us with the gains or answers sought. High technology such as improved scanners, gene therapy and smart drugs cost millions of pounds in research and governments then use taxpayers' money, to purchase these products from companies. Do we as taxpayers consider this is the best use of *our money*? Will these high technologies prevent us from looking at cheaper methods, which when fairly tested may provide better outcomes?

There is also the question of choice. It would be far fairer to issue a credit for treatment of any disease, allowing the patient to *choose* the manner in which he or she wishes to deal with it.

The majority of alternative therapies are not cancer specific, which means they are capable of curing a number of chronic conditions. Unlike orthodox methods they do not attack cancer cells, but primarily aim to raise the patients immunity and rectify any biochemical and physiological abnormalities, together with detoxification. This allows the body's natural defence systems to recover and deal naturally with any cancer cells. Because the alternative therapies seek to repair, detoxify and rebuild they are not damaging. Although there are differences between the therapies the underlying philosophy of all, is that a truly healthy body and mind would not develop cancer, since the body would be capable of eradicating cancer cells, through its own defence system.

Alternative therapists see the tumour as a symptom not the cause, where there is a deeper underlying metabolic disorder, which has caused deterioration over a period of time and where finally a tumour develops as a symptom. Cancers can re-occur even many years later, which may be through orthodox treatment where mutated radiated cells were formed. However there is less likelihood of reoccurrence when a healthy mind and body lifestyle is maintained.

Most of the alternative therapies are based upon diet, with varying degrees of expense and difficulty. Some like the Gerson Therapy are very demanding and relatively expensive, as they require organic food. Michael Gearin-Tosh calculated the two years on this organic diet in 1994, cost him in the region of £50,000. I assume he included supplements in that although I am unsure if that included help. The high cost is due to the huge amounts of organic vegetables required in the juices. The juices on the Gerson diet have to be prepared at hourly intervals in addition to 3 meals a day. But one must however when considering these therapies look carefully at what is entailed. In my case I had been warned there would be severe healing reactions, but nothing could have prepared me for what was to come. I really would not advise anyone to do the Gerson Therapy alone for that reason unless like me there is just no one to help and you have a particularly strong will. In short the Gerson Therapy is not for wimps. Gerson himself stated that the therapy requires loving friends and family to help the patient through these crises periods: as Walter Winchell stated: "a real friend is one who walks in when the rest of the world walk out". Unfortunately that is what you find in society, where illness is viewed as an inconvenience to those who just want to focus on their own lives and you are then no longer convenient to them. In my own case there was definite pressure to take the drugs and let everyone pretend it hadn't happened. For me however I knew from the start the cancer, was a huge warning and I needed to find its cause, even if that meant solutions which required life changing decisions and disruption There is no doubt about it I saw the illness as a critical crossroads.

Most of the alternative cancer therapies require reduced fat intake. Low fat diets are associated with low incidence of cancer and also heart disease. Fat reduction includes saturated and polyunsaturated fats although many people have long since been aware of the connection of heart disease to the intake of saturated fat.

Pickled, canned and even frozen foods are banned in many of the alternative therapies along with spicy food – so curry is out I am afraid. Nitrites used in the preservation of food are considered carcinogenic because they can be turned into nitrosamines, which are also carcinogenic. If you look at the back of a lot of food labels they have nitrites in them as well as the preservatives or E numbers, which are also forbidden. Coffee, tea (but not herbal tea), alcohol and of course cigarettes are forbidden. Virtually all of the alternative therapies require you to cook food from scratch, with organic ingredients.

Virtually all the diets recommend plenty of fruit and vegetables especially those high in Vitamin C and Carotene, which is converted into Vitamin A in the body. Carrots contain plenty of carotene, which gives them their orange colour. Oranges, apples, dark green leafy vegetables such as lettuce are also essential. Each diet will have its own permissible and non-permissible list. If you are in the position of not having the finances to do any of these diets, then you are going to have to be creative and think of a way round it.

As far back as the 1970s the American Senate Select Committee on Nutrition and Human Needs printed a publication entitled *Dietary Goals for the United States*. Nothing came of it and America like many other western nations, slipped into fast and highly processed food and obesity assisted by fast food companies. The physical form of people in the 1930s was very lean because most people walked or cycled, as cars were not generally available. Drugs were not generally taken either pharmaceutical or street and most meals were for financial reasons cooked from scratch using fresh ingredients, with no preservatives or additives and particularly the salt level could be monitored.

In 1976 Dr Gori who was then Deputy Director of the National Cancer Institute's Division of Cancer Causes and Prevention concluded in a statement to the Senate Committee that diet was an important factor in the causation of various forms of cancer and that it was correlated to more than half of all cancers in women and at least one third of all cancers in men. So an extra ordinary about turn occurred where diet was downgraded, whilst scientists focused on drugs and genes. By 1982 this bold conclusion was omitted from a similar report.

Virtually all of the alternative therapies emphasise a low intake of *animal* protein such as meat, eggs, milk etc.: professor Jane Plant in her book '*Your Life in your Hands*' devoted quite a bit of space, to her theory of milk as a contribute factor in cancer. In comparative studies those people, for instance California Seventh Day Adventists, who eat limited amounts of animal protein show lower death rates from cancer.

Researchers have suggested that an optimal concentration of Vitamin A is required for the energy mechanisms of the cell. Other researchers have shown that high intake of Vitamin A decreases the chances of contracting lung cancer. Vitamin A however is toxic in high doses and thus most of the dietary regimes give Carotene, in the form of carrots, which is converted into Vitamin

246

A in the body. More than 35,000 patients in Germany and elsewhere used Vitamin A alongside conventional chemotherapy and radiation, and it was found that patients with cancers of the oesophagus, bronchi, mouth, throat, larynx, penis, vagina and skin did much better than those who just received the conventional treatment. There was one study, which showed that a number of patients with squamous or flat cell carcinoma of the skin had complete remission using Vitamin A alone and without any further treatment.

Simon Martin in an article in *Here's Health'* magazine in *1988* entitled *'Six Reasons why I will not give to Cancer Research'* stated this of Vitamin A: 'Now 16 years later, the National Cancer Institute is sponsoring a double blind, placebo-controlled trial of more than 22,000 male doctors who will be monitored for five years to see whether taking 30mg of beta Carotene every other day stops them from getting lung cancer'.

Whilst it was at least a step in the right direction Martin was afraid that the researchers were only taking a single element of an entire approach and if that element alone was only successful in combination with other elements then orthodoxy could say- look see it doesn't work. Most of the alternative therapies use combined approaches, which target not just the body but mind also. Michael Gearin-Tosh used visualization and a Chinese based bone visualisation in addition to the Gerson Therapy. Professor Jane Plant took orthodox medicine, but wisely utilised psychotherapy.

It may be that these alternative methods can never be fully tested, because they only achieve positive results when all elements are combined. In science one is told one should only test one thing at a time in order to know what effect it has – it is called the fair test. Thus any test requires that only one element of an approach can be looked at and tested at a time. It might not work, unless in combination with other elements in the programme. Gerson himself stated of his nutritional programme that it was important to realise that all elements were necessary.

A great number of promising nutritional animal studies were carried out, from the 1920s to 1940s, prior to World War II, which showed that certain foods and vitamins were found to protect laboratory animals against the action of carcinogens or cancer forming agents. For example the addition of yeast, which supplies B vitamins, to the diet of rats protected them when they were fed a potent carcinogen. The B vitamins not only delayed the appearance of liver cancer, but improved the overall health of the animals even after liver cancer appeared. Penicillin discovery led scientists down a different avenue of thought in so far as if Penicillin attacked bacterial invaders, and then surely there had to be a similar chemical that could attack cancer cells. The nutritional therapies then were quietly assigned to the wilderness and only survived in the work of men like Gerson.

Most of the alternative methods of treating cancer rely on detoxification or the removal of toxic substances from the body. The Gerson Therapy uses only organic food, as Gerson believed pesticides and food additives polluted the body and the quantity of food used in the diet, would otherwise provide excessive toxic chemicals.

As I have said the alternative therapies particularly the Gerson Therapy is non-specific meaning that they can be used to treat a number of chronic diseases, which Gerson covered in his book. '*A Cancer Therapy: The Results of 50 Cases.*' During my research, I decided to evaluate the main alternative cancer therapies, in the hope that I could identify common elements and further identify what elements of those therapies were causing success and why. Having identified the common elements, it would then be easier to formulate a mechanism for cancer. It seemed to me to be a logical route that any cancer research should have taken many years ago.

THE GERSON THERAPY

The most comprehensive alternative cancer treatment at the time I looked at the alternatives was the Gerson Therapy. It is based upon nutrition and metabolic therapy; it is not perfect and as my own research shows, is acting in an additional way other than recognised.

Max Gerson was repeatedly professionally attacked, most violently by his own colleagues, and his New York clinic fought to survive for many years. When in many cases patients became cancer-free, their former doctors sometimes destroyed records confirming that they had the disease.

One of the first books I read about the Gerson Therapy apart from Gerson's own book was that of Jaquie Davidson entitled '*Cancer Winner*'. Jaquie an American was 36 years old in 1974 when she discovered a number of lumps on her body. Jaquie was determined never to have orthodox treatment and she started out on her journey, as do many survivors, by reading all she could about cancer and natural cures. Jaquie found the Gerson Therapy through a book written by a journalist entitled '*Dr Gerson a True Cancer Cure?*'[28]. The journalist had set out to cover a 'quack' type story for his newspaper, but ended up completely converted and described Gerson as a "genius".

Dr Gerson a German doctor developed his therapy in the 1920s and it became one of the most comprehensive, documented and influential treatments for the non-toxic treatment of cancer. Dr Gerson suffered over many years from the Chemical Syndicate attacks causing his methods to be rejected throughout his lifetime. The therapy still remains on the American Cancer Society's unproven methods list.

The Gerson programme is a full time occupation and is not that easy to follow. By this I mean it is very time consuming and it really is a lifestyle choice because it does change your life radically. The therapy is not just a diet it is a whole programme aimed at rectifying the patient's metabolism internally. Gerson in his book entitled '*A Cancer Therapy: Results of 50 cases*', documented 50 cases of terminal cancer patients he treated and whom survived. He produced substantive clinical evidence inclusive of X-rays. Gerson summed up his therapy by saying: 'What is essential is not the growth itself or the visible symptoms; it is the damage of the whole metabolism including the loss of defence, immunity and healing power. It cannot be explained with nor recognised by one or another causes alone'. The important point Gerson was making is that cancer is a disease that requires a number of boxes to be ticked before you actually develop the disease. This is why a whole approach is required. Some people lead very unhealthy life-styles but still do not develop cancer and it may be that they have a strong mental attitude towards life.

Gerson believed that cancer begins in the soil, which has been depleted by artificial chemical fertilisers such that it has a much lower mineral content than food grown on soil fertilised by compost (organic). Peoples that grow their food naturally without pesticides and chemical fertilisers enjoy good health. This is in direct opposition to the recent announcement in Britain in 2009 that organic food has no advantage over chemicalised food. The Japanese in their native land, eating their native food had a very low incidence of cancer, but immigrants who went to live in America and who then ate a western diet of refined foods quickly developed the statistical norms for cancer in America. I have also previously mentioned the rapid rise in cancer in China and "cancer villages" occurring due to industrial chemical pollution in the soil and water.

The soil is a complex structure where there is an ecological balance of bacteria, fungi, microorganisms, larger animals and plants, which together comprise a whole ecosystem. In a healthy ecosystem the plants are protected from disease, by the very self-balancing system: fungi and bacteria especially nitrogen fixing bacteria enable plants to make their own food, using sunlight, nitrates and water. In turn the plant food is eaten by plant eating animals and so on. When the animals and plants die they return the nutrients in their bodies back to the soil and fertilise it. Earthworms aerate the soil and certain fungi grow inside plant roots again assisting with plant growth. Organic farming seeks to protect this delicate ecosystem.

The application of chemical fertilisers may initially promote growth in plants and pesticides protect against disease, but they kill the organisms necessary to maintain the ecosystem. Consequently plants will be weaker and more disease prone. The nutrient value of such plants is poor and after many years of using chemical fertilisers and pesticides the soil becomes depleted as an ecosystem. As the soil population falls, the amount of humus the dead organic material in the soil becomes depleted and the soil cannot then retain rainwater. Finally the rich topsoil is washed away by wind and rain and you get dust like conditions, which will support only a very limited ecosystem and where food production is impossible. In the past farmers used to rotate their crops and leave one field free of food production or fallow, in order to rest it.

Gerson was very perceptive to recognise the importance of the soil as early as the 1930s. He was also very perceptive to recognise the continual destruction of food in packing where he maintained: 'the food substances are damaged as they are refined, bottled, bleached, powdered, frozen, smoked, salted, canned and coloured with artificial colouring'. He went on to describe how this weakened and adulterated food leads to systemic deterioration. He maintained that: 'cancer is not a single cellular problem; it is an accumulation of numerous damaging factors combined in deteriorating the whole metabolism, after the liver has been progressively impaired in its functions'.

The liver is known to be the major organ in the body, which detoxifies and therefore has a key metabolic role. Gerson had noticed in his own patients that impaired liver function always occurs before the symptoms of cancer appear. Today there are numerous studies, which show hepatic or liver insufficiency is present in cancer patients. Further, alcohol intake, which is known to cause liver damage and sclerosis, increased the likelihood of developing cancer. The recent rise in mouth, oesophageal, stomach and colon cancers has been suggested to be linked to alcohol consumption and smoking and I suggest, a poor diet in combination. Again a combination of factors is required for onset to occur. This is not to discount mental attitudes.

Gerson recognised the need to eliminate all toxins from the body, including the end products of poorly digested proteins and fats. Detoxification is achieved by limiting toxin intake, by eating organic food and taking coffee enemas. Potassium is also given to restore a normal sodium and potassium balance in the cells, as cancer patients show excessive sodium in the cells and very low potassium levels. Today we recognise the importance of a low fat low sodium or salt diet.

The therapy further aimed to assist oxygenating mechanisms in the cells because the tumours tend to live without oxygen using a process called anaerobic respiration or fermentation. Respiration is the mechanism by which we obtain energy from food and is not the same as breathing. It is a chemical reaction in the cells, which releases energy from food molecules, which is essential to the normal functioning of cells. In a normal healthy body fermentation or anaerobic respiration i.e. obtaining energy with reduced oxygen, only occurs in muscle cells when we exercise for some time and our oxygen consumption cannot keep up with the muscle cell demands. Normally then we don't tend to use anaerobic respiration, we use aerobic or oxygen respiration. We require oxygen to release energy from our food. Cancer cells are likely to die in the presence of oxygen, which may provide us with at least a suggestion of why lung cancer can result from smoking – decrease in oxygen to the cells, apart from the carcinogens in the tar.

Otto Warburg, two-time Nobel Laureate (1931 for his discovery of the oxygen transferring enzymes of cellular respiration and in 1944 for his discovery of the hydrogen transferring enzymes) described an experiment by Gawhe, Geisler and Lornez at Dahlen Institute:

'If one puts embryonic mouse cells into a suitable culture medium, saturated with physiological oxygen pressures, they will grow outside the mouse body in vitro' (test tube) 'and indeed as pure aerobes' (oxygen requiring metabolism) 'with a pure oxygen respiration, without a trace of anaerobic respiration. However, if during the growth one provides an oxygen pressure so reduced, that the oxygen respiration is partially inhibited, the purely aerobic metabolism of the mouse embryonic cells is quantitatively altered within 48 hours in the course of two cell divisions into the metabolism characteristic of fermenting cancer cells! If one then brings such cells, in which during their growth reduced oxygen pressure and cancer cell metabolism has been produced, back under the original high oxygen pressure and allows the cells to grow further, the cancer metabolism remains. It would appear at least then oxygen deprivation induced cancer is irreversible (in mice)' [29].

Although this tends to indicate that cancer is irreversible at least in the case of oxygen deprivation, in a later section research will show that cancer is not irreversible. However Warburg's research clearly shows that low oxygen levels could induce a cancerous state in mice.

That oxygen therapy is beneficial has been shown in another experiment. In 1957 R.A Holman of the Welsh National School of Medicine in Cardiff reported the cure in experimental models of cancer by adding hydrogen peroxide to the drinking water [30] Holman reported:

'It seemed to me, that the only effective way to destroy the malignant cells, which are already deficient in catalase and sensitive to over oxygenation, is to keep up a continued administration of an active oxidizing agent. Since hydrogen peroxide is an excellent ionising solvent and since it is formed and is obviously of great fundamental importance, in most living cells this agent appears to be one of choice...Rats implanted with Walker 256 Adenocarcinoma were treated simply by replacing their drinking water with a dilute solution of commercial hydrogen peroxide and maintaining them on a normal diet. The rate of cure was measured at on average of 50 – 60%. The time taken for the complete disappearance of the tumour was between 15-60 days'.

The treatment was used in four humans with very advanced inoperable tumours. In two of the cases there was a marked clinical improvement with a decrease in the size of the liver (which contained metastases) and progressive diminution in the blood serum polysaccharide, which Keyser had shown to be an indication of effective therapy in neoplastic states. Ozone was also found to inhibit tumour growth in mice.

It was Otto Warburg who suggested that the addition of respiratory enzymes to the food of cancer patients would improve oxidative metabolism even in malignant cells. Scientific observations confirm that all cancer cells have impaired cellular respiration. It seemed to me then, that at least researchers should have progressed in this research of oxygen therapy and support of oxidative metabolism in cancer patients.

Gerson viewed the liver as critical, because of its vital metabolic role, explaining that impaired liver function almost always predates the appearance of cancer. Dr Jesse Greenstein, former Chief of the National Cancer Institute Biochemistry Division, said in his *1954* book '*Biochemistry of Cancer*' that: 'there seems to be little doubt that hepatic (liver) insufficiency is a concomitant phenomenon of cancer'. Again it seemed to me that support of liver function in cancer patients was another area that should have received more attention and research.

Gerson saw the liver as vital because it cleans the blood of toxins and contains enzymes, which assist chemical reactions including the use of oxygen in respiration. The enzymes are re-activated in the liver. The liver also assists the pancreas with preparation of pancreatic enzymes that digest protein including

253

those that comprise cancer cells. In his book Gerson emphasised that only once the body is detoxified can the oxidising and protein digesting enzymes become re-activated, thus resulting in a metabolic environment, which helps to deprive the cancer cells of the medium for their growth. By preventing fermented processes and encouraging a highly oxidising metabolism, the cancer cells cannot grow by fermentation, a process that requires a lack of oxygen. Warburg wrote in 1966:

'During the cancer development the oxygen respiration always fails, fermentation appears, and the highly differentiated cells are transformed to the fermented anaerobes which have lost all their body functions in that they become highly de-differentiated and now retain only the useless property of growth. Thus, when respiration disappears, life does not disappear but the meaning of life disappears and what remains are growing machines which destroy the body in which they grow'.

This research at least for a scientist is stunning: stunning because the addition of highly toxic chemicals in chemotherapy, can only add to the toxic overload of an already poor liver function in cancer patients and deter the oxygenating respiration system that Warburg identifies as critical. This research would also explain why toxic chemicals in food or the environment could cause cancer. Why then are highly toxic chemicals being given to cancer patients?

Otto Warburg claimed that the prime cause of disease was impaired cellular respiration [31]. Cell respiration occurs in the mitochondria of cells, which are compared by analogy to tiny 'power plants', where the cell produces its energy in the presence of oxygen. Once food has been broken down to its simplest molecular components, this fuel travels via the bloodstream to the cells and mitochondria, which then 'burn' this fuel in the presence of oxygen to provide energy in a process termed aerobic respiration.

Mitochondrial oxidation of sugar, which requires respiratory enzymes supplied by food, produces energy in the form of ATP (Adenine Tri-Phosphate), for most energy requiring functions of the body. It is also dependent on cellar ion concentration, which provides the appropriate environment for the mitochondria to function. For example, when cellular ion (e.g. sodium and potassium ions) concentrations are altered in susceptible individuals by high sodium (salt), low potassium diets and/or toxins damage, then the production of ATP by the mitochondria will be adversely affected, which will decrease the amount of energy available. There is a dwindling cycle, whereby low ATP or energy production also intensifies the disturbance in cation association and water structuring within the cell, which then again further impairs mitochondrial function: this was described by Freeman and Cope as the 'tissue damage syndrome' [32]. What this means is that the more salt you take in, the greater ability there is to damage the internal balance in cells, which then affects the vital aerobic respiration.

In people suffering from chronic fatigue syndrome, I suspect that their mitochondrial respiratory function may be impaired, either through toxic damage, or liver insufficiency, probably both and/or some other factor. There is also a notable depression, which may depend on the psychological mechanism, I discuss for cancer.

Gerson maintained that by correcting the metabolism of the patient and assisting oxidising enzymes, which oxygenate cells and re-activating proteolytic enzymes, which then assist with the breakdown of protein, the symptoms of cancer or the tumour could be made to disappear. The therapy reduces the amount of protein in the diet to stop a build-up of poorly digested protein, when the patients' proteolytic enzymes are already challenged. In the initial months on the Gerson therapy, no protein other than the liver juices is allowed, but as the patient progresses, gradually some protein is introduced by way of cottage cheese. Also Gerson advised proteolytic enzyme supplements to further assist with protein breakdown.

Although Gerson never mentioned the mind in cancer, apart from depression during healing reactions, the re-stimulation of chronic somatics and past traumas, could cause tension in an area and therefore reduced blood flow to that area, carrying oxygen. Cells then may be forced to undergo fermentation or anaerobic respiration (without oxygen). Lymph flow carrying anti-bodies would also be reduced affecting the immune response. Further toxic waste could build up and if the diet of the individual was poor and overloaded with toxins and additives, then a cancer metabolism could develop.

Enzyme systems, which protect cells against chemical carcinogens, are depressed by refined diets. The loss of these carcinogen detoxifying enzyme systems like microsomal mono-oxygenase oxidase, means that cells run a risk of becoming malignant. Wattenberg of the University of Minnesota conducted a series of experiments revealing that a purified diet of protein, starch, corn

255

oil, salt and vitamins, depressed liver detoxification enzymes by 100%: whereas Wattenberg and his colleagues found that cruciferous vegetables such as cauliflower, broccoli, cabbage and brussel sprouts are potentiatiors of microsomal oxygenase oxidase [33]. Correct nutrition is then essential for normal cell metabolism and whilst dubious recent research appears to show no correlation between diet and cancer, there is a great deal of research that *does* show diet has profound effects on cellular metabolism. One has to scrutinise where the research comes from and who finances it.

In the 1920s Gerson experimented with the use of coffee enemas and proposed that caffeine taken rectally passes through the portal vein into the liver, where it stimulates bile flow by opening the bile ducts so bile can flow more freely. Together with the increased bile flow is the vital release of the toxins accumulated in the liver. The bile also contains many of the waste products which have been detoxified by the liver and thus in the enemas, these waste products are carried to the intestines and then out of the body. The coffee enemas together with the castor oil enemas also relieve pain and since Gerson insisted that patients had to stop using drugs including painkillers the enemas became an important way to control pain. Gerson explained the rationale behind enemas in his book by saying that when large tumours break down, the patient would be overwhelmed by the toxins these masses contain inclusive of dead tumour cells. The enemas were needed to remove this material quickly. To further detoxify patients are advised to take castor oil orally and by enema every other day.

The diet itself consists of oats or porridge organically grown as everything else, with fruit for breakfast – salad, vegetable soup or the Hippocrates soup as it is known and cooked vegetables and bake potato with salad for both lunch and then again for dinner. Protein was provided in the liver juices and later in the therapy by a little cottage cheese. Reduced protein intake Gerson considered was essential to allow the liver to rid itself of toxins produced by tumour breakdown, rather than in dealing with any large intake of protein in the diet. In addition to load the body with minerals and vitamins and the oxidising enzymes, patients drink 13 eight-ounce glasses of carrot and apple, green leaf, or raw liver juice every hour over the thirteen hourly periods. There is also one orange juice at breakfast. Today the liver juice is omitted, replaced by concentrated liver supplements, because of the BSE infection in cattle, although the current position should be checked with the Gerson Institute.

The carrot and apple juices provide large quantities of carotene, which is the precursor of vitamin A. A study carried out in 1960 in Germany published in the *Nutritional Abstract Reviews* reported that where 218 patients received intramuscular injections of 300,000 IUS of vitamin A and one gram intravenous injections of vitamin C daily between 14 and 21 days and followed by oral application for three to six months, growth of tumours generally stopped or regressed with no observable side effects. Vitamin A has an anti-cancerous activity, but in large doses it is toxic, thus the Gerson Therapy, supplies the precursor of vitamin A – carotene, which gives carrots their orange colour. Again it would seem that carotene, would be a sensible inclusion in any cancer therapy.

The rationale for the juices being supplied hourly is to provide a high level of glucose in the blood. Cancer patients in later stages lose weight. In 1982 K. Bennegard of the University of Gothenberg [34] reported that depleted cancer patients differ from depleted (non- cancerous) controls in that the cancer cells used almost no glucose after fasting. He also found that normal tissue in cancer patients is resistant to insulin (refusing to bind it as in the adult onset of diabetes), which results in the low level of glucose uptake.

If cancer is a return to the embryonic metabolism and biochemistry of high sodium low potassium, as I suggest in my research, it is possible that growth hormone may be responsible for the inactivity of insulin as growth hormone and insulin are antagonistic in their actions. Growth hormone has a diabetogenic effect: growth hormone elevates the plasma level of protein factors that antagonise the action of insulin in vitro.

The Gerson Institute [35] state there is some indication that an intravenous injection of GKI (glucose, potassium, insulin) in advanced cancer patients has a very positive and marked effect. At the La Gloria Hospital (Gerson Clinic) there was one report of a woman brought in, in a semi- comatose state by air ambulance flight, in a last ditch attempt to save her life and who after four days was up taking herbal tea.

Dr Dimitrio Sodi-Pallares in 1981 developed GKI intravenous treatment for acute myocardial infarction and heart disease and later applied it to cancer patients [36]. Dr Sodi-Pallares suggested that the influence of GKI treatment was due to the correction of the tissue damage syndrome described by Cope [32].

Jade and Manfred F. Rajewski from the Institute for Cell Biology (tumour research) at the University of Essen in Germany, reported in *Cancer Research* [37] that tumour cells when perfused with intravenous glucose solutions became acid due to the fermented metabolism of the malignant cells. No acidity developing in normal cells. The pH of malignant cells dropped from 7.1 to 5.2 preventing further division. Unlike normal cells, malignant cells take up glucose at whatever concentration it occurs in the serum, fermenting it to lactic acid. The researchers further stated that tumours do not have a good vascular system, and therefore were unable to transport away excess lactic acid, which then generally swamps and acidically poisons the cells.

Snacks on the Gerson Therapy consist of raw fruit and vegetables, although I must admit I used to slow bake thinly sliced organic potato 'chips' – no oil of course and because only two tablespoons of linseed oil a day are allowed I would save it for a dressing for my bake potatoes and the oven bake 'chips'. Not much of a culinary delight but to me it was bliss. Linseed oil it has been discovered thins the blood, through an essential fatty acid and reduces viscosity and this has been associated with reduced metastases or spread of cancer. Although not known in Gerson's lifetime, there is new evidence which shows that linseed oil is rich in a type of essential fatty acid which reduces blood viscosity, which has been shown to be associated with a reduced tendency to metastases or spread of cancer. By thinning the blood, there may be less tendency for cancer cells to clump and form tumours elsewhere in the body, when transported by the bloodstream.

There is a strict adherence to the rationale of not using fat or the re-introduction of protein into the diet for some considerable time after commencement of the Gerson Therapy. Both foods appear to re-stimulate the growth of tumours. The therapy in striving to eliminate toxins, including the end product of poorly digested protein and fat, does not provide extra protein or fat in the diet. According to Gerson, once the body has detoxified, the oxidising and protein digesting enzymes (proteolytic) are re-activated and can then turn on the cancer, digesting and removing tumours. The oxidising enzymes acting as catalysts that help the breakdown of nutrients using oxygen in a process called oxidation prevent the fermentation metabolism associated with cancer. Dr Gerson also claimed that these oxidising enzymes are also to be found in the juices and not all are destroyed in the digestive process. The use of a special grinder and press and juicer, is to maintain the integrity of these enzymes: the electric charge produced by centrifugal juicers destroys

258

enzymes and mixes air into the juices hastening decomposition: for this reason juices must be freshly prepared and cannot be stored.

The Gerson Therapy does not allow what I call 'mucked about' foods - bottled, canned, pre-packed, no colours, no additives, no preservatives, no smoked, no frozen even. Everything is sourced and prepared fresh. Herbal teas are allowed but no regular tea and coffee apart from the latter in enemas this was because Gerson claimed the effect of caffeine taken orally was quite different, from taken rectally. Further all water even that to wash and prepare vegetables and salad, has to be distilled. I purchased mine from a chemist in large two and half litre containers, although if one could afford a high volume still that would prove cheaper in the long run.

Gerson stated: 'the food substances are damaged as they are refined, bottled, bleached, powdered, frozen, smoked, canned and coloured with artificial colouring. It is this weakened and adulterated food which leads to systemic deterioration....' and commenting further on cancer he stated: 'it is not a single cellular problem it is an accumulation of numerous damaging factors in deteriorating the whole metabolism, after the liver has been progressively impaired in its function'.

Finally Gerson gave potassium thyroid and iodine as half strength Lugol solution. Again these additions were aimed at destroying the fermented environment so necessary to the growth of cancer cells. In order to assist liver function, patients also received crude liver extract injections along with vitamin B12. Gerson also recommended niacin, a B vitamin as a capillary or small blood vessel dilator, which would assist oxidation, by allowing more blood carrying oxygen to reach target cells. Patients are further advised to take betaine hydrochloride and the enzyme pancreatin to assist in the digestion of food and particularly proteins.

The addition of potassium to the Gerson diet is based on research, which shows that potassium is an anti-cancer agent. Normally in the adult, there is a high concentration of potassium inside the cells and high sodium levels outside the cells, but as the cells age, and in degenerative diseases including cancer, the amount of sodium in the cells rises and potassium levels go down. In addition to the large supply of potassium in the fresh juices, potassium is also supplied as a supplement.

259

Clarence D. Cone a biophysicist and former head of the molecular biophysics laboratory at NASSA's Langley Research Centre in Hampton, Virginia found: 'that proliferation of malignant (and normal) cells in cultures can be effectively turned off by suitably lowering the intercellular sodium concentration while elevating the potassium concentration and the blocked cells soon die; the key factor is the lowering of the intracellular sodium level'.

Again one is left stunned by this research and the fact that cancer patients are not given potassium: so if there is another thing the cancer patient should do to maximise survival, it is to take potassium and remove salt from the diet. Enough salt is provided in normal climates by fresh fruit and vegetables.

In an excerpt from Dr Gerson's unpublished papers (August 1938), he referred to the sodium/potassium balance in development. In the course of our lives we change from sodium to the potassium animal: 'that change must be complete, definite and maintained throughout life as it is decisive for health from the beginning to the end of our existence'. The fertilised ovum or the young embryo and foetus has a sodium based metabolism, but post birth the metabolism changes to a potassium based metabolism, which Gerson felt was essential to be maintained, thus avoiding salt in the diet. Gerson went on to say: 'the sodium group accumulated in the chromosomes and genes especially iodine, seems to control the velocity of growth into a morula (ball of cells) and further into the germ layers. In general, the velocity of growth seems to depend mostly upon the amount of sodium group and its iodine: as sodium plus iodine means faster growth and de-differentiation, potassium and Iodine means slower growth and specific differentiation'.

I have to remind myself of the date on which Gerson said this - 1938! It's another stunning observation that should have been followed up and evidently was by NASSA, but has not surfaced in any orthodox advice.

As a scientist I find this information particularly interesting. It is as though the embryo is best served as it develops by sodium or salt based metabolism, which may reflect the evolution of man from the seas. In the course of a science education one comes across the theory of 'ontogeny recapitulates phylogeny'. It was first proposed as 'fact' by Ernst Haeckel nearly 100 years ago, but has been allegedly disproved. The recapitulation theory, better known as the' biogenetic law', claims that each embryo in its development passes through abbreviated stages that resemble developmental stages of its evolutionary ancestors. The gill slits of human embryos are supposed to represent the fish or amphibian stage of man's evolutionary ancestors. Most professional evolutionists no longer believe this theory. The famous evolutionist Dr Paul Ehrlich, for example, said: 'this interpretation of embryological sequences will not stand close examination. Its' shortcomings have been almost universally pointed out by modern authors, but the idea still has a prominent place in biological mythology' [38].

In his book *'The Beginnings of Life'*, embryologist Dr E. Blechschmidt reveals some of his frustration with the persistence of this myth: 'The so-called basic law of biogenetics is wrong. No buts or ifs can mitigate this fact. It is not even a tiny bit correct or correct in a different form. It is totally wrong' [39]. And yet here we have a basic piece of research to show that the embryo relies on sodium metabolism, whereas the adult has potassium based metabolism and one wonders whether in fact Haeckel was correct and the embryo does at least metabolically recapitulate its phylogeny. At least the mind appears to retain the old primitive mechanisms for survival.

Gerson and other researchers have all noted that high levels of sodium (to potassium) are present in fast growing plant and animal tissues. In order for the child to change to a potassium-based metabolism Gerson maintained depended on the child having access to a plentiful supply of fruits and vegetables rich in potassium. Organic food he maintained, grown without artificial fertilisers and pesticides contained higher levels of potassium, minerals, vitamins and enzymes. He went on to say: 'The more firmly the new potassium majority is established and maintained in the essential organs such as liver, muscles, brain, nervous system, stomach, kidney, cortex etc., the stronger is the resistance and protection against acute and degenerative or chronic diseases, one of which is the great complex of cancers and malignancies'.

Gerson also interestingly stated: 'when the general K/I (potassium/iodine) protection is lost, there is not much difference whether the malignancy generates from an embryonic remnant, where the original sodium majority is still present, or from a part of an organ where sodium is physiologically re-absorbed and accumulated. We find this biological situation in the pancreas, colon, kidneys, and lower ducts of the breast and also in the stomach walls where chloride is split off and sodium returned to the veins. Finally it is true in tissues damaged by chronic inflammation, thrombosis, ulcer formations, or

261

underdevelopment, frequent in ovary and testes. They all show the same characteristics a surplus of sodium and Iodine *locally* but more or less lost *generally*. This facilitates carcinomatous growth of cells with all its consequences'.Gerson thus gave the additional supplements of potassium, iodine and thyroid extract to redress the sodium/potassium balance.

So it is a formidable diet and as Gerson warned: 'It is advisable not to start the treatment, if for any reason strict adherence to it is not possible'. Each element Gerson maintained is important and he emphasised that for the diet to be effective every aspect had to be complied with. Even the juicer has to be a special corkscrew motion type such as the Norwalk, or Champion and they are very expensive.

Apart from the diet, there are the so-called 'flare ups' or healing reactions one goes through on the therapy. The symptoms range from flu-like symptoms, weakness, depression and feverishness to the other end of the scale of diarrhoea, nausea and vomiting. However there is no warning given over the psychological flare-ups, which can be horrendous in the first four months of the therapy. In the early stages there is also often a great deal of gas, but that passes. For my part the mental component of these flare-ups was by far the worse. A lot of patients simply give up at this stage of the therapy when it occurs around 4 months into the therapy, because they are panic driven – Michael Gearin-Tosh went through this pure panic stage accompanied with his dreams. The Gerson Institute always explains the mental component as due to toxin elimination and would not consider, at least in my efforts with Charlotte, to recognise the mechanism of the mind discussed here; although privately a doctor at the Institute told me: "I had better come to you if I really want to know how the Gerson Therapy works".

The flare-ups generally last for only two or three days, which seems a lifetime, because they can be very frightening, but they do pass if you continue with the diet and enemas. It is during the flare ups and because rest is required, that although I did it alone, I would not advise it because the experience was on the edge of what anyone is capable of enduring: as one patient stated: "If you don't have help you're not on the Gerson Therapy, you are doing something else". So if climbing Everest alone with two children on your back would not deter you, then go ahead! Many Gerson patients have friends or family who take shifts or rotas in the daily routine. Jaquie Davidson's husband Ron supported her decisions and helped to hold the family together during her many crises. One of her daughters -Ramona stayed home from school for a long time to help her mother with the therapy. Michael Gearin-Tosh had a helper to do his juices and he was able to return to work at Oxford University, through an agreement with their caterers. Michael also had friends who rallied round. Perhaps in some enlightened future, firms will provide facilities for employees who develop cancer.

Although I will leave a greater discussion of this aspect to the section on the mind and my own research, I will mention here that in my view psychological counselling is an essential part of the Gerson Therapy. I have seen patients who do well on The Gerson Therapy and then something happens, such as a family conflict or some psychological upset that they feel either they cannot resolve or overcome – the will to live just goes. Patients who did resolve psychological conflict did much better and survived, whilst the others died.

Dr Gerson immigrated to America from Germany, before World War II and opened a clinic in Nanuet, New York. He successfully treated cancer of the lung, breast, skin, brain and digestive tract, including many so-called "terminal" cases. He cured Dr Albert Schweitzer of diabetes and Mrs Schweitzer of tuberculosis. Dr Schweitzer considered Gerson to be: 'one of the most eminent geniuses in medical history'. Dr Gerson graduated from the University of Freiburg in 1907 and began his career as a specialist in nerve and other diseases. He did however suffer from debilitating migraines that his doctors were unable to cure. Gerson tried many therapies before finally turning to a fresh fruit and vegetable diet and found his migraines stopped. Gerson naturally tried this diet on other migraine sufferers with the same success. One of those patients was a young man who had lupus vulgaris a form of skin tuberculosis considered at the time to be incurable. Gerson found to his amazement that not only did the young man's headaches disappear but also his lupus vulgaris.

Because of this success in 1924, Doctor Ferdinand Sauerbruch a leading European authority on lung TB or tuberculosis contacted him. In a joint study the two men treated 450 lupus patients with the therapy and 446 of them recovered. Sauerbruch in his book 'Master Surgeon' acknowledged Gerson's work. Dr Gerson then tried his diet on a variety of other chronic diseases and found the diet was successful in the treatment of arthritis, heart disease, chronic sinusitis, ulcers, colitis, high blood pressure and psoriasis to name a few.

In 1928 a woman with inoperable bile duct cancer and with two metastases to the liver asked Gerson to treat her with his diet. Gerson at first was very reluctant because he had already started to experience orthodox antagonism to his work after his success in treating TB. The woman agreed to sign a disclaimer for the outcome of her treatment and Dr Gerson successfully treated her.

In 1933, the rise of Hitler in Germany forced Gerson to leave and he went to America in 1936 and gained his New York licence in 1938. Gerson was never short of a steady stream of cancer patients knocking on his door, many of whom had been told to go home and die, as there was nothing more that could be done for them. Gerson was quite aware of the impossibly thin line he was treading with orthodox medicine and the Drug Trust, particularly the AMA – American Medical Association, but he was a highly compassionate doctor and could not turn these people away when they had come to him as their last hope. To quote Gerson:

'The knife of the AMA was at my throat and on my back. I had only terminal cases. If I had not saved them, my clinic would have been a death house. Some of the cases were brought in on stretchers. They couldn't walk. They could no longer eat. It was very, very difficult. So, I really had to work out a treatment that could help these far advanced cases'.

Initially using the diet, detoxification and the supplements Gerson had success with some of these difficult cases that were deemed incurable. In 1944 Gerson presented five of his recovered cancer patients before a session of the Senate Foreign Relations Committee. The hearing related to a piece of legislation known as the Pepper-Neely Bill. The Bill was to authorize and request the President to undertake to mobilise at some convenient place in the United States an adequate number of the world's outstanding experts, and to co-ordinate and utilize their services in a supreme endeavour to discover means of curing and preventing cancer. Many eminent doctors testified during the three days of this hearing, including Dr Rolla Dyer, Assistant Surgeon General and Director of The National Institute of Health. Dr Rhoads, Director of New York's Memorial Hospital attended as did Dr Oughterson who was Medical and Scientific Director of the American Cancer Society and Albert Lasker a member of the Executive Committee of the American Cancer Society.

The Pepper-Neely Bill, named after Senator Claude Pepper, who was the Chairman of the Committee, was aimed at providing a minimum of one hundred million dollars a year, to mount a 'war on cancer' - mounting the same kind of scientific and political effort that had led to the development of the atomic bomb. The same suggested effort re-occurred in 1971, when President Nixon announced his war on cancer, which was to parallel the effort it took to put a man on the moon. Despite Gerson's appearance along with some of his cured patients, his request for some of the multi- million-dollar research funds available was defeated by four votes due to the efforts of the medical lobby supporting the standard orthodox package.

It was a small success for Gerson however, because it was the first time in history that the Senate had honoured a physician in this way; but as Don Mitcham wrote in 1946 in '*Herald of Health*' magazine:

'The Committee report of 227 pages, Document number 89471, gathers dust in the archives of the Government Printing Office'.

My own research paper lays collecting dust in the British Library.

A newspaper reporter, who later inquired about the report, was told there were "no copies left". Five years after the congressional hearings, Gerson was not allowed to practice at any New York hospital. He was the victim of a by-now familiar cancer blackout: the inventor is isolated; the medical journals won't publish his work; and when he or she publishes elsewhere, they say it is not scientific. My own story followed much the same course.

As Houston and Null wrote:

'Meanwhile, the graves were filling up with the frightening mutilations of operating and X-ray rooms. 'Nothing more could be done for them,' said the medical establishment. They had already had their check-ups, sent in their cheques, and travelled the same worn, one-way road to suffering and death. Gerson died in 1950. The man who cured Albert Schweitzer's wife of tuberculosis and who was totally unrecognised by the medical world was hailed at the end by Schweitzer: "We who knew and valued him mourn him already today as medical genius".'

Gerson made the fatal mistake of sticking his head above the radar screen through his successes, where the Drug Cartel and the ruling orthodoxy spotted him. Gerson then went through the all-familiar methods of the Drug Cartel and orthodoxy to suppress his work, which was also rejected by most of his orthodox colleagues who feared they would have their medical licences taken away. Throughout his career, the medical authorities challenged Gerson and in 1958 the Medical Society of the County of New York suspended him. He also had great difficulty in publishing his scientific papers and getting past the peer review system. In this respect after contacting goodness knows how many journals my own research was finally published in an alternative medical journal (3). The whole point of publication is to inform the scientific and medical community and by preventing publication, the research then remains unknown.

Dr Gerson finally in frustration, gave a talk on an all-night radio programme and was promptly suspended by the County of New York Medical Society: 'as a result of personal publicity'. A reporter named Haught in trying to find out why the American Medical Association opposed the Gerson therapy was told: 'Although Dr Gerson had been requested to do so, he has failed or refused to acquaint the medical profession with the details of his treatment'. Believe you me I have many of these insane 'catch 22' letters in my files. Changing the facts is another method of the Syndicate and after years of dealing with these spiritually bankrupt types you just walk away to save your own sanity. One scientific magazine, told me they could not look at work that was not published even though I sent them a copy of the published scientific paper!

Gerson of course *had* managed to publish his work. The American Cancer Society made its position quite clear when in a July 8th 1957 edition of their Journal they stated: "There is no evidence at the present time that any food or any combination of foods specifically affects the course of any cancer in man". As America and many other western nations now show increasing nutritional related diseases and problems such as obesity, this can only be laid at the Drug Cartel's door and the Medical hierarchy as their lackeys. In 1976 the U.S. Senate Select Committee on Nutrition and Human Needs with Senator Mc Govern as Chairman held hearings and produced a highly commendable report entitled *Dietary Goals for the United States*. The report emphasised the importance of reducing the dietary intake of salt, sugar, fat, white flour and other highly processed foods, agricultural chemicals, chemicalised food, additives and other substances considered harmful. The report also encouraged the increased consumption of fresh fruit, vegetables and unprocessed foods. Predictably the American Medical Association responded angrily that there was no proof that nutrition has any effect on disease. Given that scurvy, rickets, beriberi, and pellagra had long since been identified, as being caused by vitamin deficiencies, the credibility of the American Medical Association should have been questioned, but then few scientists or doctors have the sustained determination to stand up to formidable bullies.

It's not that the Drug Cartel want to kill you, because dead people don't take drugs, they just don't want lots of healthy people, because they don't take drugs. As with the Pepper Neely Bill, which was not passed, the Drug Lobby got to work and Senator Mc Govern's report died a quick and silent death, presumably along with millions of Americans who carried on believing their western diet was healthy. As a result America is with other westernised nations now suffering the consequences.

There are quite a lot of medical studies mainly carried out before the 1980's, which provide adjunct evidence in support of Gerson's theory of how the diet works. Vitamin A is taken in large doses as carotene from carrots on the Gerson Therapy. Researchers going back to the 1920s have found that tumour growth is inhibited with high levels of vitamin A. A documented study was reported in 1960 in *'Nutritional Abstracts and Review'* where in a group of 218 patients given vitamin A and C, their tumours regressed or ceased and there were no reported side effects. Vitamin A can be toxic if given in large quantities, so it is generally given as carotene, which forms Vitamin A in the body and this negates toxicity.

In a nineteen-year study of 1,950 employees of Chicago's Western Electric Company, researchers at Rush-Presbyterian-St. Luke's Medical Centre, found that there was significantly less lung cancer in those whose diets were high in carotene than in those who ate low levels of carotene. The 488 men who ate little carotene had 14 cases of lung cancer, whereas the group that ate high levels of carotene only had 2 cases of lung cancer. Further this research has been repeated in Norwegian and Japanese studies where the protective effect of vitamin A has been noted.

It seems that whilst vitamin A has side effects in large amounts, carotene when taken in through carrots has no side effects and certainly in the two years I was on the diet I suffered no side effects, other than initial carotenosis, which passed after 4-5 months on the diet. Dr Hildebrand explained this effect to me as the liver coming to a balance, whilst one orthodox doctor fairly frothed at the mouth claiming I would die unless I stopped. I followed Dr Hildebran's advice and the carotenosis did pass, by following the complete Gerson regime. I think it would be wise to point out, that I have no results or evidence on the intake of large quantities of carotene alone, outside of the Gerson regime protocol, other than the couple I met at the Health Exhibition, where the man took a quart of apple and carrot juice daily, without side effects.

The sodium – potassium balance is central to my own research and when I discuss the research in the section on the mind, I will be returning to the potassium sodium balance. In an article in the January 25th 1980 '*Journal of the American Medical Association*', Dr Regelson unusually for such a publication had this to say: 'We may shortly have to ask if Gerson's low sodium diet, with its bizarre coffee enemas and thyroid supplementation, was an approach that altered the mitotic regulating effect of intracellular sodium for occasional clinical validity in those patients with the stamina to survive it'. Again this is another important part of my own research and which I will return to later, but here at least was recognition of the role of the sodium/potassium balance in cancer cell growth: Sodium appearing to turn on growth or mitotic cell division and potassium appearing to turn it off.

So why didn't the medical profession at least give potassium, vitamin C and carrots to their cancer patients? Well potassium is a cheap chemical and there's no money for the Drug Cartel there. Why don't they warn women of constipation, because even as far back as the 1970s researchers have found a link between breast cancer and constipation: constipation merely allows toxins to remain in the lower gut. Petrakis and King two epidemiologists at the University of San Francisco reported a study where women who are severely constipated have a greater number of abnormal cells in their breasts. Petrakis and King as adjunct research quoted surgeons who commented on the frequency with which they found chronic cystic breast disease and breast cancer in women who were constipated. In my own view obviously faeces when not eliminated tend to form a toxic environment generally and when the body cannot eliminate those toxins adequately they are likely to be stored in fat inclusive of breast fat. Constipation however does have causes one of which is lack of fresh vegetables and fruit and thus the cause may lay deeper as poor diet and lack of vitamins especially vitamin C.

Maurice Natenberg in his book *The Cancer Blackout* (*1959*) stated:

'At the time Doctor Gerson testified (at the Senate Hearing) he was on the staff of the Gotham Hospital of New York. Today he is not on the staff of any hospital, once he instructed his associates in his method of cancer therapy. Today he finds it impossible to secure medical assistants. Approaching the age of eighty, he now practises alone. For over 30 years he has demonstrated excellent results in treating cancer, his approach is on a highly scientific level, and his credentials are the finest. Yet he has never received a penny (from Government) to aid his research...despite the fact that the Gerson Therapy is based on authentic physiology, discoveries in biochemistry and nutrition, the medical journals will not publish his work'.

I certainly found the same, where there was difficulty in getting anything published and in the end I financed the research out of my own pocket, together with a £400 donation, having failed to get a penny from the government or cancer funding bodies. Dr Gerson died on March 8th 1959. His work might have ended there had not his devoted daughter Charlotte taken up the baton. Charlotte Gerson-Strauss carried on Gerson's work for many years across the border in Mexico, because of the legal position in America. The Gerson Institute and Sweetwater Terrace Retreat are now also in California, but the main clinic is still in Mexico.

As with all pioneers many of Gerson's basic ideas have been adopted without having his name acknowledged as source. This is a familiar method of orthodox science, because they really don't want anyone to know that most if not all innovative scientific thought comes from lone pioneers who are attacked by orthodoxy as heretics throughout their lives. The orthodox hierarchy would like the public to think that brilliance emerges from universities and research institutions including the charities, so that such bodies can keep receiving taxpayers' money and donations. They really don't want the public to know that the history of science is one of extreme suppression of any new idea, which stands to threaten the Syndicate or the 'secret society' as Bluchel claimed. They also suppress scientists who they think are not politically correct. It is astounding that Gerson was not able to engage in scientific research or teach in the land of the supposed free. Why didn't they make Gerson a Professor of nutritional medicine? That to me would have been the sane response to Gerson's work.

In the 1980s Dr Peter Lechner at Graz hospital in Austria sent me a report of his study using a limited form of the Gerson therapy in cancer patients who were also receiving orthodox treatment of surgery, radiation and chemotherapy. It was the first and only real modern attempt to appraise the therapy apart from the debacle of The Bristol Clinic trials, which I will come to. Despite the fact that he did not apply the full therapy and his patients were also being treated with toxic drugs, both actions Gerson would have denounced, Dr Lechner achieved favourable results. In a preliminary report Dr Lechner showed: 'Gerson patients with certain cancers, particularly adeno-carninomas of breast or colon, live longer and have a better quality of life than conventionally treated patients'. For political reasons Dr Lechener was only able to apply a highly modified version of the Gerson programme and not the full therapy, in conjunction with orthodox treatment, which Gerson would have rejected.

The Gerson therapy is the most scientifically documented alternative therapy but there are others and it is helpful to look at these therapies to find a common thread in their successes, which lead me to my own theory of the mechanism in cancer.

LAETRILE - B17

Laetrile is a trademark for an unstable, short-lived compound. It is a naturally occurring nitriloside containing cyanide. Anything sold, as laetrile is not laetrile at all, but probably amygdalin. It is claimed that when the patient takes amygdaline, it is broken down to produce laetrile, which is further broken down to produce two substances - cyanide and benzaldehyde, which then act at the tumour site. Laetrile then is a concentrated form of a compound similar to amygdaline or vitamin B17. It is derived naturally from a number of vegetarian sources particularly apricot pits, plum, apple peach and pear seeds. If you have ever eaten apple seeds, the taste is that of laetrile.

The use of certain fruit kernels in the treatment of cancer goes back to the Emperor herbalist Shen Nung in the 28th century BC. The Great Herbal of China an ancient pharmacopoeia dates between 2,800 and 2,500 B.C and refers to the "sacred seeds". 'Bitter almond water' features in the writings of the physicians of ancient Egypt, Arabia, Rome and Greece. Celsus, Galen, Scribonious Largus, Pliny the Elder, Avicenna and Marcellus Empiricus all used preparations based on the seeds of the bitter almond, apricot, peach etc.

In 1952 the American biochemist Ernst Krebs PhD proposed that cancer was a deficiency disease. He identified the deficiency substance as part of the nitroloside groups specifically amygdaline; a cyanogenic glycoside first isolated, from the bitter almond, prunus amygdalus amara, in 1830 by the French chemists Robiquet and Boutron-Charland. Its chemical structure is D (1)-mandelonitrile-B-D-glucosido-6-6-B-glucoside, as recorded in the Merck Index, 1976.

Toxicologically (according to US Reg. of Toxic Effects Chem. Subs. 1976), for amygdaline falls between Class 1 and Class 2, which means that it is virtually non-toxic. This compares with saccharin, between Class 3 and Class 4 and most chemotherapy is Class 6 or super toxic.

There were cultures that remained almost entirely cancer-free. The Abkhazians, the Azerbaijanis, the Hunzas, the Eskimaux and the Karakorum all lived on foodstuffs rich in nitriloside or vitamin B17. Their food consisted variously of buckwheat, peas, broad beans, lucerne, turnips, lettuce, sprouting pulse or gram, apricots with seeds and berries of various kinds. Their diet provided them with as much as 250-3,000 mg of nitriloside a day. Ernst T Krebs Jr., the pioneer of vitamin B17 research studied the dietary habits of these tribes and stated: 'Upon investigating the diet of these people, we found that the seed of the apricot was prized as a delicacy and that every part of the apricot was utilized'.

John Diamond, the late husband of Nigella Lawson a TV chef, developed cancer and then used his position (up until he died) as a journalist to spread rather vitriolic messages on alternative cancer therapies: whilst he underwent orthodox treatment. Unfortunately he was not a scientist and certainly being ill he was in no position, to judge. In his article in *The Observer* newspaper *'Quacks on the Rack'* (*3.12.2000*) he summarily dismissed what is arguably one of the most famous of the natural anti-cancer treatments – Vitamin B17. Without conducting any detailed research Diamond was to inform readers: 'Supporters of Laetrile (vitamin B17) and Essiac in particular, made so much noise about their miracle cures that both have been through the research mill on numerous occasions and found to be useless'. The statement was not true; nether-the-less *The Observer* printed the story, without question. Diamond had taken his view based on the 'doomed trials' which set out to encourage people like Diamond, to disseminate these faulty results to the public and so 'doomed trials' become points of 'fact' even nearly half a century later.

In fact Dr Dean Burk, the former head of the Cytochemistry Department of the National Cancer Institute, and one of the co-founders of this famous American medical institution, had worked on Vitamin B17 personally. He described this substance in very different terms: 'When we add laetrile to a cancer culture under the microscope, providing the enzyme glucosidase is also present, we can see the cancer cells dying off like flies'. In fact the enzyme glucosidase, was required to break down laetrile into its components, one being cyanide and this acted as a natural chemotherapeutic agent. The reason why Laetrile attacks the cancer cells, whilst apparently not damaging normal cells, is that the naturally occurring cyanide is only released by the high content of the enzyme present in cancer cells.

I will discuss the apparent resurrection of laetrile by drug company Antisoma later, but it is true to say that if there is a profit to be made then the drug industry is ever vigilant. Dr Ralph Moss PhD served as the Assistant Director of Public Affairs at America's most famous cancer research institution, Memorial Sloan Kettering, in Manhattan. Moss knew the cancer industry very well and in his book '*The Cancer Syndrome*' (*1980*) said this of the effectiveness of laetrile:

'Shortly after I went to work (at the Sloan Kettering Cancer Institute), I visited the elderly Japanese scientist, Kanematsu Sugiura, who astonished me when he told me he was working on Laetrile (B17). At the time it was the most controversial thing in cancer, reputed to be a cure for cancer. We in Public Affairs were giving out statements that laetrile was worthless, it was quackery, and that people should not abandon proven therapies. I was astonished that our most distinguished scientist would be bothering with something like this, and I said, "Why are you doing this if it doesn't work?" He took down his lab books and showed me that in fact Laetrile was dramatically effective in stopping the spread of cancer'.

Moss was then asked: "So this is verified, that laetrile can have this positive effect?"

Moss replied: "We were finding this and yet we in Public Affairs were told to issue statements to the exact opposite of what we were finding scientifically".

Unable to sit on this information, Moss later called a press conference of his own and, before a battery of reporters and cameramen, charged that Sloan-Kettering officials had engineered a massive cover-up. He provided all the supporting documents and named all the names necessary to validate his case. The following day he was fired for: 'failing to carry out his most basic job responsibilities'.

Similarly, in his book '*World without Cancer*' (*1974*), cancer industry researcher Edward Griffin noted:

'Every Laetrile study had been tarnished with the same kind of scientific ineptitude, bias and outright deception... Some of these studies openly admitted evidence of anti-cancer effect but hastened to attribute this effect to other causes. Some were toxicity studies only, which means that they weren't trying to see if Laetrile was effective, but merely to determine how much of it was required to kill the patient'.

Laetrile is another cancer therapy on the unproven list. When Laetrile started to show some positive effects, it immediately hit the radar screen of the authorities and so like many other alternative therapies was only thereafter to be found across the border in Mexico. Dr John Richardson had a clinic in Berkeley California when he first used Laetrile. The sister of one of his nurses had advanced malignant melanoma on her left arm and had been advised by her physician that she had six weeks to live and should have immediate amputation. Dr Richardson applied Laetrile therapy and after two months the arm was normal.

Thus it was on June 2nd 1972, the black cars arrived at his clinic carrying 9 officials and policemen, with guns drawn. Dr Richardson was spread eagled up against the wall in front of his patients, one of whom died 3 days later – perhaps they shattered her last hope in Dr Richardson. Dr Richardson was then marched out in handcuffs. Of course this was all filmed for media consumption along the lines of the 'quack bust' story. As with Gerson his licence to practise medicine was withdrawn. He was then forced to attend 15-minute court hearings some 600 miles away in San Diego, where many of the hearings were cancelled at the last moment. They kept this up for 6 months at weekly intervals. Dr Richardson claimed that juries and judges were rigged and with that kind of mental, financial and professional pressure it might have broken him.

The same fate had occurred to one of the first doctors to use Laetrile –Dr Maurice Kowan. He ended up in court in Los Angeles. The prosecutor told the jury: "This is not a kindly old man. This is the most thoroughly evil person the imagination can concoct...This man has to be stopped. He is very dangerous. The way to stop him is a guilty verdict". Dr Kowan was heavily fined and at the age of 70 sentenced to two months in prison.

In fact the justification used by the cancer cartel to attack Dr Kowan was a falsified report produced by two doctors, Garland and MacDonald in 1953. These two doctors were employed in conventional orthodox treatment of cancer i.e. surgery and radiation. They also had links to the tobacco industry and promoted them as a health measure! The two produced a report, which stated they found no evidence of anti-cancer properties in the use of Laetrile and yet no such tests or trial had been conducted. This report however was retained as gospel by the cartel and quoted in legal cases and in refusal of grant funding.

Although by the 1940s the Drug Cartel had 300,000 names on its 'quack' list, the case of B17 or Laetrile was always a particular threat because it was cheap and simple. The Cartel went into overdrive, not only creating fraudulent test reports, but also hired banner-carrying pickets to protest outside any clinic offering Laetrile. This was in addition to rigged juries in any trial, media character assassinations and dismissal of employees who would not toe the line.

The FDA sent out 10,000 posters and thousands of leaflets warning of the dangers of Laetrile, which was described as highly toxic and poisonous, playing on the cyanide component. Most FDA employees were part of the 'revolving door' and at the time it was discovered that 350 FDA employees had shares or links to pharmaceutical companies.

In order to prove their claim that Laetrile was poisonous the Cartel had to find deaths and after sifting through thousands of cases that had taken Laetrile the best they could come up with was two women who had swallowed vials of Laetrile meant for injection only. The other case was that of a baby who they claimed had ingested 5 (500mg) tablets of Laetrile meant for her father who had cancer. The mother however in an article in *Acres Magazine USA* (*August 78*) claimed the child had not ingested the tablets and died when the hospital administered an anti-cyanide antidote.

The scare stories on Laetrile distributed by the FDA soon crossed the pond to Britain. The Department of Health aided by Gwyneth Dunwoody MP, promoted these hysterical claims of 'cyanide poisoning' justifying the removal of apricot pit powder from health shops and in March 1984 the UK government brought in, 'The Medicines (Cyanogenetic Substances) Order' 1984. This required preparations which: '...are presented for sale or supply under the name of, or as containing amygdaline, Laetrile or vitamin B17 or...contain more than 0.1 per cent by weight...' of the 'cyanide producing substances' were to be controlled by the 1968 Medicines Act and thus unavailable to the cancer sufferer.

The figure of '0.1 per cent' was significant because bitter almond kernels are around 2 per cent amygdaline and certainly many foods containing almonds were not subjected to the witch-hunt on toxicity. Neither were grocery stores told to stop selling cherries, apples, pears, plums, peaches and apricots. All these vegetables farcically contravened the Order. Presumably Antisoma's new cyanide-based drug will not be subjected to a witch-hunt either.

Laetrile however was a therapy that did not go away and due to public pressure (which does work by the way, provided that voice is heard, which so often it is not); the ban on Laetrile was lifted and the Food and Drug Administration started a doomed trial as a counter measure. I think that the Drug Cartel smelt a profit here and that's the only reason they lifted the ban. Laetrile might be considered as natural chemotherapy and the Drug Cartel presumably thought they could bottle it and sell it. However the trick was to erase the history of the natural product and then having cut research and development costs use Laetrile as a starter for the development of a new drug. In the last section bringing you up to date, this is perhaps what has happened.

In addition to the falsified report by Garland and Macdonald the Cartel relied on experiments such as force-feeding large amounts of cyanide extracted from amygdaline directly into dogs' stomachs. In Laetrile therapy only small doses are used and further, the cyanide component is only released from amygdaline by an enzyme in cancer cells.

How did the Food and Drug Administration then finally erase the natural product? They used another familiar method of the 'doomed trial'. They *set out* to make the trial fail. Again I will come to more recent cases of this in the last section. The FDA in conjunction with the National Cancer Institute – NCI studied 200 patients over a two- year trial period using Laetrile. They deliberately chose very advanced cancer patients who were beyond any hope of cure or therapy known to extend life expectancy. In drug trials for the pharmaceutical industry, normally early stage patients are selected. Further the chemical used was not Laetrile but a less effective compound. No strict vegetarian diet was implemented and patients were allowed to eat animal products and the usual junk diet. Successes with Laetrile had only been obtained when it was used in conjunction with a dietary regime. As Gerson pointed out it's a whole approach, not just one specific item. Just to make sure it did not work, the injections of Laetrile were discontinued after 3 weeks instead of 3 months that Laetrile doctors recommend.

D. Dean Burk, head of cytochemistry at the NCI for 34 years later revealed the method of keeping the public deceived of any new alternative advance:

'Once any of the hierarchy so much as concede that laetrile anti-tumour efficacy was indeed once observe in NCI experimentation, a permanent crack in the bureaucratic armour has taken place that can widen indefinitely by further appropriate experimentation'.

Dr Ernesto Contreras in Mexico and Dr Hans Nieper in Hanover were working extensively with Laetrile in the 1980s and produced statistics based on 30,000 cases. They showed that in patients who have no metastasis or spread they achieved an 80% recovery rate. If the cancer had spread they achieved a 40% recovery and for terminal patients they obtained a 17% recovery rate. The results then if they are true, represent a better response than orthodox medicine. However it is important to note that Laetrile was not used alone in their programmes and was always combined with a diet, which was very similar to Gerson's in so far as it was low in protein, high in raw natural foods; and where pancreatic enzymes and certain protein dissolving or proteolytic enzymes were taken orally or injected into the tumour site, or used with the solvent DMSO as a poultice for external tumours, and coffee given as retention enemas. Vitamins particularly A and C, minerals and glandular extracts were also used. The programme itself is now known as metabolic therapy.

Dr Ernst Krebs Sr. and his son found that Amygdaline reduced some mice tumours and became interested in the work of John Beard a Scottish embryologist and Professor at Edinburgh University before his death in 1924. Beard being an embryologist was working with very early cells in embryo development called trophoblasts, which are the outermost layer of cells of the blastocyst that attaches the fertilized ovum to the uterine wall and serves as a nutritive pathway for the embryo.

Thus trophoblasts are basically a bunch of cells occurring after fertilisation, which under the action of oestrogen grow rapidly and then dissolve part of the uterine wall so that the fertilised egg can attach itself thus receiving the mother's nutrients and oxygen via the blood stream. The attachment eventually develops into the umbilical cord. What was extremely interesting to me was that Beard noticed the similarity of the cancer cell to the early trophoblast cells and he wondered whether the cancer cell could be a misplaced trophoblast cell or in other words a bunch of embryonic cells. These cells then lie dormant if you like in the body until they convert to cancer cells by some trigger, perhaps sodium. I have taken a different viewpoint on it, which again I will come to in the section on the mind.

Here however to me when I was researching in the 1980s this embryonic origin was a very interesting point: that cancer cells are similar to embryonic cells. In my file notes of the time I note I asked: 'so how does a cancer cell become embryonic?' I then noted a reference to Dr Regelson's work and his view of the mitotic regulating effect of sodium and another arrow in my notes lead to Gerson's view that cancer cells don't like potassium and that was his rationale in giving Lugol's solution. There is another note which reads: 'Cancer cells are embryonic, they have *reverted* to an embryonic metabolism for *some reason*!' In my research paper in 1989 I did suggest a reason and tied that to the mind. Embryonic cells are also more fermentive or can survive with less oxygen as might be expected when the baby is gaining its oxygen via the bloodstream through the umbilical cord and not the lungs. Cancer cells in biochemical comparison are also fermentive requiring less oxygen. Any therapy I concluded should be aimed at restoring the mature metabolic function of the cells, which clearly do not have the same metabolism as the cells of the embryo. In large words I wrote in my diary:

'CANCER CELLS RAPIDLY DIVIDE AND GROW AND SO DO EMBRYONIC CELLS SO IS THE CANCER REALLY JUST A REVERSION TO EMBRYONIC GROWTH?' *(Appendix 3)*

My mind had settled on the idea that reversion or 'going back to' was a key mechanism in cancer – the question became then how was this mechanism of reversion of mature adult cell to inappropriate embryonic growth brought about – what triggered this reversion? Things started like a jigsaw to make sense, a bigger picture of cancer was emerging, but I still had not quite worked out how mature cells suddenly revert or de-differentiate to an embryonic state. Was it really just an overload of salt in the diet, or lack of oxygen, but that did not fit many cases – there had to be something more and that something more I eventually found was *loss* and *a mind*.

Beard maintained that the *potential* trophoblasts do not all become trophoblasts or viable embryos, but mature to become sperm or ova. The terminology has changed a bit since Beards day and it's not worth going through terms; the point here is that many of the *potential* trophoblasts or early cells some 20% to 30% according to Beard are dispersed throughout the body.

I had to ask myself at the time whether they were the potential 'time bombs', just waiting for the right milieu or conditions when they would be activated to form cancer or if my theory is correct mini embryos of fast dividing cells. It may answer why the hormones oestrogen and testosterone have an effect upon cancer incidence. It might also suggest why recent research has shown that success in breast cancer treatment depends on when in the woman's menstrual cycle surgery is performed. How many women know about *that* research and insist their surgery is timed to their menstrual cycle?

Beard proposed that these embryonic pre-trophoblasts could under the influence of oestrogen develop into tumours. In pregnancy the trophoblast according to Beard multiplies rapidly until the fifty sixth day, when the foetal pancreas begins to secrete enzymes and then it stops. Beard reasoned that if the trophoblast could be stopped then he might be able to stall cancer growth with pancreatic enzymes. His work however, whilst showing some success was not conclusive. Significantly the Gerson Therapy and a number of other alternative therapies apply pancreatic enzymes.

Dr Krebs and his son started using proteolytic enzymes and also Amygdaline or Laetrile in their research. They theorised that Amygdaline was once a part of mans' diet but since grains of millet and buckwheat containing Laetrile or Amygdaline were not eaten now, then the natural ability to control cancer had been lost. They concluded that cancer was a vitamin B17 and vitamin C deficiency. Krebs in looking for some adjunct research to support his theory, pointed to the Hunzas in the Himalayas. Their diet, which used to consist of as many as 30 to 40 apricot kernels a day, was Krebs maintained, responsible for the fact that they showed little incidence of cancer. As another peripheral source of evidence Krebs also pointed to the Eskimos before they ate refined foods and where they showed virtually no cancer. One of the major foods of the Eskimo was caribou and when the Eskimos killed it, they would slit the stomach and eat its contents. The caribou eat a lot of arrow grass, which has a high level of Amygdaline in it.

Krebs in the 1950s teamed up with Dr Harris in Los Angeles, who had studied embryology under John Beard in Scotland and these men had good successes. In 1952 Harris invited the Chairman of the California Cancer Commission, which was part of the California Medical Association to come and review 44 cancer patients. In 1953 the Commission declared Laetrile had been investigated and was found to be worthless. This of course was the faulty

279

study. Further doctors were threatened with legal proceedings if they used it. As you will note later, this hasn't stopped laetrile being resurrected in current drug research – the tracks dusted of course.

Dr Guidetti in 1954 reported from the University of Turin in Italy that Laetrile applied to growths in the uterus, cervix and rectum, caused the cancers to dissolve. In 1963 Dr Morrone a surgeon at Jersey City Medical Centre reported in '*Experimental Medicine and Surgery*' that: ' the use of Laetrile intravenously in ten case of inoperable cancer, all with spread or metastases provided dramatic relief of pain, discontinuance of narcotics, control of fetor' (the noxious odour of advanced cancer),' improved appetite and reduction of adenopathy. The results suggest regression of the malignant lesion'.

Unfortunately no follow up studies were printed after Morrone died. In 1963 the FDA denounced Laetrile as ineffective and California State Public Health Department banned it. Despite this, Laetrile still refused to go away and by 1977 some 50,000 cancer patients were using Laetrile. By 1980 it was found some 2,000 patients a month went across the border to Mexico to obtain it. Laetrile was only legalised in some States after the Committee for Freedom of Choice took up the case of Laetrile. The faulty study by the NCI however had killed Laetrile; where they used terminal cancer patients, limited application of laetrile, wrongly sourced laetrile and thus without diet and all other elements of the holistic approach it was bound to give poor results. In fact the Report by the NCI claimed that 90% of the patients had growth of their cancers and half the patients died within 5 months with only 20% alive at eight months. As Krebs acidly put it: "They're not going to raise the dead, of course". Later it was claimed by Krebs that the material used in the NCI study was not the compound laevo-amygdaline produced by Krebs but another potentially toxic substance called racemic amygdaline.

The position with Laetrile then is confusing because of the doomed trials and not enough data, but I do note recently it is being resurrected in another incarnation, as a cyanide-based drug, which is one of the products of the breakdown of Laetrile in the body. However it is important to point out that most metabolic therapists also use diet. It seems that even in 1972 through to 1976 that Laetrile was still being researched, this time controversial experiments were being carried out at Sloan-Kettering by Dr Kanematsu Sugiura. Initially the research was withheld but under public pressure the results were eventually published in 1978. The report denied that Laetrile had any activity, although this contradicts Dr Moss's account earlier where Dr Sugiura obtained promising results with laetrile. Perhaps pressure was placed on Dr Sugiura to denounce laetrile's effectiveness. As if to confuse things further, the conclusions were rebutted in another report entitled *Second Opinion* and also in a paper called *Special Report: Laetrile at Sloan-Kettering*. It seems that the confusion arose because the findings actually showed that Laetrile reduced metastases in mice, which would have provided significant support for Laetrile to be further researched in clinical trials.

It seems that laetrile is a natural chemotherapeutic agent, but cannot alone miraculously provide a cure in the patient, where metabolism of cells is not addressed. It seems success was obtained in some cases when a whole approach including diet was undertaken.

HOXSEY

The story of Hoxsey and his fight with the medical establishment over unorthodox cancer treatment is another important historical episode in the development of alternative medicine in the 20th Century.

William Hoxsey and his son John lived on a farm in Madison County in the U.S and owned a rather lovely Percheron stallion. In 1849 the horse developed and open sore on its right leg, which developed into cancer. The vet recommended shooting the animal, but Hoxsey was reluctant to do that and so he put it out to grass. The animal's leg to Hoxsey's surprise started to improve, so Hoxsey watched what the animal ate. The horse every morning would go to the same pasture and graze. Eventually the tumour shrank enough and dried up, so that Hoxsey was able to cut it off with his knife. Hoxsey set about making various combinations of the herbs and plants the horse had eaten and then tested his results on other sick horses. He finally formulated a liquid, a salve or ointment and a powder. He successfully cured numerous horses and upon his death he passed his secret formula to his son John who passed it to his son Harry.

By 1901 Harry's father had been treating human cancers and did have successes. Harry continued this work, where his clinic became very successful and the largest independent clinic of the time. Hoxsey had put his head above the radar screen and was bound to come to the attention of the orthodox authorities. Dr Malcom Harris Chief Surgeon at two hospitals in Chicago and later President of the American Medical Association became interested in Hoxsey's medicine. Harris told Hoxsey that his medicine opened up a whole new area of treatment and that a large-scale trial should be conducted to look for possible side effects and to determine the effectiveness of dosages. Hoxsey was at first in total agreement, but then Harris hit him with a legal contract, which required Hoxsey to turn over the formulas to Harris and give up all future claims. Hoxsey under the agreement would mix and deliver the medication and train one doctor under Harris to deliver the medications. Further Hoxsey was to close his clinic, never treat patients again and during a period of 10 years he would gain no money, but after which he would receive 10% of net profits. Harris would set fees and receive 90% of the profits.

Hoxsey was not really money focused or an entrepreneur, both his father and grandfather had never turned anyone away who had no means to pay. In fact he had promised to continue the tradition. Hoxsey refused to sell the formula in a percentage deal and after that he was subjected to a familiar campaign of lies, slander, and deceit, vicious even by the American Medical Association's standards. Their aim was to force Hoxsey to close his clinic. The AMA utilised their own media circus through a Hearst newspaper beholden to them; they carried an article and a cartoon type drawing of a poor woman on a couch of pain surrounded by grief stricken children and a dog. She was handing over her last few dollars to a beaming caricature of a quack dressed in black coat tails and razor sharp trousers with a fancy scarf with a big diamond stickpin and white spats. The text ran: 'All the other wicked medical fakes, firing hope and darkening to despair, pale beside the savagery of the cancer charlatans. They look like men, they speak like men, but in them, pervading them, resides a quality so malevolent that it sets them apart from others of the human race'. Well that's going back to 1901 but we see in readers' letters to *The Times* in 2003, the idea of the charlatan when it comes to alternative cancer therapies is still alive and kicking which is more than one can say of billions of past cancer patients.

Hoxsey at the time of the article was treating a patient of Hariss's - a man called Thomas Mannix, who had been diagnosed with terminal cancer. Hariss refused to let Hoxsey treat the man after Hoxsey refused to sell the formula to him. Hoxsey however treated the man privately and he recovered and died 10 years later of heart disease. Hoxsey was an optimist and not deterred, opened up a new clinic in 1925 in Taylorville. Hoxsey had no formal medical qualification and thus worked with Dr Washburn, who was a local doctor. The clinic charged a maximum of 300 dollars and accepted all patients whether they could pay or not. The Taylorville Chamber of Commerce began a campaign to publicise the clinic, which of course came to the attention of the American Medical Association. On January 2nd 1926 an article denouncing Hoxsey appeared in the American Medical Association Journal and the editor of the journal a Dr Morris Fishbein forwarded the article 'helpfully' to the Taylorville Chamber of Commerce urging them not to support Hoxsey. This did not convince the Chamber of Commerce in Taylorville and so the State Medical Board tried to serve Hoxsey with a warrant for practising medicine without a licence. The Sheriff refused to serve it, as many people in Taylorville owed their life to Hoxsey including the sheriff who at the time was being treated by him.

Hoxsey also survived a claim by his siblings for a share in the formulas. When he spoke to them he discovered lawyers who intended to sell the Hoxsey formulas to the same AMA group who under Harris had tried to gain the formulas before. Hoxsey however was forced to sell his clinic, because he was now in debt, but his luck had not yet run out. He was approached by a number of wealthy men in Girard, the town where Hoxsey was raised, who offered a donation to open a new clinic there. So it was that in 1929 Hoxsey and Dr. Millar as clinic director opened up a clinic again. I think in Hoxsey's case it was not just the AMA battles, but Hoxsey because he was not qualified in medicine seemed to surround himself with men who would only damage his reputation. The smell of money in Hoxsey's medicine seemed to attract such men, which meant that the label of quack was always going to hang over him. Despite this Hoxsey still continued to fight to have his treatment recognised and accepted by orthodox medicine and undoubtedly he did have many successes with patients.

In 1946 Hoxsey met with Dr Spencer, then chief of the NCI – The National Cancer Institute and three congressmen and four doctors. It was agreed Hoxsey would send the records of fifty cured cases along with microscope slides of biopsies to prove his patients actually had cancer and following this the NCI would investigate. Hoxsey however couldn't supply the biopsy slides. because as Hoxsey stated: 'the AMA doctors, hospitals and laboratories refused to furnish them' to him. He had just encountered the classic 'catch 22' - he could not obtain the evidence they wanted because the AMA would not allow the laboratories and hospitals to release the evidence. Hoxsey tried to get around the impasse by giving the NCI the names of doctors or institutions where the slides could be obtained by the NCI themselves had they ever wanted to check. The NCI then discounted Hoxsey's treatment justifying that, by claiming there was no biopsy proof, for half the cases. Dr Gerson in a similar action was accused of not publishing, when journals under advice and policy from the orthodox establishment refused his work for publication. I went through the same process.

Despite Hoxsey was warned he would never be accepted by the AMA it is surprising that he pursued acceptance for so long and that must in some way have been because he lacked a medical degree. Hoxsey continued to cure patients and when he cured a young boy of Hodgkin's disease – cancer of the lymph, the boy's father was so overjoyed that he contacted Senator Thomas. Thomas visited Hoxsey's clinic and examined records and interviewed thirty cancer survivors and afterwards he wrote to the Surgeon General urging him to investigate Hoxsey's treatment. The Surgeon General replied by sending a copy of the AMA journal article denouncing Hoxsey. Senator Thomas finally wrote to Hoxsey saying: "It seems that the medical fraternity is highly organised and that they have decided to crush you and your institution, if at all possible. I have had a few rounds with the heads of all medical organisations as well as the Public Health Service here in Washington, and it seems that the Public Officials are afraid if they make any move, or say anything antagonistic to the wishes of the medical organization, that they will be pounced upon and destroyed". In this statement we see Kurt Bluchel's secret syndicate at work, where all services are provided by a monopoly.

Many people spoke of Hoxsey as a charismatic character, who by sheer force of personality could 'will' people to live. As with many successful alternative treatments one cannot discount the personality of the healer and the confidence they give to their patients. Gerson was like that and so was his daughter Charlotte. Unless a patient develops that will to fight their fate is uncertain. Gerson was also described as having great faith in his own ideas and that was transmitted to his patients. However faith in another may be tied up in loss and the psychological component I describe in the section on the mind. A healer may provide unconditional love and support the person has failed to find in life.

After repeated requests a group of ten independent medical doctors investigated Hoxsey's therapy and in 1954 issued a statement:

'This clinic now has under treatment or observation between four and five thousand cancer patients. It handles approximately ninety patients per day. Approximately 100 new patients per week come to the Clinic seeking relief, and the evidence we have seen indicates that approximately 90 percent of these are terminal cases.

Over the years the Clinic has accumulated more than 10,000 case histories, photographic studies and X-ray studies from all over the United States, Canada, Alaska, Mexico, Hawaii, the Central Zone and elsewhere.

We find as a fact that the Hoxsey Cancer Clinic in Dallas, Texas, is successfully treating pathologically proven cases of cancer, both internal and external, without the use of surgery, radium or X-ray...

Some of those presented before us have been free of symptoms as long as twenty four years, and the physical evidence indicates that they are all enjoying exceptional health at this time...We are willing to assist this Clinic in any way possible in bringing this treatment to the American public. We are willing to use it...on our own patients.

The above statement represents the unanimous findings of this Committee. In testimony thereof we hereby attach our signatures'.

(S. Edgard Bond M.D. Willard G.Palmer M.D. Hans Kalm M.D. A.C. Timbs M.D. Frederick H. Thurston M.D.D.O.E.E. Loffler M.D. H.B. Mueller M.D.R.C. Bowie M.D. Benjamin F. Bowers M.D. Roy O. Yeats M.D)

The AMA failed to stop the therapy and the Food and Drug Administration were brought in. FDA agents raided patients' homes and confiscated Hoxsey's medicine from them. Finally, the FDA padlocked all 17 clinics on the same day. Hoxsey felt unable to take legal action on this scale and gave up.

Mildred Nelson, a Hoxsey nurse, took the therapy to Tijuana, Mexico in 1963 and changed the name of the clinic to 'BioMed. Patients'. The majority of alternative cancer clinics were forced over the border into Mexico.

So what was in Hoxsey's black liquid? The liquid contained *potassium iodide*, and was combined with liquorice, red clover, burdock root, stillingia root, bar beris root, poker root, cascara, aromatic USP 14, prickly ash bark and buckthorn bark. The herbs are mainly those, which aid detoxification and support metabolism. The potassium iodide is startling because it was central to Gerson's dietary regime and which has implications in the embryonic- cancer cell link discussed. Potassium was found to turn off cancer cell growth and iodine stimulates the thyroid gland and speeds up metabolism thus increasing the production of energy in aerobic respiration. So was Hoxsey able to get results just by using potassium iodide and some detoxifying herbs and where he managed at least to give patients the will to live by sheer force of his personality?

The yellow powder and red paste that Hoxsey used on external cancers were corrosive materials and contained sulphur as arsenic sulphide and pure sulphur packed up with talcum powder. Sulphur has long been known to have medicinal properties when applied externally as was Hoxsey's powder and paste. The red paste contained antimony trisulphide, zinc chloride and blood root in trichoroacetic acid. Hoxsey claimed the yellow powder worked only on malignant tissue and so would not harm healthy tissue, whereas when he used the red paste, he had to protect surrounding tissue with Vaseline or zinc oxide cream. Arsenic like cyanide would seem to have natural chemotherapeutic properties and sulphur has long been known in hot springs to be beneficial to skin conditions. Interestingly cyanide and arsenic are known to block enzymes in respiration and may therefore act by cutting off oxygen and respiration in cancer cells, causing their death.

Hoxsey's diet for his patients differed from Gerson's in that it was less strict, but still required whole fresh foods with no salt, sugar and alcohol. Further no carbonated drinks (presumably because they lower blood oxygen levels through their carbon dioxide content), pork, tomatoes, vinegar or highly seasoned foods were allowed; because Hoxsey claimed it interfered with the medicine.

Dr Lugo a former chief physician at the Bio-Medical Clinic said this of Hoxsey's therapy: 'It changes the metabolism of the body, extracting large amounts of sodium from the cells, and introducing potassium and Iodine. The formula and the diet help the normal cells to regain their balance that they are supposed to have and the bad cells, the cancer cells; well they don't have anything to feed on. It's like anything else. These things don't have anything to reproduce or to feed from, so they die'.

It's an easy way to explain it, but essentially at the core of Hoxsey's therapy was medicine that contained potassium and according to the theory discussed returned the sodium based embryonic biochemistry of the cancer cell to its mature state of potassium biochemistry. Hoxsey also recommended drinking large amounts of grape juice, which contains potassium in addition to its detoxification properties. Organic grape juice would be required to avoid insecticide spray.

Hoxsey died in 1974, having spent most of his life fighting the lawsuits of the AMA and in trying to gain acknowledgement from them. Hoxsey's story is interesting, because unlike Gerson he had a product – a medicine, which Harris thought he would gain the rights to and when that did not happen, he outlawed Hoxsey.

If one considers the similarities between Hoxsey's approach and that of Gerson, the successes that Hoxsey gained, must at least have been due to the inclusion of potassium and Iodine which Gerson gave as Lugol's solution, along with detoxifying herbs and the application of a fresh fruit and vegetable diet: in addition to the charismatic personality of the healer.

WILLIAM KELLEY

Kelley will forever be remembered in the annals of alternative medicine as the brave man who took on Steve Mc Queen the Hollywood actor. Actually Kelley was an orthodontist, who had worked out a nutritional programme to treat cancer. Mc Queen had metastasised mesothelioma, a rare and nearly always fatal form of lung cancer. Newspapers reported in 1980 that Mc Queen was being treated at the Plaza Santa Maria Hospital in California. Stories focused on the unusual aspects of his treatment, which included the compulsory coffee enemas, nasal flushes with vitamin C and essentially an almost raw food diet.

Mc Queen was already in a bad way when he went to the Plaza - he was very thin with by that time, one lung almost completely covered with tumours, which had metastasised to his stomach and neck. He was by all accounts in a lot of pain. Mc Queen stayed at the Plaza for around 4 months and then according to reports went to a hospital in Mexico to have his stomach tumours removed. Following the surgery he was reported to have died of a heart attack.

Kelley was warned not to take on Mc Queen, because his cancer was advanced and if he died, Kelley would receive the backlash of publicity. Kelley felt he could not turn down Mc Queen but when he died the inevitable backlash occurred and of course it was seen as a failure of the nutritional approach. But you have to ask the question whether Mc Queen wanted to live, because Kelley claimed that Mc Queen did not want to do the coffee enemas and continued to smoke cigars and ate copious quantities of ice cream. Dr Gerson would have been horrified, but then I suspect Mc Queen was not a man you ordered about. Kelley however claimed that despite Mc Queens' lapse approach to the programme, that after eight weeks the tumours had stopped growing and that he was off painkillers and had put on some weight.

The decision to send Mc Queen for surgery was apparently taken because the tumours in his stomach were putting pressure on other areas including the urinary tubes, which take urine from the kidney to the bladder and thus made urination difficult. Kelley was also concerned at the size of the tumours and their potential toxicity. Dr Gerson of course got around toxicity with the castor oil and coffee enemas, which with the high vitamin C content in the diet also reduced pain and toxicity.

Kelley later claimed that he was present during surgery and that there were three large tumours, where two were already dead and could be lifted out and the third was barely attached to the base of the liver. Whilst Mc Queen initially survived surgery, the surgical team were anxious that he might be haemorrhaging internally and decided to give him a blood-clotting agent. Kelley later said it was over cautious and there was no need for it. Kelley always maintained it was actually a blood clot that killed Mc Queen. Whatever the case here, Kelley inevitably suffered as a result of bad publicity.

Kelley was another alternative practitioner whose dietary regime is on the unproven methods list of the American Cancer Society. Kelley claimed to have cured himself of metastasised pancreatic cancer using a dietary approach. Like Hoxsey he was not qualified as a medical doctor and practised dentistry, which lead to him being arrested in 1962 for practising medicine without a licence. In 1976 the Texas State Dental Board even suspended his licence to practise dentistry for 5 years.

Kelley's dietary regime was very similar to Gerson's and he also claimed it was non-specific in that it was able to cure a number of diseases. Charlotte Gerson maintained that most if not all dietary approaches to cancer stemmed from her father's work. Whereas Gerson's diet was a one fits all approach Kelley tailored the diet to each individual patient and their metabolism. Patients had to answer a 3,000 questionnaire nutritional survey, which was then analysed to identify which metabolic type the patient belonged to. Kelley had devised a sophisticated metabolic typing classification programme, which he maintained targeted specific metabolic insufficiencies which allowed him to tailor the diet not only to cancer, but to multiple sclerosis and even schizophrenia.

Kelley claimed he first became interested in nutrition through the practise of dentistry, where he recognised the link between poor nutrition and decayed teeth. The diet he developed seems familiar to other nutritional programmes for cancer. It is mainly vegetarian, based as is the Gerson therapy on low protein intake and where a small amount of yoghurt in the morning and 10 almonds at breakfast and 10 almonds at lunch were allowed to provide some protein if not amygdaline. By limiting protein intake to a six-hour period Kelley theorised that eighteen hours would be left in a 24- hour period to break down tumours. Similar to the Gerson therapy and other nutritional approaches coffee enemas were given to detoxify along with large quantities of citrus juices. Unlike other programmes and especially the Gerson therapy, fasting was utilised, which represents perhaps some ancient medical knowledge in religious texts. Dr Gerson held a different viewpoint and claimed the patient had to consume large quantities of juices, but also insisted on 3 meals a day.

Kelley's patients did however go through the same healing crises that the Gerson therapy produces. As with the Gerson therapy there were spectacular successes and then those who did not do well, which Gerson stated was due to non-adherence to the whole programme. Kelley maintained that those who did not do well required an individual approach, because each individual had different biochemical needs based on their type. On might describe his programme as having an anthropological approach based on the evolution of the dietary types.

Kelley explained the use of coffee enemas in a similar rationale to Gerson by claiming that in addition to activating bile secretions, the enemas also activate liver enzymes. He also claimed that they were important in activating the immune system, by clearing out toxins, which depress immune function.

Kelley's classification system for metabolic typing was based on the activity of different parts of the ANS or autonomic nervous system. The ANS is comprised of the sympathetic and parasympathetic nervous systems. The sympathetic system speeds up body metabolism and the parasympathetic slows it down. Kelley maintained that each person has a unique inborn balance of the two where one is more active than the other and any diet should take account of this. For this reason he claimed that sympathetic types tend to do best on a vegetarian diet and are more susceptible to cancer, because of the under reacting parasympathetic system, which includes the immune system. Parasympathetic dominance Kelley maintained caused the meat eaters. Kelley then went onto further classify metabolic types into ten sub types and each of those sub types required a different diet.

Kelley explained his metabolic typing this way: 'We would suspect that the forerunners of the human species displayed a balanced type of metabolism, ideally suited to a hunter-gatherer life-style. These prehistoric humans evolving in a temperate ecosystem would have had access to a wide variety of vegetable foods, nuts, seeds, occasional meats and fish. A flexible physiology, capable of utilising a variety of foodstuffs, would have most definitely been an evolutionary advantage'. The earth having experienced serious climatic changes e.g. the ice ages would mean that according to Kelley's theory, some humans were forced to turn to meat, when vegetation was sparse.

Professor Jane Plant in her book was convinced that the western dietary intake of milk was causative in cancer. Those humans that survived these climatic changes would have been those whose metabolism was capable of adapting to eating meat. According to Kelley the sympathetic types, the vegetarians were those who 10,000 years ago survived on a diet of grains, berries, fruits and very little in the way of meat or milk products, such as the people in the Middle East.

Apart from this metabolic approach Kelley claimed as did Gerson that cancer patients and those with chronic diseases were severely depleted in vitamins and minerals and that large doses of supplemental nutrients were required for the rebuilding of the metabolism and to induce healing. Gerson mainly relied upon the diet to provide the vitamins and minerals, whilst Kelley used supplements in addition to the diet. It seems that Kelley may have built on Gersons's work because he held a similar view in that he claimed the nutrients were no longer in the food through agricultural practise and where since 1945 there has been widespread use of chemical fertilisers and pesticides: for this reason Gerson used only organic food.

The current orthodox view at least in the U.K is that chemicalised food is just as nutritious as organic food, which provides no greater advantage. Medical science also seeks to warn of the harmful effects of high doses of vitamins arguing that water-soluble vitamins for example B and C are excreted in excess anyway, whilst excess oil soluble vitamins such as A, D, E and K are stored in the body fat and for which reason excess storage could be toxic.

Kelley like Gerson used digestive enzymes such as pepsin and hydrochloric acid, which occurs naturally anyway in the stomach and aid protein digestion. The addition of these to the diet is aimed at assisting digestive metabolism, particularly proteins and also to help clear the build- up of mucous coating in the intestine, built up over time through a poor diet. The mucous covers the small hair like projections in the intestine, which are called villi and it is here where most absorption of nutrients takes place. Any excessive mucous coating would greatly deter digestion. Dietary products particularly hard cheese often cause increase in this mucous coating.

Kelley did have the accusation of profiteering aimed at him, because he manufactured his own supplements and enzyme preparations, which were quite costly. In his defence Kelley said that he only extracted his supplements from naturally occurring sources and they contained no synthetic or chemical products, which in turn made his products costly.

Unlike Dr Gerson who published his work in 54 scientific papers and articles dating from 1907 to 1958, the Kelley programme when I looked for an alternative did not have as much in the way of published data, although it did have recorded successes.

LINUS PAULING AND EWAN CAMERON -VITAMIN C

The surgeon Ewan Cameron working in Scotland in the U.K carried out a study with cancer patients who were given Vitamin C. Cameron's patients showed an increased quality of life and longer survival times, requiring less pain relief. Cameron did not present Vitamin C as a cure, but clearly in the nutritional therapies I have discussed Vitamin C is common to all and through the vegetables and fruits are given in quite high quantities naturally.

Researchers at least from 1951 had found that people with cancer usually had very low levels of vitamin C in their blood, and experiments confirmed this finding over and over again for the following thirty years. It wasn't until 1976 that two very well regarded scientists decided to conduct a clinical trial of vitamin C.

In 1976 Dr Cameron and two-time Nobel Prize winner Dr Linus Pauling published the results of a controlled study of 100 patients at Cameron's hospital in the Vale of Leven Scotland UK; all Cameron's patients were deemed untreatable by at least two doctors or surgeons. The patients received no other treatment but received 10 grams of Vitamin C a day. The control group against which these study patients were matched contained 1,000 patients also deemed untreatable, who received no Vitamin C. The patients in both groups were matched for age, sex and the same primary organ and histological tumour type.

The results showed that those patients who had received Vitamin C, had a survival time 4.2 times greater or more than 210 days compared to controls of 50 days. Thus Vitamin C had prolonged the survival times of patients. Interestingly enough the researchers found a small group or 10% of the Vitamin C treated patients who had a survival time of more than 20 times that of non-treated patients. I say interesting because this hard core or what I call the 'ten per centers' is a group that crops up in other therapy studies. A few patients – around 10% seem to do well on therapies, despite their very poor prognosis whilst others who have a better prognosis do not in some cases seem to do as well. I will return to this point in the section on the mind.

294

In the insane world of cancer, you could have predicted what would happen to Cameron and Pauling, once they announced this success. Yes that's right, they put their head above the radar and the Drug Cartel no doubt felt alarmed, since Vitamin C is a cheap compound available at any chemist. Their study was criticised and so Cameron and Pauling repeated the experiment two years later in 1978 and gained the same if not improved results. Predictably then came the 'doomed trial' – as one of the Drug Cartel's main methods of discrediting any promising alternative approach.

In 1979 the Mayo Clinic in the U.S concluded in a study, which claimed to repeat Cameron and Pauling's work that vitamin C did not prolong the lives of terminal cancer patients. When Pauling and Cameron examined the method the Mayo Clinic study had used they discovered that the trial patients were receiving chemotherapy *and* vitamin C, whilst Cameron and Pauling's patients only received vitamin C. It seems obvious that vitamin C assisted patients in detoxifying and neutralising toxins from the tumour in the absence of chemotherapy, but it was insufficient to carry out that role *and* detoxify the chemotherapy. Further Pauling argued that the chemotherapy destroyed patients' immune mechanisms and the vitamin C was being used to rebuild what the chemotherapy had destroyed. The idea of an apple a day or orange a day to keep the doctor away, surely repeats the age-old knowledge that vitamin C increases immunity and wards off infection.

In fact the Mayo Clinic patients with advanced colorectal cancer were given 10 grams (10,000 mg) of vitamin C per day. The study then reported that: "high dose vitamin C therapy is not effective against advanced malignant disease". The Cartel as another method of invalidation of alternative research then set about gaining wide publicity for the conclusions in the media. Patients with no training in science would merely rely on the media and not recognise as a scientist would, that the results were meaningless as the study was flawed, because the method Cameron and Pauling used, was not repeated in the Mayo study.

Another important difference between Pauling and Cameron's study and that of the Mayo Clinic study was that in the Mayo study the patients were not kept on the vitamin indefinitely, as were Cameron's patients. Instead, vitamin C dosage was discontinued as soon as 'there was evidence of marked progression of the malignant disease'. In fact in the Mayo study, patients were kept on vitamin C for a median time of only 2.5 months (range from one day to 15.6 months), whereas Cameron's patients were never taken off the 10 gram per day dose of vitamin C and one patient was still surviving thirteen years later. Thus the Mayo study meant it neither accomplished its objective of checking Cameron and Pauling's findings, nor supported the conclusion that high dose vitamin C therapy has: "no advantage over placebo therapy with regard to either the interval between the beginning of treatment and disease progression or patient survival". Instead, it only showed that high dose vitamin C therapy should not be administered to patients for several months and then suddenly stopped.

Pauling was at least proven correct in 1976 when researchers at the NCI in the States found that Vitamin C is a potent stimulator of lymphocyte production. Lymphocytes are cells that play an important role in the immune defence mechanism, which also destroys cancer cells, when functioning properly. Our first line of defence against infection - phagocytosis, is also reliant on ascorbic acid or vitamin C. Phagocytosis is the 'gobbling up' and digestion of invading bacteria in the blood stream and tissues by white blood cells or phagocytes. Under normal conditions, with a good supply of ascorbic acid in the blood serum, any injury or bacteria getting into the tissues attracts hordes of white cells to the area: and they immediately go to work swallowing and digesting the bacteria and foreign material. In the process of phagocytosis, the number of bacteria ingested and digested is directly related to the blood serum levels of ascorbic acid (vitamin C). When the ascorbic acid levels are low or absent, phagocytosis stops and the bacteria grow and reproduce in the tissues, and a full blown infection develops.

The Pauling Institute were reduced to advertising in the Wall Street Journal for funds: Von Hoffman in 1976 stated: 'Our research shows that the incidence and severity of cancer depends on diet. We urgently want to refine that research so that it may help to decrease suffering from human cancer. The US government has absolutely and continually refused to support Dr Pauling and his colleagues here in this work'.

Dr Pearce an oncologist, in response to my research in the 80s sent me a private communication, relaying a theory of leukaemia. He suggested that people with leukaemia are not killed by the neoplastic disease itself, but by haemorrhage and infection. Both lack of resistance to infections and haemorrhaging are pathognomonic symptoms of scurvy, a disease connected directly to low vitamin C levels. Leukaemics Dr Pearce suggested, were suffering from uncorrected hypoascorbemia or severe chronic sub-clinical scurvy in addition to leukaemia; and they require high levels of ascorbic acid amounting to many grams per day to conquer their severe hypoascorbemia – low vitamin C levels. As Dr Pearce pointed out to me: ' if one could prevent them from dying of the manifestations of scurvy, it may be found that leukaemia itself may not be such a serious fatal disease at all'.

Some basic work has been done on this, but only low doses of vitamin C have been given; from 100 milligrams or 200 milligrams a day to 900 milligrams per day. On these low doses, variable and uncertain clinical results were obtained. In the one-recorded case where complete remission was achieved and maintained in myelogenous leukaemia, the patient took 24 to 42 grams or 24,000 to 42,000 milligrams of ascorbic acid (vitamin C) per day.

Dr Pearce gave me a report of one patient in 1954; it related to a 71-year old oil executive who was first seen for alcoholic hepatic cirrhosis (alcohol related liver damage) and polycythemia. Previously he had developed symptoms of chronic rheumatic and arteriosclerotic myocarditis (heart problems). He was hospitalised and passed a large uric acid bladder stone, and a few months later a diagnosis of chronic myelogenous leukaemia was established. He also had intractable pyorrhoea (gum disease) and his remaining 17 teeth were extracted in one operation. The history so far was indicative of severe chronic sub-clinical scurvy, but it appears that no one bothered to look into the ascorbic acid status of the patient.

On his own initiative, the patient started taking ascorbic acid at the rate of 24 to 42 grams (24,000 to 42,000 milligrams) a day, because as the case history stated: "He reported that he felt much better when he took these large doses". His physician stated: "The patient has repeatedly remarked about his feeling of well-being and has continued his vocation as an executive of an oil company. On two occasions, on my insistence, the ascorbic acid was discontinued as an experiment. Both times his spleen enlarged to the brim of the pelvis, became soft and very tender. When the ascorbic acid was again started, his signs and symptoms were greatly improved, his temperature becoming normal within six hours".

Dr Stone also outlined a similar position when he stated:

'Hypo-ascorbemia...is caused by humans carrying a defective gene for the production of the liver enzyme L-gulonolactone oxidase...(due)...to a mutation occurring in a primate ancestor of man. The lack of this enzyme in the human liver... prevents us from synthesising our own ascorbic acid...This defective gene is common to all mankind, therefore chronic hypo-ascorbemia is now our most prevalent disease...it is possible that the chronic sub-clinical scurvy, existing in the victim since infancy, may be a factor in initiating the leukaemia...It is a hard clinical fact that leukaemics have pathologically low levels of ascorbic acid in their blood plasma...what kills most leukaemics is ...haemorrhage and infection...Both...are pathognomonic symptoms of scurvy. In the one case where complete remission was achieved and maintained in myelogenous leukaemia, the patient took 24 to 42 grams (24,000 – 42,000 mg) of ascorbic acid per day...'.

Dr Stone stated: 'I wrote ...a paper in an attempt to have the therapy clinically tested. I sent the paper to three cancer journals and three blood journals. It was refused by all...two...without even reading it...I cannot help wondering how many lives could have been saved and how much suffering could have been avoided had the editors...permitted publication'.

A pity because I note that even after seven years and post Gerson Therapy, Michael Gearin-Tosh noted on page 186 of his book that he still had depressed haemoglobin: 'Carmen calls me 'sub-anaemic' –and my immune system is disordered'. Michael may have had sub-clinical scurvy.

It is inconceivable that no one appears to have followed this up, in any of the thousands of cases of leukaemia, which appear each year. However given the resistance Cameron and Pauling encountered, perhaps someone did try at one time to get a grant to conduct a trial, but was turned down and perhaps even threatened. You might say well perhaps, one doctor could have recommended his patients take it, but then even today, doctors are suspended or struck off by the GMC (General Medical Council) for deviating from any policy, which governs the treatment of every disease including cancer. That policy is invariably geared towards big Pharma medicine.

Dr Pearce, a cancer consultant stated of his research in a similar position to my own research: 'For years now it has been collecting dust in my files and I cannot help wondering how many thousands of lives could have been saved and how much suffering could have been avoided had the editors and reviewers just read the paper with an unbiased mind and permitted its publication'. His letter more than anything convinced me that I was not alone in my experiences, even though my research too would end up languishing on dusty bookshelves. He suggested that leukaemia is not a single disease, but a combination of a neoplastic blood disease and severe biochemical scurvy: massive daily dosing with ascorbic acid or sodium ascorbate could alleviate the scurvy. The secret it seemed was in applying between 25 to 100 grams of vitamin C. However, the theory needed properly testing in double blind controlled trials and I certainly having already funded the cancer research involving the Gerson Therapy and psychological counselling, could not undertake any more trials, without funding.

Thus without the severe underlying biochemistry of scurvy, leukaemia may be a relatively benign, non-fatal condition, but the Mayo study has more or less made vitamin C therapy a no go area for researchers and certainly as government agencies retain these faulty trials, then every time someone applies to do a trial with vitamin C they will be turned down for grant funding, with evidence quoted on the faulty Mayo study given as the reason. So let us say that some post-graduate medical student wants to give vitamin C research a go, having seen this book. His professor or mentor will suggest he give it up (knowing how the system works) and if he persists and the university hospital department applies for funding for the trial, then the university department may be threatened elsewhere with funds being withdrawn, or the postgraduate may be dismissed. I will recount later another case where exactly this scene occurred.

Ascorbate, in large doses, is the only non-toxic non-specific natural virucide (anti-viral) known and therefore may have other applications in viral infections – perhaps even AIDS patients. The Gerson Therapy provides the large vitamin C doses through the juices naturally and avoids then any imbalance in other vitamins caused by vitamin C application alone. There is also a potential danger of stopping abruptly a large vitamin C intake. According to Swedish studies at Karolinska and Umeo Hospitals, vitamin C in large doses can be an effective prophylactic against cancer. It has been shown that abnormal metabolism of the amino acid tryptophan, with the consequent oxidation of its metabolites, can lead to the development of bladder cancer. Vitamin C, by blocking the oxidation process, can prevent cancer development; and Swedish researchers suggest that vitamin C can be used as a general cancer preventative agent. Doses up to 5 grams (5,000 milligrams) a day or more however, are needed for effective protection. Recent research has also shown that vitamin C contains flavonoids, which lower the mortality rate in animals that received radiation, which might indeed suggest that vitamin C should be taken when receiving radiation. At least it might provide some protection.

The synthetically produced antibiotic chloramphenicol (chloromycetin) was tried out for a long time on dogs and found to produce only a transient anaemia, but fatal results were found to occur in human use. Keith Lasko reported in his book *The Great Billion Dollar Medical Swindle* (*1980*):

'Even one capsule of chloromycetin could cause...leukaemia...I remember a child dying of aplastic anaemia after a general practitioner had prescribed chloromycetin for a cold...For a cold – a virus infection! The parents were crying the kid was bleeding. I was warned by several physicians that grave consequences would befall me if I told the parents that their beautiful child was dying because of a doctor's mindless prescription'.

Cameron expanded his theory of how Vitamin C works by explaining that it helps to maintain the integrity of the inter-cellular fluid – the fluid between cells. Vitamin C is the most potent anti-toxin known and therefore would be beneficial in maintaining the integrity of cells by detoxifying inter-cellular fluid. This ground fluid is made up of water and electrolytes such as sodium and potassium. It also contains metabolised substances from the cells and gases such as oxygen and carbon dioxide. Trace elements, vitamins and enzymes along with carbohydrates, fats and proteins are also found in this fluid.

During cell division, when more room has to be made for the dividing cells, the enzyme hyaluronidase is released which breaks down the gel-like substance of the inter-cellular fluid. To avoid continual division of cells an inhibitor called hyaluronidase inhibitor or PHI for short, stops the over production of hyaluronidase. Cameron thought that the actual contact with other cells stops cell divisions and the cells are only restrained from constant growth by the correct composition of the intercellular fluid and PHI production. Cameron claimed that Vitamin C is needed to make both the PHI inhibitor and collagen, which is another vital component of the inter-cellular fluid and which helps to structure the fluid. Cameron pointed to scurvy, a disease caused through lack of Vitamin C, where the collagen in the body breaks down and certainly hypoascorbemia may be a mechanism in leukaemia as discussed.

I cannot fully go into my own research on this inter-cellular fluid, because of its technical complexity for the non- medic or scientist, but briefly my research shows that this inter cellular fluid and its integrity is vitally important to maintaining potassium and sodium balance inside and outside cells. Briefly I stated in '*The Second Millennium Cancer Report*', which accompanied my Petition to the UK Parliament through Tim Rathbone MP:

'In cancer as in many other degenerative diseases, including Ischaemic Heart Disease, there is a high certainty that all body cells and particularly cancer cells are suffering from the tissue damage syndrome; whereby the cells become abnormally swollen with water and contain high levels of sodium. These abnormal cells no longer function normally'.

I concluded that not only was the balance of sodium and potassium critical but also the water inside and outside cells was not free liquid or a 'bag' of water; it was fully structured in much the same way as an ion-exchange resin works in water softeners. In short in healthy mature cells if by analogy the ion-exchange is working well then sodium will be passed out and potassium will enter the cell. This ionic state is the normal state in *mature* cells. In cancer cells however the process seems to reverse and sodium accumulates *inside* the cell, which causes the cell to swell up. This would have disastrous effects on the healthy metabolism and biochemical reactions inside the cell. Thus the water inside and outside of cells becomes de-structured and sodium seeps into the cell, which becomes cancerous, resembling an embryonic cell in so far as they also have high sodium levels and rapidly divide. Most of the anti- cancer diets forbid salt intake. I think also these changes would cause a fermentive and non-oxidising environment which is the milieu in which cancer develops rather than the oxidative one that occurs in mature healthy cells. Of course also the embryonic cell is mainly non-oxidising or fermentive.

Despite the fact that Linus Pauling had received two Nobel Prizes, when he applied five times to the NCI – The National Cancer Institute and the ACS – The American Cancer Society for research grants to study Vitamin C, he was turned down each time. Vitamin C is a cheap compound and of no interest to the Drug Cartel. In my own journey down that path I think I tried around 30 grant funding organisations, for a slice of the solid gold gravy train of research funding and despite being registered as a charity, I was turned down by all and eventually funded it myself, along with a £400 donation. I certainly gave up the idea of ever setting up a centre, where some of these alternative approaches could be researched. As Martin Luther King stated "I have a dream" – or at least I had one, but broken down by years of legal battles, destruction of one's career and financial duress, one simply walks away in a case of self-survival. Even from my own research, I realised that the constant losses were a risk to my own health.

OTHER ALTERNATIVE CANCER THERAPIES

Some cancer patients have used more unknown and little researched therapies, which although they have successes, are not considered all-inclusive enough to be seen as alternative approaches to cancer. Such therapies may have some value in non-chronic degenerative diseases and maintaining general health.

Dr Anne Wigmore a doctor of divinity and naturopathy developed a nutritional therapy based on juicing wheatgrass. In a similar story to Hoxsey, she observed nature to find out which plants animals ate when they became sick or diseased; observing many of them ate wheatgrass. You have probably noticed cats eating grass, when they are off-peak. Wheatgrass is full of vitamins and minerals.

Wheatgrass is easily grown from seeds or wheat berries and is obtainable from most health stores. It can be grown in trays and then juiced in a special juicer. I did try doing this, but the taste was quite strong for me. The dark green juice is loaded with chlorophyll, which is a pigment that makes plants green and is very similar in composition to our own blood pigment – haemoglobin. Wigmore claimed that chlorophyll is a detoxifier and cleanser and protects the body from carcinogens. In addition to the wheatgrass juices, Wigmore's diet is based totally on raw foods, uncooked to preserve the enzymes. No animal protein or products such as meat, milk, eggs or fish are allowed. Protein is supplied by a combination of nuts, seeds, grains, sprouts and vegetables. In addition large quantities of wheatgrass and Rejuvelac, which is the liquid in which the wheat berries, have been sprouted is drunk. Coffee enemas are also used.

In alternative circles the diet is recognised as not being inclusive enough for cancer, but is viewed more as a general detoxification programme and for less serious chronic diseases. There are however people who have survived cancer using this diet – for example Eydie Mae who wrote '*How I conquered Cancer Naturally.*' The wheatgrass also contains many of the vitamins needed in a healthy diet and so Wigmore tried to introduce her programme in Africa as a way of providing good nutrition at low cost and to my mind, was an excellent idea.

Another less well-known diet is the Dr Cornelius Moerman diet, which you can research if you are interested and the rather better known macrobiotic diet based upon ancient eastern teachings.

George Ohsawa was one of the macrobiotic diet's earliest pioneers, developing his therapy from Chinese, Japanese and Indian philosophy and medicine, where balance and harmony is a pivotal experience. Ohsawa visited Dr Albert Schweitzer at his hospital in Africa in 1955 and discovered a cure for deadly tropical ulcers. Dr Schweitzer and his wife had been treated for TB and diabetes by Dr Gerson and it is unclear how much of Dr Gerson's diet and philosophy were to contribute to George Ohsawa's teachings on the physical aspects of disease.

The idea of conflict is alien to macrobiotics, where everything becomes part of a whole on the universal ying and yang principle. Ohsawa in his book entitled: 'Cancer and the Philosophy of the Far East', wrote: 'cancer is in reality a profound benefactor of mankind. It is cancer that slows down the catastrophic speed of our civilisation – which is hurrying pell-mell toward the very extremities of dualism'.

I am sure the idea of cancer as a benefactor, will seem alien to most cancer patients, but I can see some truth there. I have known people who say: "oh I just want to take the chemo and then get on with my life". They take chemo and work, to take their mind off the cancer and they eat out of the canteen at work and then they are so tired, they can't take time to prepare the nutritious food they need. Cancer is a warning sign that some heed and others don't. If you remember, I jumped off the express train and wandered off into the meadows with flowers, where I had time to think. I shut my door on the world for two years, whilst I did the Gerson Therapy and it certainly slowed my social life down to zero. I remember thinking when I was diagnosed with cancer, that by analogy I had let my cupboard run bare, I looked in it and there were no reserves, nothing there to survive or fight a long cold and hard winter with. I was just kind of horrified and thought how could this happen? So there was a time to heal and replenish my cupboard and if it took two years, then it would have to take two years, but not one moment do I regret the healing time; in true healing one finds oneself.

In America Michio Kushi who wrote *The Cancer Prevention Diet* in *1983*, maintained it is a dualistic mistake to view cancer as an enemy to be destroyed. He took the view of many alternative practitioners that the cancer or tumour is a *symptom that all is not well in your life,* your body is out of balance and in my view that extends to the imbalance in your emotional life, which I will come to in the section on the mind. Cancer is a symptom a warning sign and if one is wise, one will take that warning seriously and act upon it. The view of orthodoxy that *the tumour* is *the cause,* simply encourages people to believe that they can continue with their lives, once they have had surgery, radiotherapy or chemotherapy, but so often find the cancer returns in many cases more aggressively and often too late they turn to alternative therapies, when it is much harder to achieve results in late stages, particularly when the immune system has been damaged in toxic chemotherapy.

IMMUNE THERAPIES

We have already seen that the alternative therapies for cancer mainly aim at detoxifying the body, which will help to increase immunity and strengthen the natural defence systems in the body. The immune therapies base themselves on the rationale that a healthy body and immune system, will act to destroy cancer cells, when they arise. Unknown to us it is probable that this process occurs constantly and in a healthy individual no tumour arises. Whilst the dietary approach aims at strengthening the immune system, immune-therapy seeks to directly involve the immune response.

It has been noted that children who suffer some form of immune-deficient disease present with a higher incidence of cancer. In patients who have had transplants or received immunosuppressive drugs to reduce organ rejection there is a higher incidence of cancer.

Dr Mc Caskey noted in 1902 in the '*American Journal of Medical Sciences*' that an injection of tuberculin, which is a tuberculosis vaccine, caused regression of cancer in some patients. The whole purpose of a vaccine is to give the person a weak form of the disease, or inject a dead form of the disease, which then creates an immune reaction in the body. The body thinks it is under attack and will use its immune defences to kill the invader. If the body actually comes into contact with the real disease at a later time, then the body remembers this invasion and can rapidly respond by using its remembered immune defences and thus the infection will not be so severe. This is the whole rationale behind vaccination programmes.

Returning to the Dr Mc Caskey's experiment then it appeared that by injecting the BCG (Bacillus Calmette-Guérin) vaccine into cancer patients, the immune response, which activates the immune system, had been triggered and in turn then attacked the cancer cells. Bearing in mind that this research dates back to 1902 then had current researchers looked through the alternative therapies, this interesting bit of research from D. Mc Caskey would have come to light much sooner. Certainly had the British government not buried my cancer report containing this observation in 1997, some further studies could have been carried out.

In 2010 Dr Vincent Tuohy reported in the journal *Nature Medicine* that he had developed a vaccine for breast cancer. The research naturally hit the front pages of national newspapers: 'A revolutionary jab that could both prevent and treat breast cancer has been developed. Its creator Dr Tuohy an expert in the workings of the immune system from one of America's top hospitals, the Cleveland Clinic in Ohio claimed: "the effects could be monumental," explaining that the drug targets a protein called alphalactalbumin, present in breast cancer tumours. Having the jab revs up the immune system, priming it to destroy the protein as it appears and stops the tumours forming'. The research was carried out in rats and has yet to be tested on humans. No doubt Dr Tuohy received funding, since the drug companies see mass vaccination on the horizon.

Researchers such as Dr Morton at UCLA Medical School had good success with tumour regression when using BCG on skin tumours, such as malignant melanoma. Fourteen studies showed that an average of 58% of patients reacted positively by either having remission or longer survival times. Bernice Wallin in her book '*I beat Cancer*' (*1978*) was on the programme at UCLA and received the BCG injections. On reading her book one cannot dismiss her sheer determination to live. You see that is the 'ten per center' again the 10% of survivors who are bloody minded enough to do whatever it takes.

The research posed by Dr Mc Caskey was extremely interesting to me. Why did the body's immune system not recognise cancer as an invasion and yet recognised BCG as a foreign invasion? Again I look in my research notes of the time and see my conclusion:

'CANCER MUST BE A NATURAL CONDITION REMEMBERED OR RECOGNISED BY THE BODY AS A NATURAL PROCESS AND NOT ALIEN -THAT IS WHY THE IMMUNE SYSTEM DOES NOT AUTOMATICALLY RECOGNISE IT.'

My conclusion was fairly startling to me at the time, because the whole of orthodox medicine was dedicated to destroying cancer as an alien condition, which had to be fought in some kind of medieval battle. "What if"- I reasoned in my notes:

'CANCER SLIPS UNDER THE BODY'S RADAR DEFENCE SYSTEM, BECAUSE THE BODY VIEWS THE **CANCER AS A SURVIVAL MECHANISM** AND **NOT AS A NON-SURVIVAL MECHANISM?**'

In that moment, which I have to say was one of those giant bounds of eureka moments for a scientist, like the apple falling on Newton's head, I suddenly realised that cancer is a reaction of the body and mind to a non-survival situation, where no matter how irrational that is, the body and mind **views the cancer as a survival mechanism**. Now I suspect that you will have to run that statement past yourself many times and read the sections on 'the mind and cancer' and 'cancer as an evolutionary throwback,' to fully understand what I believe is the mechanism of cancer.

As a scientist I am sorry, but I have to say it's a sublime piece of miss wiring and it really does humble one, in that cancer is a reminder of the evolutionary tree and how we have come to this. Now I will have to leave this thought with you, that cancer is a survival mechanism, because I intend to pick it up in further chapters. So hold that thought, that cancer to your body and mind is seen as a survival mechanism and thus the whole rationale of orthodox medicine is wrong in its assumption that this disease can be cured by attacking it, with high technology – you can't attack an in-wired survival mechanism. As insane as it sounds, your body and mind is actually trying to help you survive, by producing a tumour. It is doing that because you the driver so to speak of the car, has jumped into the back seat and handed all control to a body and primitive mind that is following a road map of *evolution*. So ironically if you the driver have passed responsibility to the evolutionary road map, then that is how your problems will be solved, according to primitive evolutionary mechanisms – **a tumour is a primitive evolutionary survival mechanism in response to loss.**

You remember the 'ten per center's', those who against all the odds, often with poor prognosis who actually do very well - they all had certain characteristics and one of which is that they took control of their lives and took away responsibility from the evolutionary survival mechanisms. They fought, they questioned, they found new goals, they were determined to live, they resolved past conflicts, they completed therapies, they found reasons to live, they overcame grief, they overcame loss, they found it within themselves to take control over their lives, they also identified the situations that had lead them to cancer, where they passed control to their body, when they literally gave up.

COLEY'S TOXINS

Dr Coley was born in 1862 and was chief of the bone cancer unit for Memorial Hospital in New York and was also professor of clinical surgery at Cornell University. Dr Coley noticed that when one of his patients developed a severe bacterial infection his cancer disappeared. Coley then decided to inject another cancer patient with the same infection of erysipelas a Group A haemolytic streptococci and he found that the cancer disappeared in less than two weeks. Despite these initial successes Coley suffered a series of failures until he grew the streptococci with another dead bacterium thus producing a more virulent form of the streptococcus, which he then used. This was called Coley's toxins, which he injected into a man with inoperable stomach cancer with metastasis to the pelvis and bladder. After several months of injections Coley could find no trace of the tumour.

A trial of Coley's toxins by Dr Johnston in the 1960s produced some improvement in a number of patients but surprisingly nine were cured. The use of toxins was removed from the American Cancer Society's unproven list in 1975. It seems the Drug Cartel could see a profitable product as a vaccine.

Some rationale was put forward for the action of the toxins – such as the beneficial production of a fever: cells are damaged at high temperatures and as far back as 1918 Dr Geyser was using a diathermic current to heat tumours on the body surface where at 108 degrees Fahrenheit the cells would die. He managed to gain some promising results and then in 1976 Dr Le Veen at the Medical University of South Carolina started using hyperthermia or a high temperature approach and in 1980 achieved tumour regression in eleven of thirty-two inoperable and untreatable lung cancer patients. Six of the patients became disease free. Dr Le Veen reported that: 'there was dramatic systematic relief in 27 of 32 cases with return of appetite, weight gain, strength and in general considerable improvement'. He also remarked that pain relief was achieved in 21 out of 25 cases.

Other approaches using hyperthermia in conjunction with ultrasound or radiation have been used although results vary. Later interferon and monoclonal antibodies were other approaches that have been tried.

In my own view as covered in the last section on immune therapies, I believe that the cancer is not recognised as an invader, but a survival mechanism and thus is not immediately attacked by the immune defence system, just as an embryo would not be attacked even though it is a fast growing entity. Once you give an infection to the patient, the immune system is then stimulated and will attack the cancer cells. No doubt also the low immunity of cancer patients, will also contribute.

In the programme '*Superhuman*' (*BBC1 October 17th 2,000*) Dr Robert Winston related the remarkable story of Salome, a prostitute in Nairobi. She had been a sex worker for 20 years, offering full sex without any protection to an average of eight or nine men each day. Despite the fact that at least one or two of the men she serviced each day would be infected with HIV, she never developed the full blown AIDS disease herself. There are about 200 Nairobi prostitutes like Salome, all of whom statistically should by now be dead, but whom appears to be disease-free. It seems to be the case that her immune system recognises and deals with the virus, having been primed many times to recognise it. As soon as women like her give up prostitution and they are no longer exposed to the virus – they become as vulnerable as the rest. They appear to lose their immunity.

Asthma also is a decreased immunity resulting in hypersensitivity. Such decreased immunity can and often does arise in asthmatics from stress, or re-stimulation of Level 1 traumas. In my own case I never developed asthma until after being tied down in hospital, which created a Level 1 trauma. Research using the tuberculosis-like bacteria – mycobacterium vaccae which stimulates the immune system, has been used with success in chronic asthmatics. There is some evidence to suggest that over hygiene conscious parents who do not expose their children to dirt may be weakening their children's resistance. Certainly the rise of asthma in children is probably also related to stress, poor nutrition and other polluting environmental factors including pet cats, which recent research has posed as a contributed factor.

DR. JOSEF ISSELS

Dr Issels used hyperthermia and anti- cancer toxins or vaccines along with a low protein, largely raw food diet including detoxification in his programme. Unusually he was adamant that any sites of on-going infection such as teeth and tonsils should be removed. I would think the rationale here is that low-level infections constantly challenge the immune system and weaken it. Like many of the alternative practitioners he was a charismatic personality and inspired hope and confidence. Dr Burkitt who discovered the form of lymphoma that was named after him, had studied Issels work and the man himself and stated that Issels had come to the excellent conclusion that a patient is more than a case. He agreed with Issels that love and trust and never giving up hope count far more than peering down a microscope.

By the 1980s Issels had treated more than 8,000 terminal cancer patients. Dr Audier from the University of Leyden in Holland visited Issels in 1958 and verified the cures Issels had made. Dr Audier examined the case histories of 252 patients with different metastasised cancers, all untreatable by orthodox medicine and confirmed that Issels had achieved cures in 42 or 16.6%. That is pretty impressive considering these patients had been told there was nothing more to be done for them and terminal cases are very difficult to turn around. The figure I note is close enough to that interesting 10% value of the hard core survivors. Those who refuse to take no for an answer, read everything they can, find a therapy, stick to it, have full confidence in the therapy and the practitioner and approach the mental component of their illness. It seems then that Issels perhaps by sheer force of character and the confidence and care he gave to his patients had managed to cure a further 6% over that 10% figure. Had these results been achieved by orthodoxy, they would have made banner headlines.

Issels in his book entitled: 'Cancer – A Second Opinion' (1952) explained his rationale in treating cancer: 'the body is rather like a swimming pool whose water is not being filtered, whose drain has become clogged, the water will simply get dirtier and dirtier'. It's a good analogy and even Gerson in his own life time up until his death in 1959 noted it was becoming more difficult to treat patients, because of the rise in toxicity in their body. He put this down to the chemicalisation of food and the rise in prescription drugs, which would include street drugs from the 60s onwards.

Like many of the alternative nutritional diets for cancer, Issels diet stressed the importance of raw or live foods, making up to one half or two thirds of intake. Proteins came from sour milk products e.g. buttermilk and cottage cheese, the latter also being allowed after a while on the Gerson Therapy. He warned his patients against meat.

Dr Audier a Dutch statistician published Issel's five-year survival figures for inoperable and incurable cancer patients in 1958. You can almost guess what would come next; when a cure rate of 16.69% hit the scanners of the medical orthodoxy who it must be remembered had thrown all of Issel's patients out to die as incurable. Predictably then Dr Audier's paper was rejected by almost every medical journal in Germany and Bavaria where Issels practised. The 'cancer blackout' mechanism that prevents publication was described by the editor of one journal when he told Dr Audier that it was *policy* to reject anything connected with Issels and his clinic Ringberg, because to quote: 'it would have meant seriously upsetting some powerful men in the German Cancer world'. Here you have The Syndicate that Reusch and Bluchel described operating as a monopoly on publication, research, grants and provision of cancer services. When Dr Audier finally managed to get the paper printed in a medical journal, physicians from other European countries became interested in the therapy, they were then informed by the ruling orthodoxy that Dr Audier had not checked the records of patients properly and they never had cancer to begin with.

These events lead to Issels being arrested in 1960. He was charged with five pages of accusations including defrauding 4 patients and manslaughter by negligence of two. Issels was not given bail and ended up in solitary in a prison in Munich. His clinic was then raided and his records taken, whereupon he was then charged with four cases of manslaughter, where it was claimed in court papers that he had kept patients from surgery that orthodox doctors claimed would have saved their lives. At the trial witnesses confirmed that it was the *patients themselves* who refused surgery when Issels had strongly urged it in all 4 cases.

Issels was cleared of fraud and was found guilty of 3 charges of manslaughter and given a one-year sentence. Issels appealed in 1962 gathering more witnesses and leading cancer experts were sought for defence and prosecution. The original physicians of the patients testified that all patients had cancer when they went to Issels and none when they left his clinic. The prosecution claimed that either the diagnosis was wrong or that the orthodox treatment they had before going to Issels was responsible for the cure. Issels was finally found not guilty of manslaughter. Thus Issels had been cleared of both manslaughter and fraud, but the orthodoxy knows that labels stick.

Like Hoxsey, Issels was not deterred and re-opened his clinic in 1965. In 1968 the BBC – British Broadcasting Corporation in London sent Dr John Anderson, a professor of physical medicine at Kings College Hospital to see Issels. Anderson was a World Health Organisation consultant and a doctor who had worked with cancer patients. He was also an expert on computerised medical statistics and was familiar with Dr Audier's paper on Issels cures. Gordon Thomas in his book entitled: '*Dr. Issels and his Revolutionary Cancer Treatment*' stated: 'Without doubt Issels is a remarkable man doing something which is much needed. He is undoubtedly producing clinical remissions in patients who have been regarded as hopeless and left to fall back on their own resources. I also accept that even when he cannot produce a long remission he aims to allow the patient to live out his life in a worthwhile manner with more quality than would be possible otherwise'.

When the BBC tried to gain opinions from other experts in the U.K they were reluctant, because the American Cancer Society had put Issels on its blacklist – the unproven methods list – but they had failed to even visit his clinic or look at his work before they did so.

Houston and Null maintained in their investigative journalism article:

'Files on unorthodox therapies are kept by various medical agencies as lists of taboo areas to guide funding and policing policies. The American Cancer Society, the Vatican of the cancer establishment, maintains the central Index of heretics. ACS Inc. appears to conceive its mission to be that of axing discoveries that seem too good to be true. As a protection agency for the status quo, the Society issues a widely circulated blacklist, entitled 'Unproven Methods of Cancer Treatment', defaming approaches that have dared to deviate from the standard cut-burn-poison school of healing.... It seems odd that an organization supposedly devoted to encouraging research, by definition the study of the unproven, should use 'unproven' as a pejorative and promote the cardinal error in science of confusing 'unproven' with 'disproven'. If unproven avenues are blocked what remains is what is already known and progress is foreclosed'.

314

The BBC did film secretly and the programme called '*Go Climb a Mountain*' was due to be broadcast in 1970, but the powers that be in the cancer world blocked its scheduled screening on March 17th 1970. *The Observer* newspaper found out about the programme and brought pressure to bear on the BBC to show it. The BBC was forced to screen it on prime time TV on November 3rd 1970. Fourteen million people tuned in to watch it. Sir David Smithers an expert on cancer, who advised the British Government's Department of Health, was wheeled out to attack both the BBC and Issels therapy. In a sane world, any success in pulling terminal cancer patients through, would be considered as an approach to be researched and looked into, however as I have explained even in my own story, I realised that the journey through cancer was one of insanity and I say that as a scientist.

Lillian Board an Olympic medallist sprinter, who was suffering from an advanced rectal cancer, had already had a colostomy when she was taken to Issels clinic. Like Steve Mc Queen, who went to Kelley, Issels took on Lillian putting her before his reputation. She was in an advanced state and when Lillian died a few weeks after her arrival, the medical establishment and the press, despite the fact that orthodox medicine had failed to cure her, no doubt courted the publicity.

Because of the publicity and resulting public pressure the Cancer Research Campaign, The Imperial Cancer Research Fund and the Medical Research Council in the U.K were forced to investigate Issels methods. Naturally they sent two of Issels greatest opponents – Sir David Smithers and Dr. Harris. John Anderson was refused because he had given a positive report of Issels work. Gordon Thomas in his autobiographical book, *Issels: Biography of a Doctor (1975)* claimed Smithers and Harris wrote a report on Issels work on the second day after they arrived at the clinic, when they could not have undergone any serious fact finding. There was no statistician on the team and with interpreters who spoke German but had no knowledge of cancer. The facts were no doubt along with the results lost in translation. The report entitled: '*A Report on the Treatment of Cancer at the Ringberg Clinic, Rotach-Egern Bavaria*' was not published by the British Government and attacked everything but the psychological support and nursing care delivered. Perhaps in the section on the mind, which I will come to, they really underlined the true source of Issels success in attaining a 16.69% survival rate in so-called incurable and terminal cancer patients. Let me put that figure in perspective for you – out of every 100 so-called incurable cancer patients, Issels cured 17 of them who had been told by orthodox medicine to go home and die. Issels did write a refutation of the report, but the British Government had safely preserved the status quo.

Gordon Thomas's pro Issels biography had been published in the United States in 1973, but the BBC who objected to the history of the programme 'Go climb a Mountain' deterred the U.K. publishers. The U.K. edition of Thomas's biography of Issels did not occur until sections of the book were removed, predictably the BBC controversy and Dr Denis Burkitt's pro-Issels statements. Dr. Burkitt was a leading cancer specialist.

Not surprisingly given my own experiences of New Scientist magazine David Smithers was allocated page space in the April 1975 edition to seriously slam Issels book, perhaps to satisfy the powers that be in cancer and make sure that everyone was 'singing from the same song sheet.' Surprisingly however almost as a matter of conscience, Dr Bernard Dixon then New Scientist's Editor in the May 1975 edition pointed out that it was necessary for medical science to be open and fair minded about new and controversial ideas and their initiators. Dixon to his credit went on to refer to opponents of Issel's treatments as: 'vicious intolerance of an unorthodox outsider'. Well amen to that and my own treatment and what a pity Dixon was not around at New Scientist, when I sent in my own theory of cancer. It looks to me as though Dixon had his hands tied by advertising or the Drug Cartel and medical establishment, but wasn't happy about it and thus his after- thought – but too late Issel's work was consigned as with Dr Gerson's work to the dust shelf, along with other promising research.

One of Issels reported cases was of great interest to me. Thea Dohn was 19 and very ill with cancer when she went to see Issels in October of 1952. He discharged her in December of 1953. Her tumour was still there, but dormant and not growing. However in 1954 she had a re-occurrence and Issels was interested to know what had caused the new growth. Thea had fallen in love and she and her fiancé had set the wedding date. The man however had changed his mind and within two months her cancer symptoms had re-appeared. This time she seemed to accept the cancer. When I read the obituary of Michael Gearin-Tosh, the same thing came to mind – what had happened in Michael's life to make the tumour re-grow? I will cover the mechanism of the mind shortly, but the point here, is that one must even in the mechanism of the mind, find the cause, otherwise cancer becomes a case of management. Cance a case of loss and if one does not deal with the source of loss, the mechanism of the mind is a powerful predictor of any future re-occurrence. Loss however on Earth is a problem man will never solve, whilst predators prey on mankind for profit and power and people are so nasty to each other. I believe even *The Bible* talks of a 'great sore' that emerged on Earth.

It seems that Thea gave up the will to live when she encountered a considerable loss that devastated her and then her cancer returned. She returned to the caring Dr Issels and although we don't know how he persuaded her, the story now lost, she did go back on Issels therapy and no doubt by contact with the caring man himself, she survived and then married in 1957 and from what I can gather was still cancer free 10 years later. Michael Gearin-Tosh whilst given only 6 months to 3 years life expectancy survived 10 and then suddenly, he succumbed and the question to me is what happened psychologically that caused the cancer to re-occur?

There is at least one alternative cancer therapist who stuck two fingers up at the whole scene of cancer: unlike Hoxsey, Issels and Gerson Dr Burton with a doctorate in experimental zoology, treated patients in the Bahamas with immuno-augmentation therapy. Patients arrived at his clinic in the morning, had their blood tested for its immune status and the five immune factors that Dr Burton had identified as necessary in fighting cancer. Patients returned in the afternoon and picked up their injectable serum, which contained any missing factors that were not found in their blood taken in the morning. No diet or any other approach was advised. Dr Burton was an arch cynic on the cancer establishment and despite being American, had no intention of returning, publishing his results, or seeking to have his therapy acknowledged by the cancer establishment. I can see from my own journey how one might end up an arch cynic, when you have run the insane maze of cancer.

Even if one has no scientific or medical background, one can easily pick out elements in all these therapies, which are common to each and if one was to enhance one's chances of survival then it seems rational to at least look at those elements, which have helped terminal patients to survive. There is no point just considering the outward therapy that a patient took be it orthodox or alternative, you have to actually look at *what survivors did* in a holistic approach and many of them not only undertook the nutritional and detoxification programme but also overcame loss.

317

THE RELATIONSHIP OF THE MIND TO ILLNESS AND CANCER

After the map of the human genome was presented to the world in 2001, psychiatrists had high hopes for it. The psychiatrists as with doctors are still mesmerised by the 19th century mind-set of Newtonian mechanics. They were hoping for molecular evidence as the cause of mental illness: 3D holographic wave theory was beyond them. The Drug companies looked forward to a whole era of massive profits to be made from drugs aimed at these solid Newtonian molecular 'blips' or faulty genes. Just as there is little part played by genes in determining why one sibling, social class or, ethnic group is more likely to develop cancer, genes will provide no answer to mental health problems and certainly will not play a part in answering the question of how *loss* is a psychological indicator in cancer.

Craig Venter, one of the key researchers on the Human Genome Project, had warned previously that because we only have about 25,000 genes, they could not determine psychological differences. It boils down once again not to genetics or nature and that cruel twist of genetic fate, but nurture and the environment of an individual that is not only critical in cancer, but in mental illness. Just as there are no individual genes for the vast majority of mental health problems, then the role of genetics in cancer is minimal. As Oliver James author of '*How Not to F*** Them Up*' (*2010*), in an article for *The Guardian* (*13.10.2010*) pointed out: 'This February's editorial of the Journal of Child Psychology and Psychiatry was entitled 'It's the environment, stupid!' The author, Edmund Snuga-Barke, stated, 'serious science is now more than ever focused on the power of the environment...all but the most dogged of genetic determinists have revised their view'. Equally in the case of cancer, I could remark – 'its LOSS stupid!'

The Drug Cartel is quick to publicise however any tenuous link to 19th Century Newtonian mechanics - solid bodies and genes. A heavily publicised study by Anita Thapar, of Cardiff University in 2010, claimed a genetic link to ADHD – Attention Deficit Hyperactivity Disorder. As Oliver James pointed

318

out: 'Although she claimed to have proved that ADHD is a "genetic disease", if anything, she proved the opposite. Only 16% of the children with ADHD in her study had the pattern of genes that she claimed causes the illness. Taken at face value, her study proved that non-genetic factors cause it in 8 out of 10 children'. In other words the children who show ADHD are more likely to develop this through their environment. However much drug money is tied up in drugging the young, where it is necessary to show that the environment is not to blame but some cruel genetic twist of fate. This seems to me to be an important question to answer as much money is used by a State at tax-payers' expense, in funding additional support in the classroom to children who are 'statemented' with various medical tags such as ADHD and therefore qualify for classroom support, which means that a classroom assistant on a salary is employed. This is in addition to free medication again at taxpayer's expense.

Oliver James stated:

Worldwide, depression is least common in south east Asia. Yet a study of 29 nations found the variant (genes) to be commonest there – the degree to which a society is collectivist rather than individualistic partly explains depression rates, not genes. Politics may be the reason why the media has so far failed to report the small role of genes. The political right believes that genes largely explain why the poor are poor, as well as twice as likely as the rich to be mentally ill. To them, the poor are genetic mud, sinking to the bottom of the genetic pool. Writing in 2000, the political scientist Charles Murray made a rash prediction he may now regret. "The story of human nature, as revealed by genetics and neuroscience, will be conservative in its political [shape]." The American poor would turn out to have significantly different genes to the affluent: This is not unimaginable. It is almost certainly true'.

Such right wing views are quite incapable of observing that a poor person does not have the resources to cope with the emotional losses that not only induce mental illness but also in my own theory here, play a part in the mechanism of cancer. Undeniably cancer is more prevalent in lower socio-economic groups in individualistic societies.

Oliver James stated: 'Instead, the Human Genome Project is rapidly providing scientific basis for the political left. Childhood maltreatment, economic inequality and excessive materialism seem the main determinant of mental illness. State sponsored interventions, like reduced inequality, are the most

319

likely solutions'. Such an approach may also assist the case of cancer, where I consider LOSS is a major psychological factor in the onset and progression of the disease and loss, is more likely to be experienced by lower socio-economic groups. The political stratagem of detecting the disease early, in order to improve cancer survival statistics is a cynical tilt at all scientific evidence to the contrary; avoided by successive governments in order not to confront the blazing problem of inequality and how to enable the lower socio-economic classes to rise out of poverty and a sub- standard education.

In Britain 0.6 per cent of the British population owns 69 per cent of the land – and they are mostly the same families who owned it in the 19th century: 103 people own 30 per cent of Britain. Twenty members of the current conservative government are male millionaires and many were educated at Eton and Harrow or Westminster – top public (private) schools in the UK, which feeds Oxford and Cambridge universities, which supply the next political leaders and governments. As school fees at top universities move beyond the reach of the poor but bright, the inequality is bound to remain or worsen for many years to come. We find virtually no women in the conservative government and their cuts in these austere times are we are told unfairly aimed at women and children.

In developed nations, women and those on a low income are twice as likely to be depressed as men and the wealthy. As many women now struggle with children, after abandonment, with often no income or variable income from the fathers of these children, it is outrageous that successive governments have avoided the simplest solution. Money should be automatically withdrawn from a man's salary or benefits, instead of forcing women into the indignity and humiliation of having to chase money for food for their children from these disgraceful men. One can however rely on right of centre governments, whenever they grab power, to hit those socio-economic classes and especially women first and where one can almost predict a rise in the rate of cancer. When DNA is tested in large samples, neither women nor the poor are more likely to have the variant (genes).

I spent some time in the 80s disseminating the role of the mind in cancer to any organisation that had a role in this field. I would like to think at least Dr Forbs then medical director incorporated my research at the Bristol Cancer Help Centre in the UK. In the late 80s I forwarded the data on the mind to him, emphasising that it is not stress in itself but more how we deal with stress, or do not deal with it that affects the course of cancer. Dr Forbes even went as far as telling me that in cases of cancer that do not respond, he felt the cause was "karmic".

Following Dr Forbes, Dr Rosy Daniel was medical director of the Bristol Centre until 1998, where she reported that: "the emphasis in cancer now, is on the mind-body connection". She pointed out in an article in *The Daily Telegraph* (*03.08.2001*) that: 'we have to face the fact that medicine is not working with cancer. After spending 70 years and billions of pounds on research, we are still only producing a cure in three relatively rare cancers'. She went on to comment that Sir Richard Doll and Sir Richard Peto have found that 81.5 per cent of cancer deaths in the West relate to the way we live, with diet and smoking accounting for most of this figure.

I have already discussed the lowering of immune function by lack of ascorbic acid or vitamin C. However the studies of psychoneuroimmunology or PNI, show that long-term stress and depression can lead to reduced immune function and a depletion of oxygen levels in red blood cells. Repeating my own research of the 80s Dr Daniel stated: 'What PNI scientists are telling us is that it is not stress or distress per se that is the problem, but how an individual reacts to it'.

Some patients undergoing the Gerson Therapy who had a poorer prognosis than others, survived, whilst some with a good prognosis succumbed. The question I asked myself at the beginning of my research, was why do some patients even with advanced cancer survive and yet others with early diagnosis die? Charlotte Gerson and her father Dr Gerson explained these cases, by saying that some people did not adhere strictly to the therapy. This on the face of it seemed a reasonable explanation and was a similar explanation to the one given by Kelley when he said that Steve Mc Queen indulged in ice cream and cigars and would not do the enemas, when undergoing Kelley's programme: however one could not simply dismiss those who adhered strictly to the diet and yet did succumb.

In my research notes, I see that I pondered at first Kelley's rationale where he believed that it might be possible to crack the individual's metabolic code, and then boost the glands and organs. If this was done he argued to anywhere near 100% the body would cure by itself. His aim was to find the perfect food for each cancer patient. The logic seemed faulty as the Gerson therapy is a 'one

321

fits all' and still attains successes – in other words the diet did not need to be that tailored or specific. Like the current hope of gene technology, it seemed to me not to answer very basic observations I had made concerning the psychology of cancer and its link to the embryonic biochemistry.

When many years later I turned to Michael Gearin-Tosh's account of his time on the Gerson Therapy, I noticed he went through the psychological crisis that usually occurs at around 4 months into the therapy and which I reported in my published research paper. Turning to page 90 of his book [1] he stated: 'My dreams about the French Cancer Professor and the Nazi trains are starting to get worse. *I must not go back* into that again' (*author's emphasis*). By not going back into it, he had in fact given the driving seat to the primitive mechanisms, which control tumour growth. I have stated elsewhere that 'going back' or reversion is a key mechanism in cancer, both psychologically, physiologically and biochemically, where cells revert to an inappropriate embryonic biochemistry.

Michael was not involved in the holocaust this lifetime and thus one might ponder why this dream as he admitted drove him to panic. Let me quote this passage on page 96: 'Rachael and I are sitting in the garden. Suddenly she says, 'Michael, your fury is a world apart from your panic.' Where does this come from?' Michael thought and going on to say: 'It is obvious, no doubt that I am angry, but I have never said a word to Rachael about 'panic' about the French Cancer professor or the Nazi trains. But in understanding my state of mind she is bulls-eye: The French professor and the trains made me panic, my fury is a fight back'.

If I had been counselling Michael, I would have probed him about the French cancer professor and the Nazi trains, because having seen the psychology in many patients, there was a key, critical and underlying psychological event (trauma) there, which needed to be dealt with and resolved. The French professor during Michael's early search for a decision on which path to take i.e. alternative or orthodox had said "Do not ever use the word cancer again". Michael admitted the remark had driven him mad, but like the man who had an accident with his nose that I recounted in the introduction, this was a mere *trigger* and it drove Michael mad, because it stirred up the panic (a past Level 1 and/or 2 trauma) of the Nazi trains. I suspect that it was a similar enough phrase to: "Don't ever use the word holocaust again", for it to stir up Nazi trains. The decision to write this book, emerged from the thought I had when I

322

read Michael's account – 'does the suffering have to go on?' Michael had survived a long time for a person with his diagnosis and I can only wonder what psychological event occurred to make the cancer re-occur and whether that re-occurrence was linked to his failure to identify the true source of loss (Level 1 trauma) and its connection to 'trains' and 'Nazis.' The heart-breaking thing is that the trauma had presented itself and just needed an experienced counsellor to help him access it.

Michael so poignantly stated on page 96: 'If you cannot tell the truth, if you cannot express deep worries, is not that equivalent to a lobotomy?' It is the deep worries and losses that stir in the mind of cancer patients and the Gerson Therapy is capable of bringing the emotions of the losses to the surface.

On page 104 Michael stated: 'Rachael plans to stay with friends in Wiltshire and I am to go to Scotland. But will I have to travel alone, and my car is up north. Can I face the train? I am not having bad dreams, but has the French cancer Professor really gone? Will a train bring him back? I am scared'. Outwardly to the rational and analytical mind this fear of travelling to Scotland by train seems ungrounded, just as my own fear and terror seemed to come from nowhere, but the real loss that Michael felt lay in the primitive mind and was not accessible to him in detail, even though its emotion of fear and panic was. The mere thought of having to travel on a train stirred up the 'Nazi' trains in his dreams and re-stimulated the Level 1 trauma, presumably of a previous life. That it was a Level 1 trauma is obvious from the A=A=A computation or 'Nazi trains' = all trains.

On page 236 Michael stated: 'Newton's discovery of the law of falling bodies is all very fine, but that doesn't mean that a Mother's discovery of how to hold a baby isn't important too'. It seems that Michael's childhood although financially sound, carried with it some upset from his stepfather and certainly if I had been counselling Michael this was an area that needed to be explored and resolved.

I note too that before Michael's cancer returned, his friend Rachael Trickett, who he was obviously very attached to and with whom he had shared a home for twenty years, although there was no relationship, died in 1999. As Michael admitted on page 187 'There is a huge void in my life' – *loss*.

I quote here the summary to my scientific paper published in *Complementary Medical Research Spring 1989, Volume 3, Number 2.* The paper entitled '*A Theory for Cancer, using the Gerson Therapy in Conjunction with Psychological Counselling*' (*Appendix 1*).

'In the course of observing the psycho-physical profiles of cancer patients undergoing the Gerson Therapy we have uncovered a specific psychology, which we propose is directly linked to traumas received before the age of six months postnatal. In the process of reversing embryological metabolism the Gerson Therapy causes biochemical cellular conflict, which is registered by the unconscious mind and is experienced by the Patient as negative emotional and psychological states. Unless this conflict is resolved by counselling a patients progress is seriously impaired'.

The fear and panic experienced by patients undergoing the Gerson Therapy at around 4 months into the therapy, is caused by the surfacing of traumas held in memory in the primitive mind, which are not accessible to the Patient in their content, but manifests as emotional content of the traumas: for example if the trauma has an element of panic or fear in it, this will be the emotion that presents in present time. In my own research I have found that only regressive counselling *without* the use of drugs and hypnotism is effective in gaining access to these traumas and resolution. I did note however that Professor Jane Plant [27] gained great relief from psychotherapy as a coping mechanism.

In my notes of the time in 1987 I asked the question whether the embryonic trophoblasts of Dr Beard present a link between early trauma, the similarity of embryonic cells to cancer cells and the potassium-sodium balance which I have discussed in prior sections. Again quoting from the introduction to my research paper I stated:

'Dr Gerson maintained that during the course of development from embryonic to adult metabolism a change from sodium to potassium metabolism occurred Sodium and Iodine seeming to control the velocity of growth into a morula" (or ball of cells) "and further into germ layers i.e. fast growth and differentiation. High ratios of sodium to potassium are present in fast growing tissue of animal embryos, plants and cancer cells, therefore to increase the potassium/Iodine group further potassium and Iodine are given'.

If you remember from prior sections, potassium turns off growth and sodium turns on growth through rapid mitotic cell division. In the majority of alternative diets for cancer, we have seen that potassium and Iodine are given. Even in Hoxsey's formula the main ingredient was Lugol – a potassium/Iodine solution to which Hoxsey added other detoxifying herbs. In 'The Second Millennium Working Report on Cancer' compiled to accompany the research paper, when seeking funding, I did give a more technical area that would benefit from further research, which is the structural content of intercellular water which may be very important in maintaining a high level of potassium inside mature healthy cells, keeping sodium out. At the time the sodium pump was thought to be responsible, but in my view could not be considered a serious or correct theory, when ion exchange occurs even if the so-called pump was disabled. These matters are too technical to continue with here.

So embryonic cells are biochemically similar to cancer cells, in that they are fast growing, contain sodium instead of potassium, a position that changes entirely in the mature adult cell, which grows in a controlled way and contains a high level of potassium inside the cell. My own research led me to conclude that the reason cancer is not recognised in the body as an invader, is because it is seen by the body as a *survival mechanism*, where the cell reverts to a high survival embryonic state and that appears to involve and be underpinned by the subconscious presence of early psychological traumas involving loss.

Dr Lawrence Le Shan in the 1980s studied 400 patients and in more than 100 hours of psychotherapy found that 72% of patients lost a primary relationship or job before the onset of their cancer. Dr F Levenson a psychotherapist working with terminally ill cancer patients, using a form of regressive therapy was able to approach in a very basic way long held traumas, with good success.

While Carl Simonton was completing his residency in oncology at the University of Oregon Medical School, he found lung cancer patients who continued to smoke, liver cancer patients who continued drinking alcohol and patients who continually failed to make appointments. These patients he concluded seemed not to care. Conversely, Simonton found a small group of terminal patients who stayed alive for many years. These patients he discovered had specific goals that kept them going, a positive attitude, a will to live and a belief that they would survive. Simonton noted in his research that a positive attitude towards treatment was a better predictor or response to that treatment than was the severity of the disease. Simonton on the basis of his research went on with his wife Stephanie a psychoanalyst, to develop what became known as the positive visualization approach. I note that Michael Gearin-Tosh used this therapy, which involves using positive mental images of powerful immune defence mechanisms conquering weak and feeble cancer cells. Michael's imagery was both elaborate and amusing as one might expect of an Oxford don in literature and one of the few men brave enough to write a book about his experience. Michael's images of borsch being handed out in Russian field kitchens with armed soldiers perhaps also had a connection to his Nazi trains, but we will never know now.

The Simonton's opened a clinic and explained their methods in the book entitled: *'Getting Well Again'* first published in 1981. Since Dr Simonton used his visualization techniques in conjunction with orthodox therapy i.e. surgery, radiation and chemotherapy, despite his approach was unusual for the time in the 80s, he was never subject to the attacks that alternative practitioners experienced. Dr Simonton was a trained oncologist and radiologist and thus was not considered a threat even if he was using an adjunct method.

There were many objections however even from cancer patients to the work of Simonton. The author Susan Sontag, herself a cancer sufferer objected to Simonton's point of view in her book: *'Illness as Metaphor'* (*1978*), where she claimed that emotions have been implicated in cancer only because its underlying cause and therefore a reliable cure have not yet been discovered.

In my own observations of cancer patients and even those with chronic disease, there can be real reluctance to look at life issues that are painful and emotional for them. However as I concluded in my cancer research paper, all those who underwent counselling in our study survived, whilst those who did not take counselling for whatever reason died. It must be emphasised however, that the patient does not consciously know the most damaging traumas, Level 1 traumas, because they lie in the primitive mind and are only contacted through regression.

The objection to Simonton's view which emphasised responsibility for the illness must be part of the therapy and healing process, was that patients should not be made to feel guilty and that somehow they brought it all on themselves. The Simonton's in their book never said this, despite this and how people chose to interpret it they repeatedly underlined their goal was not to

326

make people feel guilty, but to help them recognise self-destructive behaviour patterns and to use this knowledge in their own therapy and healing. In my own view some self-destructive patterns may be obvious but often the underlying cause is not obvious to the patient and must be sought in regressive counselling. How can one be responsible for something one does not know about? In my own case I made it my goal to find out. As the saying goes "Healer heal thyself". Certainly very damaging traumas in my case existed in early childhood, but also there were damaging past life traumas and perhaps this is where Michael Gearin-Tosh's 'Nazi trains' lay.

However a lot of patients I spoke to in my research, can see a clear connection between their present lives and the onset of cancer. What caused the patient to make the choices they did however, is a less easy task for the patient and only comes slowly over a period of time and may only be approached when the patient is physically improved; because the choices we make are often dependent on the dictates of Level 1 traumas. There is no point approaching painful life issues when a person is physically unwell and only light counselling should be undertaken focusing on positive goals etc. More in depth counselling can occur when the patient is more himself or herself and the medical condition is improved.

The Simonton's maintained that since emotional states contribute to illness they could also contribute to health. By acknowledging your own participation in the onset of the disease, you acknowledge your power to participate in regaining your health and you have also taken the first step forward in getting well again. Anyone can see truth in this statement. Consider the person in a loveless cold relationship and they develop cancer, remaining in that relationship is a serious risk to re-gaining health. One can either handle a situation that is creating a negative emotional state, but if one cannot then the only way to re-gaining health is to completely disconnect from it.

Let's go way back now to 1701 when the physician Gendrona in his treatise entitled: *'Enquiries into Nature – Knowledge and Cure of Cancers'* noted that cancer occurred in grief situations. You might remember the story of Thea John whose cancer re-occurred when the young man she became engaged to, eventually told her he did not want to marry her. The loss that Thea experienced was significant enough to cause her cancer to return or become active again, until Issels managed to instil in her the will to live again.

Doctor Hyle Walshe in 1846 in his treatise entitled '*The Nature and Treatment of Cancer*' noted that there was a link between cancer and personality. What I believe he meant by personality was an *emotional state* and my own research shows cancer develops in low emotional states such as when a person experiences grief, constant anxiety, fear, and apathy. As a person recovers they become more themselves and are in a better psychological mood, which the Gerson Therapy contributes to, but also as they start to recover they feel more confident about taking control of their lives and addressing those negative elements. Emotional states are dictated by the emotion content of Level 1 and 2 traumas. If for example a person is stuck in a *past* Level 1 trauma containing the emotion of fear, then their personality in *present* time will be fearful.

Doctor Willard Parker in 1885, noted that out of 397 breast cancer cases he studied in America, many of these women had been subjected to grief, which they had not been able to deal with effectively. Often a situation arises which is not seen as a significant trauma at the time, but it can trigger underlying traumas, which then affect the person through the subconscious or primitive mind in present time.

Professor Jane Plant in her book entitled: '*Your Life in Your Hands,*' took the orthodox route of surgery, radiation and chemotherapy, but she also admitted she took psychotherapy, which she found very beneficial and prior to that counselling. She mentioned an unresolved grief situation involving a child that had been in the background of her life as an emotional trauma. Based upon my own experience of cancer patients I would be virtually certain that before her cancer appeared there was another perceived loss in her life, which triggered the former trauma. On page 197 of her book she refers to the book by Louise Hay entitled '*You can heal Your Life*' [40]. I am familiar with the book and personally know a lot of people who have benefited from it.

The book by Hay gives a list of diseases and their probable psychological causes. In the case of cancer the probable cause Hay gives is: 'deep hurt, long standing resentment, deep secret or grief eating away at the self, carrying hatreds, what's the use'. The advice or combative psychology that Hay gives is to develop new thought patterns such as 'I lovingly forgive and release all of the past. I choose to fill my world with joy. I love and approve of myself'. To quote an exasperated Professor Plant who as a scientist herself when at the time trying to deal with her own cancer stated: 'Fine, but I prefer a more rational approach which seeks to remove cancer-causing chemicals from my life!' However Professor Plant did go on to receive psychotherapy and myself, I did feel some truth in Hays estimation, but as with the exasperated Professor Plant who felt counselling was irritating when she was constantly asked "How do you feel?" there are events in one's life that can only be approached by access to the subconscious primitive mind, where the real losses are stored as memories not accessible to the conscious analytical mind.

Returning to Lawrence Le Shan's book: '*You Can Fight for Your Life.*' Le Shan an American psychotherapist, worked with over 200 cancer patients and according to Le Shan, the typical personality of a cancer patient is one that had a deprived youth, followed in later life by a period of fulfilment in an intense relationship or through all-involving work, followed by the loss of that relationship or work at which time the cancer occurs. The other main characteristic is the person's inability to express anger, particularly in his or her own defence. Others often describe such a person as being like a saint. Le Shan believed that the pattern fitted 76% of his patients, with only 10% of a control group showing this pattern. Professor Plant denied the description fitted her or anyone else she knew with breast cancer. However, the mechanism is not so simple as to be summed up in this way. Even threat of loss of job, or a perception that one's work is not meeting a level expected, or a change in a close relationship can be experienced as a loss. Several women I met developed cancer when their children left home and they were left with that loss. One woman, developed cancer when she found out her husband was having an affair. Another person developed cancer when they lost a parent. One person told me she could not think of a trauma or grief situation in the 12 to 18 months before the onset of her cancer, but as a producer she had experienced money problems over a period of time and had worried excessively about her retirement. This would be a slow drip feed of loss, but she did eventually go on to resolving the trauma that had been triggered by her money problems, which related to her early childhood.

Of course many people experience losses, but not all will go on to develop cancer. In cases where cancer develops, it is combination of a number of factors including an inability to resolve the loss, coupled with factors such as diet and life style choices and past life memories.

Sometimes authors of a biography on surviving cancer are not completely honest in telling readers the whole story. No one wants their private lives held out in public and so often the psychology is not referred to in any great detail, along with private issues in their life: it's as though they can't admit or look at those aspects of their lives. However, if one looks at the success stories each survivor has evaluated their lives in some manner and resolved issues. I have chosen to be honest in this book, because I can't think that sharing such moments diminishes one in any way and it certainly helps others who follow.

Professor Plant admirably said: 'I have to say that I found counselling of the type which is based on trying to release any pent-up emotions far less helpful than the psychotherapy sessions, which were intellectual and analytical and gave me new understanding and insights into situations so that I could develop clear, simple coping strategies'. The regression therapy that I prefer, seeks to resolve rather than achieve simple coping strategies and the reason for this, is that so often in counselling the emotions of the trauma or situation are churned up but since the details of the trauma lie in the subconscious and are not accessible, then the real nature of the trauma is not addressed but merely brought to the surface and left unresolved. As Professor Plant said: "'the analogy I would use about my counselling sessions is that of a pond in which the emotions had settled to the bottom and the water cleared, and every week I was encouraged to put in a large stick and stir it around until I became upset'.

The counsellor was merely re-stimulating level 1 and 2 traumas and the emotional content, without accessing the nature of the trauma itself. This is actually quite damaging and is not at all to be recommended, as it would actively keep the condition of cancer active. The problem is that many therapists simply do not understand the mechanism of the mind. Any psychotherapy must be aimed at resolution *not* re-stimulation. The other problem I have found is that emotional problems may result from association with family members or even friends or relatives. The patient may be unable or unwilling to confront this and one patient said to me: "Oh I could not possibly upset my husband and family by talking about this". Another woman said: "Oh I could not divorce him, he would leave me penniless – he's like that". Unfortunately both women died. The important point here is that both women failed to resolve the situation of loss.

Elida Evans research in 1926, was a precursor of Le Shan's work, where in a psychological study of cancer patients, she found that the patients seemed to place a great deal of importance in one relationship or job and when that was lost, the patient had no resources with which they were left to cope. You may

330

remember that metaphorically at the time of my own diagnosis, I looked in my cupboard and it was bare, there were no resources left with which to cope, having spent them by remaining in a highly damaging and negative environment and importantly by not dealing with it. Evans also noted that cancer patients often present a strong and positive image to the world, which belies their real and true feelings, which verge on misery. Such misery however is I find the thought that the situation cannot be resolved and a well of loss that knows no bottom. Such feelings only arise from not resolving the underlying Level 1 and 2 traumas and the nature of the environment which re-stimulates those memories.

Dr Caroline Thomas in 1974 working on a study with cancer patients at Johns Hopkins University found unexpectedly that these patients were generally placid, not aggressive, and were not close to their parents, particularly their fathers. The cancer patients seemed to exhibit on a test score, low anxiety, low anger and little depression which at first sight appears contradictory, but if remembered, that the cancer patient tries to present a positive face to the world, covering their inner turmoil, then obviously the best answers are mocked, in an attempt to hide their true feelings, which they cannot communicate.

With loving, safe and trained guidance, patients can start to communicate feelings and they can start to identify the areas of their life, which have contributed to their illness. To resolve such issues may require a certain upheaval in their life and even the prospect of starting again and the cancer patient has in some way given up that hope. In my initial frantic search for a therapy, at some point near rock bottom, I visited a famous reflexologist in London, who told me I was a "beautiful rose" that had "not been cared for and had been allowed to wither and die", it was that comment that impinged deeply and seem to stir some ancient memory that finally lead me to Greece where I not only connected the dots, but recovered a personal historical memory. One never knows in one's healing journey where the signposts will arise.

Dr Millar in 1977 at the 29th Annual James Ewing Lecture to the Society of Surgical Oncology in America stated in his speech entitled: '*Psychosomatic Aspects of Cancer*' that patients who are apprehensive about their disease, almost always do badly and die rapidly, even when the cancer is treated at an early stage. Conversely the patient who denies the implications of cancer

331

usually does well. Even in my experience the patients who became totally involved in their treatment, read all they could and received counselling or better still regressive therapy did much better, than those who leave their treatment totally to someone else and fail to look honestly at their life.

Dr Snow carried out the first statistical study connecting cancer to emotional states. In his study he found that 203 patients with breast or uterine cancer, out of a group of 250 had a history of emotional distress – 85% in other words. Now that is too large a percentage to be ignored. Other researchers have noted the same background, where the disease developed when patients felt hopeless, helpless and alone, soon after they had experienced a major loss as in a relationship, job, career, or loved one. The will to live was lost. It was felt that after this loss they could no longer go on. There was no perception of a future. I have found that loss can be a 'drip drip' over a long period and then something happens, where it becomes the final straw. An antagonistic relationship, or a cold one, constant denigration and loss of self-esteem, loss of job and career expectations – loss is accumulative and given the state of today's world and the callous actions people inflict on others, when they could not survive such actions themselves, it is not surprising to me that cancer is on the increase.

Even such techniques as the Simonton's used had good success where with just adjunct visualization in conjunction with orthodox treatment, 240 incurable patients they treated between 1973 and 1979 had a median survival time double that of the national averages: and 10% of their patients had a dramatic remission where the cancer disappeared. There is that interesting 10% figure again, the awkward squad, who refuse to take no for an answer, refuse to die, find new goals, complete every aspect of their therapy, read all they can about cancer, take positive life steps and confront past negative patterns. They also have complete faith in either their practitioner or therapist, or the therapy itself. You find this 10% figure in so-called incurable cases on a number of the therapies.

The Simonton's method though was a coping mechanism. They studied self-help courses such as the Silva Mind Control and Mind Dynamics programmes and Biofeedback, which were programmes that emerged in the 1970s aimed at coping with stress. At the time transcendental meditation became popular as another feedback coping method. As the Simonton's pointed out the visualisations had a number of benefits in so far as in addition to helping patients focus on healing, it reduced the fear that results from feeling out of control. As patients change their imagery, it gives them more confidence that they can change the course of their disease. The feeling of loss of control and chaotic thoughts arose a lot in the patients I spoke to. I steeled myself to the chaotic emotions through reading books on the warrior's code. The Gerson Therapy with its strict regime provides immediate order and this gives the patient control, where the mind is occupied with the daily round of survival. The body in an evolutionary sense is tuned to bio-cycles in nature and any predictive cycle offers order at the physiological and psychological level.

Edmond Jacobson in the 1920s found that when experimental subjects pictured themselves engaged in a physical activity their muscles fired as if they actually were performing the activity. As a scientist I have no problem with accepting that thoughts are capable of changing matter. Turn to physics and you will discover that when you get down to the tiniest particles that comprise matter, they are not particles but packets of energy and waves. We can think about our bodies and even a tumour as energy – chaotic energy. Thoughts too are just energy, which incidentally you can pick up on an NMR scanner and so why shouldn't they be capable of changing matter, which is really just a slowed down form of energy? I did have a computer programme that showed on the computer screen the energy patterns created by thought simply by using an 'electronic glove'. So you could think bad thoughts, negative thoughts and then positive ones and watch the wave patterns and colours change. Again this could provide the basis of future research.

The Simonton's were quite aware that a positive outlook and determination to succeed were essential for success and thus only took on patients who showed this determination. They also requested that the Patient bring their spouse or close family member, in order that they would be able to provide support at home. In my view this would also eliminate antagonism that is likely to cause a barrier to re-gaining health. It is absolutely necessary for patients to remove or disconnect from any source of antagonism or hostility. The Simonton's also encouraged patients to engage in regular exercise, because it is well known that exercise has a positive effect on mood and gives an enhanced sense of well-being: apart from the beneficial effect of an oxidising metabolism as discussed.

Franz Alexander in his book: '*Psychosomatic Medicine*' which was published in 1950 maintained that: 'all our emotions we express through a physiological process; sorrow, by weeping: amusement, by laughter; shame by blushing. All emotions are accompanied by physiological changes, fear by heart palpitation; anger by increased heart activity, elevation of blood pressure and changes in carbohydrate metabolism'.

The evolutionary survival mechanisms e.g. where fear causes adrenaline release, preparing the animal for flight in the 'fright and flight' response, are based upon cause and effect in a biofeedback system. The animal is frightened the body prepares the animal for fleeing by releasing adrenaline. The animal flees and adrenalin production ceases. This is the desired outcome, where the *fearful situation is resolved* – the animal runs away from the source of fear and threat and finds a safe place or alternatively in a fight defeats the opponent. What happens in continually fearful situations where the person may not be able to identify the source of the fear or panic? Their environment is threatening, but they can't resolve it and so the metabolism of fear is prolonged where adrenalin and cortisone production continues with potential damaging physiological and biochemical effects, which then also lower immunity.

Man has inherited by way of evolution a primitive set of behavioural and physiological responses to fearful situations. He is built to either run away or fight in a threatening situation or at least resolve the situation which creates fear and panic. Let us take modern man perhaps in a fearful relationship with a bully, job or suffering from money problems, he would like to run away, but finds he has responsibilities such as a mortgage, children and job etc. So he has to sit in his fearful situation and it doesn't get resolved and so he applies coping mechanisms, which normally involve avoiding confronting the source of his problems altogether. If these don't work, he believes there is no way out and he drops on the psychological scale to apathy where thoughts of death reside. The person will develop a series perhaps of acute minor illnesses and will feel depressed and lethargic – if the situation continues to be unresolved acute illness will become chronic. The emotional tone will be one of fear, grief, hostility, anger and apathy etc.

Helping to explain why heavy smokers sometimes do not contract lung cancer Dr David Kissen of the University of Glasgow in the U.K. in 1962 discovered that heavy smokers, who contract lung cancer, have fewer emotional outlets than those who don't. He concluded that the more repressed the smoker the less smoke was needed to precipitate lung cancer.

Dr Vernon Riley in 1975 used a strain of mice, which normally develops breast tumours between 8 and 18 months. Riley insulated their cages, eliminated loud noises and kept the temperature even and generally provided a stress free environment for the mice. Usually 90% of these mice develop breast cancer by the age of 13 months, but in Riley's study only 7% developed cancer. This seems to suggest that even pre-disposition to a disease through genetic make-up is not predictive of whether the disease will develop, however environment is predictive. This would have implications for genetic research, where the argument again is nature versus nurture.

Stress then plays an important part in the course of chronic disease and in one study by Dr Ramirez in London in the 80s, it was found that women breast cancer patients subjected to stress were more likely to develop secondary's and die than those women who experienced no stress. It is my experience that patients who start to recognise destructive patterns in their lives can make a start to recovery. Once a person begins to see formerly insurmountable problems in his or her life can be resolved, they begin to regain hope and expectation that they can have some control over their life again and the belief that one can **do something** about the condition is important. The act of doing something, means the driver – *you* is still in control. The danger comes when the person does nothing and thus hands the driving wheel to the irrational primitive mind, which will solve the problem along primitive lines even though that solution in a modern context is irrational. This is the case of cancer – it is a primitive survival mechanism.

From a scientific viewpoint it is difficult to test faith, hope or belief. Attempts have been made to assess how thoughts and beliefs can bring about physical changes. The researchers Drs Jon Levine, Gordon and Fields gave placebos or ordinary sugar pills to patients in pain. The patients believed these pills were painkillers and a large number reported pain relief. In this case belief brought about physical changes. I have already pointed out that belief in a therapy, belief in a doctor or therapist can be a significant indicator of survival.

There are some scientists who have suggested that the history of medicine is actually the history of the placebo effect: the belief being more important than the medicine. Dr Benson of Harvard University in 1975 and 1979 noted that during the last 200 years every medication used for angina pectoris (chest pain) was effective 70% to 90% of the time when it was first introduced. However, its effectiveness would fall to 30% - 40% as soon as a newer therapy appeared. The belief being that the old drug was not as effective as the new one. We have seen that many alternative therapists are charismatic individuals who inspire hope in their patients and provide it might be questioned a will to live: as Einstein once stated: 'Science without religion is lame, religion without science is blind'.

Dr Hutspnecker as far back as 1951 in his book entitled: *'The Will to Live'* stated 'Today we are beginning to recognise that the first danger to the length of life may not be the invading germ, nor any physiological process beyond our control, we are beginning to understand that the first line of defence is our emotional health. If we are emotionally sound, we will be physically sound. Body and mind are one. When we truly want to be well, to live long and in health, we have the power to do it'. Dr W Greene studied patients with leukaemia and lymphoma and found that in 9 out of 10 cases, the disease developed when patients felt helpless and hopeless, and alone, generally soon after they experienced a loss of some significance.

I have seen almost reluctance especially in women, to express the anger they feel. Dr Stephen Green at King's College Hospital in London in 1975 found that women who either suppressed anger and even those who turned it against themselves, were far more likely to develop breast tumours than women who are easily able to express anger. We should consider Louise Hay's psychological evaluation of the causation of cancer here and the resentment that is held in cancer. Resentment if suppressed becomes internal anger which bubbles and boils below the surface. If allowed out the patient fears a Krakatoa type eruption – and the whole issue of 'must confront', 'can't confront' and 'must do something' and 'can't do something' is set into motion. This leaves the situation unresolved. Sometimes I have asked a patient to fill in two columns one column headed reasons to live and the other headed reasons to die. It soon becomes apparent where the source of anger and loss comes from. It is my belief that any illness at least in its psychology is a cry for love and if love is not extended then an illness develops, because sympathy has at least an element of affection in it. People (if they are human) are generally not nasty to sick people and the illness then has some survival value to it. Perhaps I was lucky I can't say I had one person who even thought whether to enquire whether I might need help and support, except Sheila with all the beauty of the Irish about her. A child becomes sick, gains sympathy and therefore the illness has some survival value and if in future the child experiences any lack of love (loss), they will subconsciously draw in the illness, with its survival value of sympathy, which although not love does have some affection as sympathy. Thus there must be no rewards or gain from being ill.

Dr Bathrop in *The Lancet* in 1977 showed a link between loss of immunity during periods of grief and bereavement. We have all experienced this, we have some upset and then we get a cold. I mentioned Dr Amanda Ramirez at the Breast Cancer Unit at Guys Hospital in the 1980's who connected stress and re-occurrence of breast cancer, by concluding that patients subjected to high levels of stress were more likely to develop secondary's and die. If that were entirely true, I can't say that I would be alive today. As I fought cancer, I was dragged through heavy legal proceedings, selling off the furniture in a crumbling mansion, along with clothes and jewellery to pay for the Gerson Therapy. It is how you *deal* with stress that is important. As I have stated you have to be able to *do something* about the situation or be at *cause over it*; it is only dangerous when you are in a situation that you think cannot be resolved and become the *effect of it*. It is not that vague word stress that causes your boat to capsize, it is the ability to start, stop or change any situation, especially those, which create negative emotions. British cancer specialist Dr Jan de Winter corroborated this by saying the crucial factor in the development of cancer is the suppression of feelings and the inability to express those feelings. *Communication* is therefore important and *is* effective therapy.

Other researchers have also observed a link between stress and immunity. Hans Selye famously in the 1950s and 60s showed that mammals when placed in stressful situations transmitted this stress to the hypothalamus a part of the brain most directly associated with emotions. The hypothalamus then floods the body with hormones via the adrenal glands and these hormones then markedly depress the T cells of the immune system.

Penn State psychologist Howard Hall used hypnosis to boost white blood cell activity. Hypnosis is basically giving a person a visualization or perception as a command, which is not known to them analytically. It might be considered as another form of visualization in so far as when the suggestion is made it will evoke the visualization of the required response. Using this method he could obtain a 40% increase in white blood cell counts among younger and more responsive subjects, thus increasing their immunity against cancer.

Over the years of my research and in the time I have observed cancer patients I realised that it's not the actual personal grief, severe emotional blow or the stress that comes from a situation that causes onset of disease, or its deterioration. It is the patient's reaction to that stress, or rather the lack of it. It's the failure to communicate those feelings, which is determinant with the result that those feelings are bottled up and the loss becomes to the patient insurmountable and unable to be resolved. The loss is viewed as a death experience, and the patient gives up. Those people who survive change their attitudes and life patterns by removing undesirable elements. This may even require large upheavals and not every person feels able to do that. Men particularly are reluctant to communicate feelings and losses.

One woman I spoke to who had breast cancer described an unsatisfactory marriage, which had only just held together when the children were at home, but after they departed she experienced bereavement in their loss. She was left with her uncommunicative husband who avoided her through golf. Within 12 months of the departure of her children she developed breast cancer. She had never really had a career and thus felt that she would never be able to manage on her own. She was quite unable to get her emotionally closed husband to communicate. She just had no will to continue and it did not surprise me to later learn, she had developed secondaries and had died. There is I believe such a thing as a cancer-relationship, or often a cancer marriage. Loss of love is particularly perceived as a great loss, because love is a high survival emotion. If partners are unable to give and receive love, where feelings are not mutually shared and where one partner is continually forced to suppress their feelings then that person is at risk, particularly also if other stress factors are present. The answer is to establish mutually satisfying relationships where the problems and stresses experienced in each individual's life are communicated and shared and not bottled up. Both partners should communicate and above all respect each other's feelings and life goals. Where one partner is being denigrated and their identity belittled by the other, then that person is at risk.

During observations of cancer patients, I noted that in nearly every case there had been a loss in the 12 to 15 months prior to the onset of the disease. The loss may not even have been perceived as significant but acted in some cases as a trigger for earlier losses, which *were* significant. There are high-risk times in everyone's life especially during periods of bereavement or divorce and children need extra support during these times. One woman with advanced cancer recounted to me the scene as a child where her mother had just left without telling the children. She recounted how in a threadbare kitchen they had sat around the Formica kitchen table in silence with their father, eating a bowl of cereal. It was a scene that haunted her and when her marriage failed she developed cancer. She never knew why her mother left, her father never spoke of it and she always had the feeling that she wasn't loved and that perhaps it was her fault that she was abandoned. She allowed her husband to denigrate her and bully her, because she had shelved the past incident in the attic of her mind but retained feelings of unworthiness and low self-esteem. She could see how by not discussing the incident it had really governed her life and marriage and was clearly able to see the point at which she gave up. She experienced great spiritual peace in her last days.

Le Shan noted in his work the deprived nature of the cancer patient's childhood. This may not have involved physical deprivation but emotional. Where an adult's behaviour dominates and overshadows the child or even the whole family, then there is a risk. The late Wilhelm Reich in his treatise: '*The Cancer Biopathy,*' outlined what he called muscular armouring, a process whereby a person shuts off areas of the body, in which there are conflicts, by continually tensing the muscles around them. If these centres are shut down long enough physical changes, such as decreased blood and lymph flow will occur. This area will then have a predisposition to disease.

Ida Rolf was a biochemist and physiologist and in her work, she examined muscle tissue and cell structure in trauma. She observed that physical and emotional traumas seemed to tighten and rigidify the muscular cellular tissue. She also noted that rigid muscle and tone also established an *emotional pattern*. Further she noted: 'It is not possible to establish a free flow through the physical flesh. Now what the individual feels is no longer an emotion, a response to an immediate situation, henceforth he lives, moves and has his being in an attitude'. This attitude of course was picked up by Le Shan and described as a personality by him. The attitude of the patient will show him or her to be in fear, grief or a similar negative emotional state, where his attitude to life *will be his emotional state.*

What I mean by this is that a person in apathy will have an approach to life, which reflects that emotion. He or she will say: "Well oh well, what can be done about it...nothing I suppose, I will have to just sit here..." and so on. Their eyes look down a lot and they don't make eye contact. Sometimes if you

339

watch people they will walk stooped and they will look down at the pavement, with a blank face – that is apathy and their approach to life as an attitude.

With a person in grief, they have a sad attitude and tears come easily. The fearful person sees danger everywhere and is a pretty jumpy person to be around. Their eyes flick quite a lot in fearful expression. They might say: "Oh I wouldn't do that, this might happen..." they fear the unknown and even the known. The hostile person is tense, they are combative in conversation and tend to contradict everything you say – these people come as two groups, those who are openly hostile and where any conversation with them is exhausting and then those who are covertly hostile who usually engage in hostile remarks about you when you are not around. Covertly hostile persons are pretty dangerous to be around, since they can have a really negative effect on your life usually causing damage unknown to you and behind your back. This sort of person often crops up in employment issues. The angry person is obvious and they are actually doing better on a psychological scale than all the other types. Certainly as a cancer patient starts to rise on the psychological scale, they will pass through the emotion of anger and even rage, or as Michael Gearin-Tosh admitted 'fury' as 'the fight-back'; whereas he recognised panic was related to the' French professor' and the 'Nazi trains' and a deep seated psychological event.

Constant routine contact, for example with a family member or boss who display all or any of these negative emotions, will lower your own psychological level and at these low emotional levels, illness can and does occur. As we have seen many researchers have noted that cancer occurs in grief situations and loss, which is associated with grief. Sometimes it's easy to be fooled, because people have a false emotional tone they display when in company like a social mask to hide their true emotional tone, which they believe would be unacceptable. I guess we have all seen this perhaps in the work situation, where a manager or colleague presents themselves as very sociable and helpful and then you discover they have been secretly plotting your downfall: the real emotional level of covert hostility is then hidden by a social face or mask they present to the world. If you see anyone going up in smoke so to speak, very upset and so forth, most people would be inclined to think that *they* are the problem, but careful analysis of personalities surrounding this person, will reveal a covert hostility type, with the smiling mask who nobody would suspect as *they* appear quite reasonable. With upset children or adults, who are failing or ill, then one should look for this hidden

34